ENCYCLOPEDIA OF SPORTS SPEED

Improving Playing Speed for Sports Competition

George Blough Dintiman, Ed.D
President, National Association of Speed and Explosion
Former NFl Draft Choice, University Head Coach

Robert D. Ward, PED
Director, Sports Science Network
Former Dallas Cowboy Strength and Conditioning Coach

SPONSORS

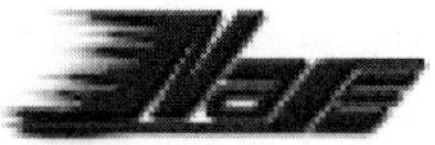

The National Association of Speed and Explosion,
P.O. Box 1784, Kill Devil Hills, NC 27948 Tel. 252-441-1185 Fax: 252-449-4125
e-mail: naseinc@earthlink.net Web Site: naseinc.com

And

Sports Science Network
Sports Science Network 11502 Valleydale Drive, Dallas, TX 75230 Tel. 214-696-663
Cell: 214-783-3984
e-mail: wardrdw@gmail.com
Web Site: www.dartfish.tv/sportsscience

Dintiman, George B., Robert D. Ward

ISBN: 978-0-938074-42-7 (soft cover)

Developmental Editor: Lynne R. Mohn

Printed in the United States of America

Library of Congress Control Number: 2008942143

Dedicated to three outstanding athletes, coaches, colleagues, and lifetime friends

Fred Caro, football teammate and Captain of Lock Haven University's 1957 undefeated, untied, championship team, multiple Wrestling Hall-of-Famer, highly successful football and wrestling coach.

Elwood Reese, former Lock Haven University running back, one of Lock Haven University's all-time best wrestlers, multiple wrestling Hall-of-Famer, highly successful football and wrestling coach.

Dr. George Colfer, football teammate at Lock Haven University, university professor, author of several books.

CONTENTS

BOOK REVIEW BOARD

PREFACE

In this modern era, the single greatest concern of athletes and coaches in most sports remains unchanged. In fact, coaches are now even more aware than ever of the importance of speed and realize that the right kind of training can produce dramatic changes in the playing speed of their athletes. The modern focus has moved to the speed of all movement in sports, including starting, stopping, cutting, accelerating; changing direction, delivering or receiving a blow, sprinting, and split-second decision making during competition. *Encyclopedia of Sports Speed: Improving Playing Speed for Sports Competition,* presented in question-and-answer form, provides the most comprehensive coverage ever written on all aspects of playing speed. Although the book incorporates the latest scientific findings of hundreds of studies, the details of complicated research design and statistical analysis are avoided. Information is presented in practical terms that are easily understood and applied to the training of athletes.

Encyclopedia of Sports Speed goes beyond helping athletes to accelerate faster and sprint faster in a vacuum or straight line. Linear velocity is correctly recognized as just one part of playing speed. On only rare occasions do athletes have the luxury of completing a long 60-100-yard sprint during competition. Text materials are designed to improve linear velocity, multidirectional movements, and skills that must be performed at high speed in sports.

Part I, INTRODUCTION, examines all aspects of speed during competition, as well as testing and basic training. Chapter 1 sets the stage for the entire manuscript and describes the key areas of playing speed in team sports to provide readers with an overview of the differences between training to improve linear velocity and training to improve speed for sports competition. Chapter 2 presents a comprehensive test battery, including sport-specific tests, to identify each athlete's strengths and weaknesses and determine the major focus points for designing an individualized speed improvement program. Sport-specific tests used in the NFL, MLB, MLS, and NBA combines are also presented, along with standards that allow athletes to compare their scores to professional athletes.

Part II, COMPONENTS OF PLAYING SPEED describes the main factors that come into play when executing short sprints. Stopping, starting, acceleration, faking, and cutting (Chapter 3), mechanics of sprinting (Chapter 4), stride rate and stride length (Chapter 5), and speed endurance (Chapter 6), cover the elements that must be understood and applied to improve speed in short sprints.

Part III, TRAINING PROGRAMS: THE 5-STEP MODEL, provides a detailed description of the specific programs designed to impact each of the factors affecting speed presented in Part II. Step 1: Foundation Training (Chapter 7) prepares athletes at all levels of competition for the comprehensive speed improvement training programs that follow. Step 2: Power Output Training (Chapter 8) describes the critical programs designed to increase ground contact force, or the pushing force against the ground on each step, that affects the start, acceleration, stride rate, stride length, and maximum speed. Detailed programs in speed-strength training, plyometrics, and sprint-resisted training are described. Step 3: Sustained Power Output Training (Chapter 9) presents sport-specific speed endurance programs to keep athletes sprinting at the same high speed throughout an entire game. Step 4: Neuromuscular Training (Chapter 10) describes numerous sprint-assisted training programs designed to improve stride rate. Finally, Step 5: (Form and Technique Training) includes drills and programs to improve starting, stopping, acceleration, sprinting, and faking and cutting.

Part IV: PUTTING IT ALL TOGETHER covers sport-specific speed training (Chapter 12), periodization, and sample workouts for the in-season and off-season periods. Chapter 13, Speed Improvement for Young Athletes, analyzes all aspects of speed and presents a modified, safe program for preadolescent boys and girls.

A list of 200 important resources are listed in the BIBLIOGRAPHY. A GLOSSARY of terms associated with speed improvement is located in the back of the manuscript to allow quick reference for readers.

ACKNOWLEDGMENTS

The authors are indebted to numerous individuals who have assisted us directly or indirectly with this book.

George wishes to thank his wife Carol Ann Dintiman for her emotional support and assistance, and his daughter, Lynne Dintiman-Mohn for her outstanding work as the Developmental Editor of this book.

Bob wishes to thank his wife Joyce for her never-ending support, and his colleagues and close associates who have contributed to his career and knowledge: Dan Inosanto, Larry McBryde, Steve Davidson, Randy White, Tex Schramm, Ralph Mann, Dr. John Cooper, Dr. Jim Counsilman, Bert Hill, Charley Baker, Todd Nadeah, and Dr. Sam Symmauk.

Special thanks to Ralph Mann for his research and dedication to uncovering the secrets of speed and playing speed improvement that can be applied to team sports; and to Tom Tellez, famed sprint coach for the direction and support he makes available with his teaching and writing.

Thanks also to John Turek, head cross country and track coach at St. Mark's School of Texas for organizing and conducting the photo sessions and to the volunteers as photo subjects: Teddy Shanahan, Wisteria Nicole Gulham, Garland Hampton, Innis Briggs, Leroy and Michell Burrell, Frank Rutherford, and Floyd Heard. A very special thanks also to Tom Roberts for use of the excellent photos.

Special thanks to the presenters at the June, 2008 NASE national conference who provided key information on speed training in their sport:

Dan Austin, Strength and Conditioning Coach, University of South Carolina
Shaun Gaunt, Strength and Conditioning Coach, West Virginia University
William Hicks, Strength and Conditioning Coach, Syracuse University
Andrea Hudy, Associate Strength Coach, Univ. of Kansas basketball
Allan Johnson, former Strength Coach at OSU and WVU
Butch Reynolds, former Olympic Gold Medalist and Speed Coach at OSU
Robert Taylor, Strength Coach, Loyola College
Tom Tellez, former Track coach, Univ. of Houston, and Olympic Sprint Coach

And finally, a huge thank you to Dr. David Hall, Hall of Fame Chiropractic, Parkersburg, West Virginia, for organizing and conducting the NASE National Conference at Marietta College, Ohio and for his contributions to the speed improvement of our nation's youth.

PART I

INTRODUCTION: PLAYING SPEED

Chapter 1

PLAYING SPEED

Athletes can improve every phase of playing speed including the start, acceleration, top speed, faking, cutting, high speed change of direction movements, and deceleration. Although genetics are important, "Heredity only deals the cards, environment and training plays the hand." Regardless of genetic make-up, every athlete can improve playing speed. On the other hand, even genetically gifted athletes will not reach their maximum speed potential unless a holistic approach is used that goes far beyond merely trying to improve linear velocity.

This chapter examines playing speed from a different perspective. It is designed to provide a more complete picture of the many hidden components of playing speed and identify aspects that may not have been considered in the past.

How Fast Things Happen

Every one of the senses provides important information for rapid decision-making on the field of play. In addition to these, the "6th Sense" offers a powerful dimension that can add immensely to the quality of performance or make up for deficiencies in other qualities.

How fast and at what level of force common sporting events happen is shown in Table 1.1. This table provides a better understanding of why attention, focus, decision-making and movements are so crucial during the game. A careful study of common events and their times of occurrence also helps clarify how critical a blink of the eye or a millisecond can be.

It is interesting to speculate about what is happening when outstanding athletes indicate that time seems to slow down during their best games even though events are obviously still happening in the physical realm at the same high speeds. This feeling of "playing in the zone," described by athletes in every sport, is a mental state that occurs through the mastery of performance anxiety and the achievement of relaxation during competition (Greenberg and Dintiman, 2009). Total preparation of the body and mind combine to produce this slowing effect and the accompanying improvement in performance.

Table 1.1 Speed and Force Used During Sporting Events

Contact event	Time of foot contact (sec)	Force (lb.)
Awareness threshold	>.0000	
Reaction	.09 to .016	
Reaction time	.090	
Sprinting	0.90	1,050
Sprinter ground contact	0.90	1,034
Sprint Master	.128	700
Sled (full load)	.175	488
Sprint load sled pulling	.175 to .195	590
Bounding	.175`	1,200
Bound	.175	1,182
High jumper .	130	1,000 - 1,300
Long jumper, takeoff	.110	1,371
Hop	.180	585
Hopping	.180	585
Cut 20 degrees	.250	682
Cut 60 degrees	.250	700
Cut 90 degrees	>.250	350
Depth jump, 16 to 100 cm	.200 to .285	945 to 1,327
Depth jump, 16 cm	.210	945
Depth jump, 40 cm	.200	990
Depth jump 100 cm	.300	585
Kicker, plant foot	.285	503
Race walker	.400	
Marathon*	<.400	
Quarterback, back foot throw	.500	364
Quarterback. front foot throw	.500	268
IMPACT Time		
Golf ball hit by driver	.001	
Baseball hit off tee	.013	
Handball serve .013		
Baseball hit from pitcher	.020	
Soccer ball header	.023	
Softball hit off tee	.035	
Tennis forehand	.050	
Football kick .080		
Striking force (boxer, martial arts)	.088	800 t0 2,000

* Marathon: + 10,000 steps X 2 X .400 sec = 8,000 sec. (133.3 min., or 2 hr. 13.3 min.

Power Output and Playing Speed

It is unusual to win one championship at any level of competition and a rare occurrence to put together a winning streak of championships. Even when teams have the same players from one year to the next, situations are different and so are the results. Let's look at the Los Angeles Lakers for a moment. What more can one ask of a professional basketball team then to win so many consecutive and total NBA championships? The author asked L.A. Lakers Trainer, Gary Vitti, what makes the Lakers tick, other than talent and a good coach, front office and fans. Gary indicated that the Lakers believe that power output, quickness, and acceleration are the key to identifying and training basketball players.

Great athletes are able to generate blinding quickness and use a higher percentage of their explosive power at various speeds of movement than the average athlete. Walter Payton, for example, would get the defender off balance by feinting, then run right over him to make extra yards, or break away for a touchdown. Other running backs, guards in basketball, soccer players, hitters, or base runners also draw on this quality when they explode from a stationary position or cut at very high speed. *Power output,* the amount of ground contact force an athlete can exert during the pushing action with each step in starting, accelerating and sprinting, is a major part of the speed training program in this book.

Gary went on to say that the Lakers measure, assess, and focus conditioning activities on enhancing the speed of the first and second steps, the first and second jumps, and sustained power output (speed endurance). Special equipment is used that is fitted with transducers to measure power output as the players do their various lifts. The Lakers are on the "cutting" edge, and we are impressed with how they train their players and emphasize the truly important areas of performance.

Old School Style

Why do some coaches still avoid the use of speed training in their sport?

Change is slow; accepting change is even slower and some individuals choose to remain in the past. A bit of history on the evolvement of speed training in sports may help.

Through the years, coaches and athletes recognized the importance of speed and quickness but were convinced that they were God-given genetic qualities that no one could do anything about. As a result, speed training did not exist among team sport coaches, but was relegated entirely to the track coach and those interested in sprinting events. Even among track coaches, the major emphasis was placed on the improvement of form and conditioning (wind sprint and other interval sprint training programs).

The idea was to produce an athlete with upper and lower-body movement in tune with the mechanical principles of sprinting. The focus was then placed on the use of repeated sprints both longer and shorter than the distance of the sprinting event. Total emphasis was placed on linear velocity, sprinting from point A to point B in a straight line. Attention to any form of playing speed, except speed-endurance training (wind sprints) was absent. At the university and professional levels, coaches recruited fast, quick athletes, rather than attempting to improve speed and quickness in athletes with superior playing skills.

American training techniques were unchallenged during a long period of US Olympic supremacy in the sprints. When Valeri Borzov of the Soviet Union won the 100-meter dash in the 1972 Olympics Games, dethroning American sprint supremacy, coaches in the United States began to realize that there was more to speed improvement than genetics and conditioning.

As early as 1963, Dr. Dintiman, Dr. Ward, and others began to test both the genetic theory and the two-prong approach to speed improvement (form and speed-endurance). Along with other researchers and coaches, the authors soon recognized that speed could also be increased by improving acceleration and training athletes to take faster and longer steps, not just by improving form, holding maximum speed longer, and reducing the slowing effect at the end of a long sprint. None of the training programs in use during the 1960s had much impact on acceleration, stride frequency, and stride length, yet these were the most important.

Bob Hoffman, one of the world's most foremost weight lifting coaches, probably had the greatest influence on our work in speed improvement and today's conditioning programs. In the 1960s, we began to focus on speed-strength and the application of force during the start and acceleration phases of sprinting. Concentrating on the start, acceleration, and stride length increases, we were unaware that increasing the force of the pushing action against the ground through speed-strength training would also increase stride rate. Regardless of this oversight, we began to analyze the effectiveness of training the neuromuscular system. *If the muscles involved in sprinting were forced to move at faster rates than ever before through methods such as sprint-assisted training, could we permanently increase the number of steps an athlete takes per second and also improve the length of a sprinter's stride?* During his speed camps in the late 1960s, Dr. Dintiman developed exciting new ways to train athletes to take faster and longer steps, towing athletes behind a motor scooter and automobile. He began publishing his early work on improving speed (Dintiman 1970; 1980; 1984), beginning a long-standing commitment and enthusiasm for investigating and developing new training programs for athletes who wanted to be faster, stronger and more competitive than others in their sport. His book in 1970, *Sprinting Speed: It's Improvement for Major Sports Competition (1970)* was the first publication to review hundreds of research studies emphasizing playing speed for team sports, which started a new era in coaching that led to a new position in sports - the speed coach. Dr. Dintiman and Dr. Bob Ward produced the first *Speed and Explosion* video for team sports in 1986, and the first of three editions of *Sports Speed* in 1988. Two editions followed in 1998 and 2003.

During the late 1960s and early 1970s, Tom Tellez, assistant track coach, was training UCLA football players under head coach Dick Vermeil. Bringing speed training to the football field was also one of the early attempts to improve the speed of athletes in sports other than track and field. Since that time, Coach Tellez has become one of the world's most accomplished sprint coaches, training the great Carl Lewis and many other world class sprinters.

In the NFL during the mid-1970s, Dr. Bob Ward joined the Dallas Cowboy program to become the first NFL strength and conditioning coach with full coaching status. Dr. Ward revolutionized how football players were evaluated and the way they concentrated on strength training, speed training, and general conditioning. Many of his special training techniques remain in use by NFL teams.

Together, in this book, *Encyclopedia of Sports Speed,* the original seven-step model has been refined to provide a "can't miss" approach to improving playing speed. The new Five-Step Model was developed from the research findings and our experiences with thousands of athletes at the high school, university, professional, and Olympic levels.

Today, genetics is considered only one factor in determining playing speed potential. It is also now widely accepted that athletes do not reach their potential unless a complete approach is followed. Athletes and coaches in practically all sports now follow the 5-Step Model or a variation. Speed coaches have been hired at all levels of competition, and the sports world is aware that, with the proper training, athletes can dramatically improve both playing speed and quickness.

Doesn't the USA still have the best sprinters in the world?

Most professionals also agree that the performances of our sprinters in the 2008 Olympic Games in Beijing, China were exceptional. Although the USA won slightly more total medals (110, 36 gold) than other countries, China (100, 51 gold) brought in the most gold. With no clear scoring system in place or on the horizon, declaring a winner is difficult. The winner is truly all countries and athletes who engaged in this competition.

Few areas, other than Michael Phelp's accomplishments in swimming, attracted as much attention as the Jamaican sprinters whose women swept the gold, silver, and bronze in the 100-meter dash. Usain Bolt set a new world record of 9.69 in the men's 100-meter dash, followed by silver medalist Richard Thompson (9.89) of Trinidad/Tobago, and bronze medalist Dix Walter (9.91) of the USA. Two other Jamaican sprinters, Asafa Powell (9.95) and Michael Frater (9.97), finished 5th and 6th and Darvis Patten (10.03) of the USA finished 8th. Usain's performance in capturing the 200-meter dash and running a leg of the gold medal 400-meter Jamaican relay team was equally brilliant. American sprinters regained some respect by sweeping the 400-meter dash, as LeShawn Merritt (43.75), Jeremy Wariner, and David Neville won the gold, silver, and bronze. The USA also won all three medals in the 400-meter hurdles.

After a country other than the USA wins the 100-meter dash and boasts the world's fastest human, it isn't long before critics imply that American sprint supremacy is over and that coaching and training technology is superior in Jamaica, Russia, Australia, or other countries. Numerous coaches even fall into this trap and search for unknown secrets to success from other countries. This assumption irritates most American sprint coaches who understand that the large majority of the world's elite sprinters and coaches have been trained in the USA.

As Tom Tellez, famed University of Houston track coach and coach of several Olympic sprinters, said during his presentation at the 2008 NASE National Conference, "the best coaching and technology is right here in the USA." This statement is in no way meant to detract from the tremendous accomplishments of Jamaican athletes and coaches. Jamaica made a commitment decades ago to develop the outstanding talent in that country, and their efforts need be applauded. This country of less than 3 million people systematically improved coaching and training methods and implemented a new system to develop raw talent at home. More than 30 years ago, former world-record sprinter Dennis Johnson took what he learned at San Jose State University in the 1960s and set up a competitive, USA-style college athletic program in Jamaica, with the goal of producing world-class athletes in track and other sports.

In the past, most high school track athletes sought scholarships in other countries. To this day, numerous Jamaican athletes can be found on NCAA track rosters. To curb this trend, Coach Johnson opened what is now UTECH, a four-year college. Operating on limited funds, he developed a highly successful program. Jamaican track athletes, like athletes in many countries, are also highly motivated and committed to rigorous training to reach their goals. Stephen Francis, coach of Osafa Powell, founded the Maximizing Velocity and Power Team in 1999, and currently is training Powell and other Olympic hopefuls.

The USA still has a group of the world's best sprinters, including former world record holder, Tyson Gay, and Dix Walter, LeShawn Merritt, Jeremy Wariner, David Neville, Shawn Crawford, Wallace Spearmon and women sprinters Allyson Felix, Lauren Williams, Muna Lee, Tori Edwards, and Marshevet Hooker. It also boasts some of the best training centers, researchers, and coaches.

Isn't a 100-meter dash nothing more than an all-out sprint?

No. The race for the title of the fastest human is not so simple. There is much more technique and strategy to the 100-meter dash. John Smith, former renowned world class sprinter and coach of many Olympic champions, describes the race and divides the 100-meters into five stages:

PHASE 1: *Reaction time* as sprinters explode to the sound of the gun and generate their first muscular movement forward out of the blocks.

PHASE 2 *The Drive phase* as runners leverage forward momentum to accelerate as quickly as possible.

PHASE 3: *Transition phase* where athletes change gears, shift into overdrive, and move into the fourth phase.

PHASE 4: *Maximum velocity* phase where athletes reach full speed, relax, and try to maintain top speed for 30 meters or more.

PHASE 5: *Final finish line phase* where the winner is the one who slows the least over the final 20 meters of the race.

Smith makes several additional points to help clarify the complexity of the 100m dash:

• An athlete doesn't have to be the first out of the blocks to win the race. The key is to execute a balanced start. Failure to do so may be evident after the first step, forcing an overextended athlete to rebalance himself, displace energy, and sacrifice time.

• Sprinters are vulnerable in the middle of the race, particularly if they push the accelerator too hard, and run out of gas the final 20 meters.

• Sprinting should appear effortless throughout all five stages of the race. This requires relaxation, proper form and technique, experience, and peak conditioning.

• Champion sprinters exert maximum power emanating from the best possible strength to body weight ratio. This enhances ground contact force during the pushing action with each step due to ideal strength/weight ratios.

• If a sprinter can stretch out the speed for the entire distance, there will be more fuel left for the finish.

• The winner is the athlete who runs the first four stages correctly and is in control of the inevitable deceleration at the end of the race. Athletes who tighten up at the finish will not be the winner.

Isn't this book more suited to sprinters than team sport athletes?

Absolutely not. Sprinters are concerned with linear velocity, which is only one part of the speed equation for team sport athletes who need to execute multidirectional moves, fakes, feints, stops, and starts, all dependent upon the action of the opponent. Unlike track and the use of a four-point stance, these sports movements may take place from a standing position, a slow jog, a 3/4 stride, or a three-point stance. In addition, changes in speed may occur at anytime and athletes must sprint varying distances over and over, not just once during a track meet. Team sport athletes must also diagnose and read the opposition and make split-second decisions about the "line of attack," then arrive as fast as possible in spite of the obstacles. Training to improve playing speed is quite different than training to sprint straight ahead for 100 or 200 meters.

How much can an athlete expect to improve?

Let's examine track and field over the past 96 years, recognizing that improvement among the world's already elite sprinters is much more difficult to accomplishment than it is with team sport athletes with varying degrees of speed. Since 1912, 100-meter world records have improved from 10.6 (Donald Lippincott, USA) to the current world record of 9.69 by Usain Bolt of Jamaica set in 2008 --a change of only 0.91 seconds or 8.58 percent. The 8.58 difference is more than it appears. Studies show that elite modern-day sprinters reach speeds of about 27.9 mph. In a race with Usain Bolt, Donald Lippincott's time of 10.6 would put him over 10 meters behind.

Obviously, improvements in 40-yard dash times do not take 96 years. Keep in mind also that most team sport athletes have never had the intense training of modern-day elite sprinters and are not even close to their maximum speed potential. Incorrect starting and sprinting form is also common among team sport athletes. The 40-yard dash used in team sports is a test of starting speed and acceleration, rather than maximum mph speed that may not be attained for 60 yards or more. After improving starting form and engaging in a holistic speed improvement program, we have seen 40-yard dash improvements in the same individual of as much as 8/10 of a second following 3-6 months of training. However, it is true that the closer an athlete is to elite 40 times, the more difficult it is to improve rapidly. Small improvements in playing speed of 2/10 - 3/10 of a second make a big difference and place an athlete 2-4 yards from the opponent.

How does an athlete improve sprinting speed?

Regardless of the sport, there are only five ways to increase speed in short sprints.

- Improve starting ability from a stationary, three-point, four-point and standing position, or from a moving posture (walking, jogging, striding) and acceleration to maximum speed.

- Increase stride length.

- Increase the number of steps taken per second (stride rate)

- Improve sprinting form and technique

- Improve speed endurance.

The first four areas are actually the only way speed in short sprints is improved while the fifth (speed endurance) allows athletes to make repeated sprints and long sprints during competition at the same high speed with limited slowing due to fatigue.

These five areas are not equally important to athletes in all sports. Basketball, soccer, rugby, lacrosse, field hockey players, and defensive backs and linebackers in football, for example, are generally moving at one-quarter to one-half speed when they begin to accelerate into a full-speed sprint, rather than from a stationary position such as a baseball player or football player in other positions. For these athletes, starting technique is not nearly as important as acceleration, stride rate, stride length, and speed endurance. For baseball and football players, starting techniques from the batting box, field positions, and turf are important.

Study Table 1.2 carefully. The key speed improvement areas for each sport, listed in order of importance, helps to clarify test scores in Chapter 2 and identifies training focus points for specific sports.

Table 1-3 identifies the training programs designed to improve each area. Improvement requires a holistic approach and each program is important and produces results when used with the other programs. A detailed description of each training program is then presented in Part III, Chapters 7 to 11.

What training programs are used to alter the five areas that improve speed?

Table 1-3 lists each of the five ways playing speed is improved and the specific training programs from the 5-step Model that impact each area.

Where can the latest information on speed improvement for team sports be found?

The NASE is the only organization with one major objective: the improvement of speed in short sprints for sports competition. Its Board of Directors, Advisory Board and Certification Board consists of the most respected coaches, strength and conditioning coaches, personal trainers, educators, and physicians in sports. The NASE is the world's leading authority on speed improvement and the only association focusing entirely on the improvement of speed in short sprints to enhance performance in baseball basketball, field hockey, football, lacrosse, rugby, soccer, softball, tennis, and track. The Association has taken a totally different approach than other organizations in their attempt to provide practical information on all aspects of speed improvement that is easily understood and applied. *Although information is based on the latest research, complicated studies are interpreted but not presented in traditional fashion to make it easier for readers to understand and apply findings to their setting.*

The NASE is also an educational organization and International Certification Agency for team and individual sport coaches (Youth Sports, Middle and High School, College, University and Professional), strength and conditioning coaches, personal trainers, and athletic trainers who seek to master the techniques of speed improvement training and become recognized for their expertise.

The NASE has directors in over 30 states: strength and conditioning coaches from Notre Dame, West Virginia University, Troy University, USAF Academy, Florida State University, Georgia State University, Iowa state University, Southern Illinois University, University of Kansas, University of Massachusetts, University of Maryland, Central Michigan University, Duke University, Ohio State University, University of Oregon, Penn State University, University of South Carolina, Clemson University, Middle Tennessee State University, University of Texas at Austin, USAF Academy, Washington State University and others.

The Certification Program offers certifying excellence in Speed and Explosion and the coaching of athletes and teams in the techniques of speed improvement. This practical program and exam involves information that can be readily applied to coaching and training at all levels of competition.

Table 1.2 Speed Improvement Attack Areas for Team Sports

Sport	Attack Areas by Priority	Comments
Baseball, Softball	1 Starting, accelerating, stopping and cutting 2 Stride rate 3 Stride length 4 Speed endurance 5 Sprinting form	A player will not approach maximum speed unless he hits a triple or inside-the-park home run. Starting ability with the crack of the bat and acceleration should receive the major emphasis for all positions. Speed endurance comes into play in base running from home to third, first to third and first to home.
Basketball	1 Starting, accelerating. stopping and cutting 2 Stride rate 3 Speed endurance 4 Stride length 5 Sprinting form	Acceleration takes place after some movement has occurred such as a jog, bounce, or slide. Maximum speed is not reached. High speed starting, accelerating, stopping, and cutting should receive the major emphasis. Speed endurance is needed to maintain speed and quickness throughout the game.
Football	1 Muscle tissue strength 2 Starting, accelerating, stopping, and starting 3 Stride rate 4 Speed endurance 5 Stride length 6 Form (start and sprint)	Starting and acceleration from a three-point, four-point, or standing start for 5 to 25 yards is critical to every position. High speed stopping and cutting is also critical. A player sprints faster in the open field by increasing stride rate and length. Speed endurance training prevents slowing due to fatigue at the end of repeated sprints and long runs.
Soccer	1 Starting, accelerating, stopping and cutting 2 Stride rate 3 Stride length 4 Speed endurance 5 Sprinting form	Soccer is a game of starting, accelerating, and cutting for 15 to 25 yards, and high speed stopping as a player approaches the ball or an opponent. Speed endurance prevents players from slowing down after repeated sprints.

Table 1.3 Speed Improvement Areas and Training Emphasis

Area of Improvement	Training Programs
Improved start, acceleration, deceleration, stopping, and cutting Muscle Tissue Strength	Speed-strength training to aid injury prevention Speed-strength training to increase ground contact force Muscle imbalance training Sprint-resisted training Plyometrics Start, stop, and cut training
Improved Starting and Sprinting Technique	Form training in the start and acceleration phases of sprinting
Improved Speed Endurance	Pickup sprints, hollow sprints, and interval sprint training Maximum effort training
Increased Stride Rate and Stride Length	Speed-strength training to increase ground contact force (pushing action against the ground with each step). Muscle imbalance training Plyometrics Sprint-Assisted and Sprint-Resisted Training Flexibility Training Form Training

Chapter 2

PLAYING SPEED TEST BATTERY

Athletes in all sports want to improve their speed and quickness. The key to success is knowing where to start and where to place the training focus. Each athlete has unique needs and exhibits different strengths and weakness that enhance or limit speed of movement. A few simple tests can eliminate the guesswork and pave the way for an effective, personalized speed improvement program. This chapter is designed to do just that by identifying strengths and weaknesses and isolating the individual factors that are preventing an athlete from starting, accelerating, and sprinting faster in their sport.

This chapter is divided into ten test areas:

1. Sprinting speed tests for all sports
2. High speed directional changes
3. Power Output (speed-strength tests)
4. Sustained Power Output (speed-endurance)
5. Quickness
6. Muscle Imbalance
7. Flexibility
8. Body composition
9. Form and Technique
10. Sports Combine Testing

The ten area test battery also includes sport-specific tests to measure playing speed. As each test is completed, keep in mind that this is not a competition. The objective is to identify the factors keeping you from sprinting faster. Eliminate all inhibitions and give your best effort in every test. Providing maximum effort at all times yields the most meaningful scores for use in preparing an effective, individualized speed improvement program. "Loafing" or "loading" (providing only partial effort knowing you will then show more improvement on a later test) makes it difficult to accurately identify weaknesses and leads to working on areas where optimum performance already exists and neglecting true weaknesses.

The first step toward getting faster is to work with a friend or coach and complete the tests in the ten general areas of the Comprehensive Test Battery. Make a copy of the Speed Profile Form (table 2.1) and place it on a clipboard or in a notebook to make it easier to record the test scores.

SPEED TESTS FOR ALL SPORTS

Is there any one speed test that provides information in key areas?

Yes. The NASE 120-Yard Dash (one sprint, seven key scores) is the single best test for team sports athletes. Although an electronic timing system with five splits is ideal, manual timing can be used to gather information that will allow a quick analysis of seven key aspects with only one all-out sprint.

The test provides information on practically every phase of sprinting speed and quickness, including the start, acceleration, maximum speed (mph, feet per second), speed endurance, and stride rate (steps per second) with just one sprint. Once the setup is complete and timers are in place, 30 athletes can be tested in less than 30 minutes; and, only one trial is needed.

For proper set up, a field or track area of 130-140 yards, five finish tapes, five handkerchiefs, four timers, and two additional helpers are needed. A handkerchief is draped over each finish tape to make it easier for timers to stop their watches on the movement of the tape as the runner crosses a finish line.

A finish tape is draped across the track at the 5-yard (Timer #1), 20-yard (Timer #2), 40-yard (Timer #3), 80-yard (Timer #4), and 120 yard (Timer #5) marks with one timer at each of the FIVE spots. Athletes assume a three-point football or four-point track stance and sprint full speed through each tape, without slowing or changing form, until reaching a point 10 yards beyond the last tape at the 120-yard mark.

Timers #1, #2, and #5 start their watches with the first muscular movement of the athlete. This prevents scores from being affected by reaction time when the stationary start is used and more closely resembles the actual activity in team sports. Timer #1 stops his watch when the runner breaks the finish tape at the 5-yard mark. Timer #2 stops his watch when the flag at the 20-yard mark moves. Timer #3 starts his watch when the flag at the 40-yard mark moves and stops the watch when the flag at the 80-yard mark moves. Timer #4 starts his watch when the flag and the 80-yard mark moves and stops the watch when the flag at the finish line moves. Timer #5 stops the watch when the flag at the 120-yard mark moves.

Table 2.1 **Speed Profile Form**

Name ______________________ **Age** ___ **Height** ________ **Weight** ________

TEST ITEM	SCORE	STANDARD	WEAK-NESS Yes/No
SPRINTING SPEED			
Stationary 120-yd.	________	Every athlete can improve these times.	
20-yd time	________		
40-yd. time	________		
Flying 40-yd.	________		
60-yd.	________		
80-120-yd.	________		
120-yd. time	________		
Acceleration	________	No more than 7/10 difference between the flying 40-yd. time and your stationary 40-yd. time.	_____
NASE First 3-Step Test	________ ________	Record the time to take 3 steps from a stationary start and the distance covered to find feet per second (fps). Norms being developed. Send your test data to the NASE.	_____
NASE Future 40	________	Your sprint-assisted towing score plus 3/10 sec. is an estimate of your potential after several months of training.	
Speed Endurance	________	No more than 2/10 sec. difference between the flying 40 and 80-120-yd. times	_____
Flying 40-yd minus 80-120-yd. time	________		
1.5 Mile Run	________	*Men*: Under 225 lb.: 10:01-12:00 - AVERAGE 8:30-10:00 - EXCELLENT, 226-300 lb.: 12:01 14:00 - AVERAGE, 301+ lb.: 14:01-15:30 *Women:* Under 150 lb.: 12:30-14:00 - AVERAGE, 151-200 lb.: 14:01-15:30	_____

Table 2.1 **(continued)**

TEST ITEM	SCORE	STANDARD	WEAK-NESS Yes/No
Stride Length	R_______ L_______ Diff. _____	Scores should be within these ranges: Males: 1.14 X height + or - 4 inches Females: 1.15 X height, or 2.16 X leg length R and L leg scores should be within 2-3".	_____ _____
Stride Rate	________	See Table 2.2. Find your stride rate using your stride length and flying 40-yard dash scores. Elite male sprinters approach 5.0 steps per second, female sprinters approach 4.5.	Every-one can improve
Directional Changes *Pro Agility Drill* *(20-yd. Shuttle)*	________	See Table 2.8, Minimum Standards by Position in football for expectations at the NFL level.	_____
Power Output (Speed-Strength) *Dead Lift*	________	2.5 - 3.0 X body weight (BW) - Excellent. 2.2 X BW - Good . 1.9 X BW - Fair. <1.6 X BW - Poor. COLLEGE and PRO FOOTBALL: Backs: 400-460, Wide Receivers - 350-400, Off/Def. Linemen/Tight Ends - 500-550 Linebackers - 450-500, Kicker/Punter - 350-400 Quarterbacks -375-450	_____
Leg Strength (Double leg press/BW Ratio)	________ ________	Multiply BW X 2.5. Leg press score should be higher.	_____
Single Leg Kickback	R _______ L _______ Diff._____	No more than 5 lb. difference between the L and R leg.	_____
Two-leg Extension *Two Leg Curl*	_______ _______ %_____	Leg curl scores should be at least 75% of leg extension scores.	_____

Table 2.1 **Continued**

TEST ITEM	SCORE	STANDARD	WEAK-NESS Yes/No
L and R Leg Extension	R _______ L _______ Diff.______	No more than 5 lb. difference between the R and L leg.	_____
L and R Leg Curl	R _______ L _______ Diff.______	No more than 5 lb. difference between the R and L leg.	_____
Standing Triple Jump	_________	Males: Jr. H.S. 20'+, Sr. H.S. 25'+ College and older: 28'+ Females: Jr. H.S. 15"+, Sr. H.S. 20'+ , college and older: 23'+	_____
R and L Leg Hops	R _______ L _______	2.5 and below - Excellent, 2.8-3.0 - Good, above 3.0 - Poor, No more than 0.3 sec. difference between the R & L leg.	_____
Sustained Power Output			
NASE repeated Sprints (10 at 25 sec. intervals, using 20, 30, or 40 yards. based on your sport)	____ ____ ____ ____ ____ ____ ____ ____ ____ ____	Difference between best and other scores should not exceed 2/10 second.	_____
Quickness *Quick Feet Test*	_________ _________	Males (middle School): 3.8 or faster; H.S.: under 3.3, College: 3.4 or faster, Females: Middle - 4.2 H.S. - 3.8, College - 3.4	_____
Muscle Balance *R and L leg Stride Length*	R _______ L _______ Diff.______	Secure your scores from the previous test sections and record here also. Right and left limb scores should be within 2-3 inches.	_____

Table 2.1 **(continued)**

TEST ITEM SPRINTING SPEED	SCORE ________	STANDARD	WEAK- NESS Yes/No
Muscle Balance (continued)		Right and left limb scores in this section should not differ by more than 5 lb.	
R and L Leg Kick Back	R _______ L _______ Diff._____		_____
R & L Leg Extension (Quadriceps)	R _______ L _______ Diff._____		_____
R & L Leg Curl (Hamstrings)	R _______ L _______ Diff._____		_____
R and L Leg Hops	R _______ L _______ Diff._____		_____
Flexibility			
Sit-and-reach	________	Above the 75th percentile in Table 2.5	_____
Practical ROM Tests	________	Successfully complete each test	_____
Body Composition			
Biceps *Triceps* *Sub Scapula* *Supra iliac* *Percent Body Fat*	________ ________ ________ ________ ________	Estimate your percent of body fat from Table 2.6. If you exceed 10% (male) or 15% (females), consult your coach or physician and follow his or her advice before beginning any weight loss program. For some positions in various sports where "push" weight is important, a higher percent of body fat may be acceptable.	_____

Table 2.1 **(continued)**

Area	Errors or Training Programs Needed	
Starting and Sprinting Techniques	Form Errors Observed:	
Starting Form	1. 2.	3. 4.
Sprinting Form	1 2.	3.. 4.
TEST AREA (from previous items)	**TRAINING PROGRAMS** (If you did not meet the minimum standard, check (√) the training program needed to eliminate the weakness.)	
Stride Rate (for all athletes)		
Stride Length	√ Sprint-assisted training √ Resisted training	√ Speed-strength training √ Plyometrics
Start and Acceleration	__Sprint-assisted training __Plyometrics	__Speed-strength training __Form training
Power Output (speed-strength)	__Speed-strength training __Plyometrics	__Resisted Training
Power Output (speed endurance)	__Speed endurance training	
Muscle Imbalance	__Speed strength training	__Resisted training
Flexibility	__Dynamic and static stretching programs	
Body Composition	__Consult a health professional	
Form and Technique	__Form Training (start, acceleration, maximum speed)	
Starting, Stopping, Faking, and Cutting	__High speed quickness drills, faking and cutting drills	

Scores in the 5-yard and 20-yard dash are also used to analyze two additional segments of the 40-yard: the start and early acceleration phase. Coaches may also find that the 5-yard and 20-yard dash times are more useful in evaluating athletes in some sports and positions than the 40-yard dash. Overall, the 120-yard dash measures seven different areas and provides an excellent first step in identifying the weakness areas in greatest need of improvement.

How are the results of the 120-yard dash analyzed?

One 120-yard dash provides the following information on each athlete:

The speed of the first three steps is determined by the time in the stationary 5-yard dash. For players at all positions in sports such as football, basketball, baseball, soccer, field hockey, rugby, and tennis, this is a critical distance and a player with the "edge" at the 5-yard mark generally maintains the advantage until play stops. The 5-yard sprint is a variation of the *First Three Steps Test* described later in this chapter that is so important in all sports.

The Stationary 20-Yard Dash Time is also a valuable test for team sports. It is the most important factor influencing 40-yard and longer distance times and in reaching maximum speed. There are relatively few times, for example, when a running back or other player sprints a longer distance. For offensive and defensive lineman in football, the stationary 5-yard and 20-yard dash are much more practical tests than the 40-yard dash. For sports such as soccer, rugby, field hockey, and lacrosse, the 20-yard dash from a moving position such as a slow jog is the best measure of playing speed.

The Stationary 40-Yard Dash Time provides coaches with the most popular measure of so-called speed that has been used for decades. Considerable data is available by player position to correlate with success in a sport. Depending upon conditioning levels, it takes about 60 meters for an athlete to reach maximum speed. Therefore, the 40-yard dash is a measure of quickness and acceleration, not maximum velocity.

Acceleration is evaluated by subtracting the flying 40-yard time (40 to 80 yard mark) from the stationary 40-yard dash time. A difference of more than 7/10 second indicates poor starting and acceleration technique and the need for improvement. To estimate how fast an athlete should already be sprinting the stationary 40-yard dash, add 7/10 of a second to the flying 40 time. An athlete who runs a 3.9 flying 40 should already be running a 4.6 stationary 40. If that is not the case, the problem lies with starting technique and lack of speed-strength.

Speed Endurance is evaluated by comparing the 40-80-yard time (flying 40) to the 80-120-yard time. If both scores differ by no more than 2/10 of a second, only limited slowing is occurring due to fatigue at the end of a long sprint. Differences greater than 2/10 second suggest poor speed endurance and the need for improvement. Ten consecutive 40-yard dashes at 25-second intervals is another excellent test to determine recovery from all-out sprints and the amount of drop-off or "slowing" after repeated sprints in a sport. The 40-yard sprint and 25-30 second rest intervals between each repetition is used for offensive and defensive backs, receivers, linebackers, and special team players in football. Athletes in other sports use the average distance and rest interval performed in their sport. Keeping all 10 scores within 2/10 of a second indicates excellent speed endurance.

Timer 1 (5-yard dash)

Timer 2 (20-yard dash)

Timer 3 (Flying 40; time from the 40 to the 80-yard mark)

Timer 4 (Speed Endurance; time from the 80-120-yard mark)

Timer 5 (120-yard total time)

Figure 2.1 Role of each timer during the NASE 120-yard dash. The 5-yard dash can be used in lieu of the First 3-Step Test

Stride rate or steps per second can be calculated by using the flying 40 time and the stride length test (length of stride in inches).

Example: Bill has a stride length of 80" and completed the flying 40 in 4.0 seconds. To find his stride rate:

Divide 1440 (inches in 40 yards) by the length of the stride: 1440 divided by 80 = 18 steps to cover 40 yards.

Divide the number of steps by the flying 40 time: 18 divided by 4.0 = *4.5 steps per second.*

A more accurate indication of the number of steps an athlete takes per second at various intervals during a sprint of 5 to 120 yards can be obtained by using a high speed video camera.

Stride rate can also be determined from stride length scores in inches and Flying 40-yard dash times using Table 2-2.

> *Example:* John has an 80" stride length and completed the flying 40-yard dash portion of the 120-yard dash test in 4.0 seconds. Find his stride length of 80 in the vertical column to the left and flying 40-yard time of 4.0 in the horizontal bold column at the top of the table. Move your finger down the 4.0 column until it intersects with the 80" stride length score. John's stride rate is 4.5 which is very good. Olympic sprinters strive for a stride rate of 5 steps per second.

Table 2.2 **Stride Rate Matrix**

Table 2.5 **Stride Rate Matrix**

Flying 40-yard dash time (sec.)

Stride length (in.)	3.6	3.7	3.8	3.9	4.0	4.1	4.2	4.3	4.4	4.5	4.6	4.7	4.8	4.9	5.0	5.1	5.2	5.3	5.4	5.5	5.6
50	8.0	7.7	7.5	7.3	7.2	7.0	6.8	6.7	6.5	6.4	6.2	6.1	6.0	5.9	5.7	5.6	5.5	5.4	5.3	5.2	5.1
51	7.8	7.6	7.4	7.2	7.0	6.9	6.7	6.5	6.4	6.2	6.1	6.0	5.8	5.7	5.6	5.5	5.4	5.3	5.2	5.1	5.0
52	7.6	7.4	7.2	7.1	6.9	6.7	6.5	6.4	6.3	6.1	6.0	5.8	5.7	5.6	5.5	5.4	5.3	5.2	5.1	5.0	4.9
53	7.5	7.3	7.1	6.9	6.7	6.6	6.4	6.3	6.1	6.0	5.9	5.7	5.6	5.5	5.4	5.3	5.2	5.1	5.0	4.9	4.8
54	7.4	7.2	7.0	6.8	6.6	6.6	6.3	6.2	6.0	5.9	5.8	5.6	5.5	5.4	5.3	5.2	5.1	5.0	4.9	4.8	4.7
55	7.2	7.0	6.8	6.7	6.6	6.4	6.2	6.0	5.9	5.8	5.7	5.6	5.4	5.3	5.2	5.1	5.0	4.9	4.8	4.7	4.6
56	7.1	6.9	6.7	6.5	6.4	6.3	6.1	6.0	5.9	5.7	5.6	5.4	5.3	5.2	5.1	5.0	4.9	4.8	4.7	4.6	4.5
57	7.0	6.8	6.6	6.5	6.3	6.1	6.0	5.9	5.7	5.6	5.5	5.4	5.3	5.2	5.1	5.0	4.9	4.8	4.7	4.6	4.5
58	6.9	6.7	6.5	6.4	6.2	6.0	5.9	5.8	5.6	5.5	5.4	5.3	5.2	5.1	5.0	4.9	4.8	4.7	4.6	4.5	4.4
59	6.8	6.6	6.4	6.3	6.1	6.0	5.8	5.7	5.6	5.4	5.3	5.2	5.1	5.0	4.9	4.8	4.7	4.6	4.5	4.4	4.3
60	6.7	6.5	6.3	6.2	6.0	5.9	5.7	5.6	5.4	5.3	5.2	5.0	4.9	4.8	4.7	4.6	4.5	4.4	4.3	4.2	4.1
61	6.6	6.4	6.2	6.1	5.9	5.7	5.6	5.5	5.4	5.3	5.1	5.0	4.9	4.8	4.7	4.6	4.5	4.4	4.3	4.2	4.1
62	6.4	6.3	6.2	6.0	5.8	5.7	5.6	5.4	5.3	5.2	5.0	4.9	4.8	4.7	4.6	4.5	4.4	4.3	4.3	4.2	4.1
63	6.3	6.1	6.0	5.9	5.7	5.6	5.5	5.3	5.2	5.1	5.0	4.9	4.8	4.7	4.6	4.5	4.4	4.3	4.2	4.1	4.0
64	6.2	6.1	5.9	5.8	5.6	5.5	5.4	5.2	5.1	5.0	4.9	4.8	4.7	4.6	4.5	4.4	4.3	4.2	4.1	4.0	4.0
65	6.1	6.0	5.8	5.7	5.6	5.4	5.3	5.2	5.0	4.9	4.8	4.7	4.6	4.5	4.4	4.3	4.2	4.1	4.0	4.0	3.9
66	6.1	5.9	5.7	5.6	5.5	5.3	5.2	5.1	5.0	4.9	4.7	4.6	4.5	4.4	4.4	4.3	4.2	4.1	4.0	3.9	3.8
67	6.0	5.8	5.7	5.5	5.4	5.3	5.1	5.0	4.9	4.8	4.7	4.6	4.5	4.4	4.3	4.2	4.1	4.0	3.9	3.9	3.8
68	5.9	5.7	5.6	5.4	5.3	5.2	5.0	4.9	4.7	4.6	4.6	4.4	4.3	4.3	4.2	4.1	4.0	3.9	3.8	3.7	3.7
69	5.8	5.6	5.5	5.3	5.2	5.1	5.0	4.9	4.8	4.6	4.5	4.4	4.3	4.3	4.2	4.1	4.0	3.9	3.9	3.8	3.7
70	5.7	5.5	5.4	5.3	5.1	5.0	4.9	4.8	4.7	4.6	4.5	4.4	4.3	4.2	4.1	4.0	4.0	3.9	3.8	3.7	3.7
71	5.6	5.5	5.3	5.2	5.1	5.0	4.8	4.7	4.6	4.5	4.4	4.3	4.2	4.1	4.1	4.0	3.9	3.8	3.8	3.7	3.6
72	5.6	5.4	5.3	5.1	5.0	4.9	4.8	4.7	4.6	4.4	4.3	4.3	4.2	4.1	4.0	3.9	3.8	3.8	3.7	3.6	3.5
73	5.5	5.3	5.2	5.1	4.9	4.8	4.7	4.6	4.5	4.4	4.3	4.2	4.1	4.0	4.0	3.9	3.8	3.7	3.6	3.6	3.5
74	5.4	5.3	5.1	5.0	4.9	4.8	4.6	4.5	4.4	4.3	4.2	4.1	4.0	4.0	3.9	3.8	3.7	3.6	3.5	3.5	3.4
75	5.3	5.2	5.1	4.9	4.8	4.7	4.6	4.5	4.4	4.3	4.2	4.1	4.0	3.9	3.8	3.8	3.7	3.6	3.5	3.4	3.4

Table 2.2 **(continued)**

Stride Length	3.6	3.7	3.8	3.9	4.0	4.1	4.2	4.3	4.4	4.5	4.6	4.7	4.8	4.9	5.0	5.1	5.2	5.3	5.4	5.5	5.6
76	5.2	5.1	5.0	4.9	4.7	4.6	4.5	4.4	4.3	4.2	4.1	4.0	3.9	3.8	3.8	3.7	3.6	3.6	3.5	3.4	3.3
77	5.2	5.0	4.9	4.8	4.7	4.6	4.5	4.4	4.3	4.2	4.1	4.0	3.9	3.8	3.7	3.7	3.6	3.5	3.4	3.4	3.3
78	5.1	5.0	4.9	4.7	4.6	4.5	4.4	4.3	4.2	4.1	4.0	3.9	3.8	3.8	3.7	3.6	3.5	3.5	3.4	3.4	3.3
79	5.1	4.9	4.8	4.7	4.6	4.5	4.3	4.2	4.1	4.0	3.9	3.8	3.8	3.7	3.6	3.6	3.5	3.4	3.4	3.3	3.2
80	5.0	4.9	4.8	4.6	4.5	4.4	4.3	4.2	4.1	4.0	3.9	3.8	3.8	3.7	3.6	3.5	3.5	3.4	3.3	3.3	3.2
81	4.9	4.8	4.7	4.6	4.4	4.3	4.2	4.1	4.0	4.0	3.9	3.8	3.7	3.6	3.6	3.5	3.4	3.3	3.3	3.2	3.2
82	4.9	4.8	4.6	4.5	4.4	4.3	4.2	4.1	4.0	3.9	3.8	3.8	3.7	3.6	3.5	3.4	3.4	3.3	3.3	3.2	3.1
83	4.8	4.7	4.6	4.5	4.3	4.2	4.1	4.0	4.0	3.9	3.8	3.7	3.6	3.5	3.5	3.4	3.3	3.2	3.2	3.1	3.0
84	4.7	4.6	4.5	4.4	4.3	4.2	4.1	4.0	3.9	3.8	3.7	3.6	3.5	3.5	3.4	3.4	3.3	3.2	3.2	3.1	3.0
85	4.7	4.6	4.5	4.3	4.2	4.1	4.0	3.9	3.9	3.8	3.7	3.6	3.5	3.5	3.4	3.3	3.3	3.2	3.1	3.0	3.0
86	4.7	4.5	4.4	4.3	4.2	4.1	4.0	3.9	3.8	3.7	3.6	3.6	3.5	3.4	3.4	3.3	3.2	3.2	3.1	3.0	3.0
87	4.6	4.5	4.4	4.2	4.1	4.0	3.9	3.8	3.8	3.7	3.6	3.5	3.5	3.4	3.3	3.3	3.2	3.1	3.0	3.0	2.9
88	4.6	4.4	4.3	4.2	4.1	4.0	3.9	3.8	3.7	3.6	3.6	3.5	3.4	3.3	3.3	3.2	3.2	3.1	3.0	3.0	2.9
89	4.5	4.4	4.3	4.2	4.0	4.0	3.9	3.8	3.7	3.6	3.5	3.4	3.3	3.3	3.2	3.2	3.1	3.0	2.9	2.9	2.8
90	4.4	4.3	4.2	4.1	3.9	3.9	3.7	3.7	3.6	3.6	3.4	3.3	3.3	3.2	3.2	3.1	3.0	3.0	2.9	2.9	2.8
91	4.4	4.3	4.2	4.1	4.0	3.9	3.8	3.7	3.7	3.5	3.4	3.4	3.3	3.2	3.2	3.1	3.0	3.0	2.9	2.8	2.8
92	4.4	4.3	4.1	4.0	3.9	3.8	3.7	3.6	3.6	3.5	3.4	3.3	3.3	3.2	3.1	3.1	3.0	3.0	2.9	2.9	2.8
93	4.3	4.2	4.1	4.0	3.9	3.8	3.7	3.6	3.5	3.4	3.4	3.3	3.2	3.2	3.1	3.0	3.0	2.9	2.9	2.8	2.8
94	4.2	4.1	4.0	3.9	3.8	3.7	3.7	3.6	3.5	3.4	3.3	3.3	3.2	3.1	3.1	3.0	3.0	2.9	2.8	2.8	2.7
95	4.2	4.1	4.0	3.9	3.8	3.7	3.6	3.5	3.4	3.4	3.3	3.3	3.2	3.1	3.1	3.0	2.9	2.9	2.8	2.8	2.7
96	4.2	4.1	4.0	3.9	3.8	3.7	3.6	3.5	3.4	3.3	3.3	3.2	3.1	3.1	3.1	2.9	2.9	2.8	2.7	2.7	2.6
97	4.1	4.0	3.9	3.8	3.7	3.6	3.5	3.5	3.4	3.3	3.2	3.2	3.1	3.0	3.0	2.9	2.9	2.8	2.8	2.7	2.7
98	4.1	4.0	3.9	3.8	3.7	3.6	3.5	3.4	3.3	3.3	3.2	3.1	3.1	3.0	2.9	2.9	2.8	2.8	2.7	2.7	2.6
99	4.0	3.9	3.8	3.7	3.6	3.6	3.5	3.4	3.3	3.2	3.2	3.1	3.0	3.0	2.9	2.9	2.8	2.7	2.7	2.6	2.6
100	4.0	3.9	3.8	3.7	3.6	3.5	3.4	3.4	3.3	3.2	3.1	3.1	3.0	3.0	2.9	2.9	2.8	2.7	2.7	2.6	2.6
101	4.0	3.9	3.8	3.7	3.6	3.5	3.4	3.3	3.2	3.2	3.1	3.1	3.0	3.0	2.9	2.9	2.8	2.7	2.7	2.6	2.6
102	3.9	3.8	3.7	3.6	3.5	3.4	3.4	3.3	3.2	3.1	3.1	3.0	2.9	2.9	2.9	2.8	2.7	2.7	2.6	2.6	2.5
103	3.9	3.8	3.7	3.6	3.5	3.4	3.3	3.3	3.2	3.1	3.0	3.0	2.9	2.9	2.8	2.7	2.7	2.6	2.6	2.5	2.5
104	3.8	3.7	3.6	3.6	3.5	3.4	3.3	3.2	3.2	3.1	3.0	3.0	2.9	2.8	2.8	2.7	2.7	2.6	2.6	2.5	2.4
105	3.8	3.7	3.6	3.5	3.4	3.3	3.3	3.2	3.1	3.1	3.0	2.9	2.9	2.8	2.7	2.7	2.6	2.6	2.5	2.5	2.4
106	3.8	3.6	3.6	3.5	3.4	3.3	3.2	3.2	3.1	3.0	3.0	2.9	2.8	2.8	2.7	2.7	2.6	2.6	2.5	2.4	2.4
107	3.7	3.6	3.5	3.4	3.3	3.3	3.1	3.1	3.0	2.9	2.9	2.8	2.8	2.7	2.7	2.6	2.6	2.5	2.5	2.5	2.4
108	3.7	3.6	3.5	3.4	3.3	3.2	3.1	3.0	3.0	2.9	2.9	2.8	2.7	2.7	2.6	2.6	2.5	2.5	2.4	2.4	2.3

HIGH SPEED DIRECTIONAL CHANGE

Starting, Acceleration, Deceleration, Stopping, and Cutting

What test measures cutting and change of direction skills?

The Pro Agility Test (Shuttle Test) used in the NFL Combine is an excellent way to evaluate the ability of athletes in all sports to start, accelerate, decelerate, stop, and execute high speed cuts. The test assesses your strength/weight ratio (relative strength) stopping, starting and accelerating speed, and the speed of lateral and linear sprinting.

With three cones placed five yards apart, each athlete assumes a starting position with both feet and one hand on the ground at the MIDDLE cone and follows these guidelines:

1. Sprint five yards to the right to the outside cone, plant the outside foot and touch the line at the cone.

2. Push off and sprint 10 yards in the opposite direction to far cone at the left.

3 Plant the outside foot, touch the line with your hand and sprint five yards in the opposite direction past the middle cone.

Key tips to Improve Your Score

Athletes can achieve better scores by following a few simple suggestions.

1. Bend slightly at the waist with the knees bent only to approximately 20 degrees.

2. Place the left hand on the ground if you are beginning the test by sprinting to the right.

3. Place very little weight on the hand. Since you will be moving laterally and not forward, weight on the hand will have a negative impact on your time.

4. Keep your eyes and head down without looking ahead.

5. Place the right arm with the elbow at about 90 degrees and the hand near your the right hip. Do not allow the hand to hang down or rest on the right hip.

6. Execute the first step by crossing over with the left leg keeping the eyes focused while staying low.

7. Avoid a "jump" stop and keep the center of gravity over the inside leg on the turn to help you "lean in" just prior to the turn. Make certain you are wearing the right shoes for the surface to avoid any chance of slipping on the plant foot.

8. Keep the hand low and try to touch the line with your hand just as the outside leg completes the plant.

9. Complete the final five yards in three steps or less.

STRIDE LENGTH

How is stride length measured?

Both under striding or over striding affects overall speed in short sprints. The key is to develop a natural, optimal stride, then focus on training programs that increase the number of steps you take per second. The same programs that favorably affect stride rate will naturally increase the length of your stride.

High speed cameras provide the most accurate record of stride length and stride length changes during a sprint of any distance. In most cases, however, coaches and athletes need to use the more practical method described below.

To find an athlete's stride length, place two markers 25 yards apart on a smooth dirt surface, such as a baseball infield, approximately 40 yards from the starting line. The soft dirt surface will allow the footprints to be seen. Runners reach near maximum speed before arriving at the first marker and sprint through the 25-yard area. Two helpers identify foot prints and measure and record stride length for two separate strides during the same trial. Measurements are made to the nearest inch from the tip of the left toe to the tip of the right toe (one stride) and from the tip of the right toe to the tip of the left toe (second stride). This provides two unique aspects of stride length and permits a comparison of the push-off power from the left foot and from the right foot to determine imbalances. A second trial is given if athletes exhibit form errors such as jumping or over striding.

The average stride length of top male sprinters is reported as 1.14 X height (+ or - 4 inches), 1.24 X height, and 1.265 X height. The average stride length of female sprinters is reported as 1.15 X height and 2.16 X leg length. Leg length is measured from inside the groin to the bottom of the heel. The length of the legs does affect stride length and obviously cannot be changed. Form and ground contact force are the two key factors that can be changed, but it is the combination of all three that results in a natural, relaxed stride. Use this information to determine if stride length scores fall within these ranges. Now compare the length of the two strides: one with a left foot push-off and one with a right-foot push-off. If one is more than 2-3" longer than the other, more push-off power is being generated on that rear foot and less on the other. This difference should also show up on the leg kickback test score measured on the Universal Gym. If a stride length is greater than this range and no over striding is observed, there is no need for change. If scores indicate over striding, the form drills in Chapter 13 will help achieve the most efficient stride length. Sprint-assisted training, form training and power output training (speed strength, plyometrics and sprint-resisted programs) will increase the length of your stride in 3 to 4 months.

The NASE First 3-Step Test

How is the "First 3-step test" administered?

One timer and two assistants are placed at the five yard mark on a track or infield where a footprint is left with each step. Both the time and distance covered for three steps are recorded. Timing begins with the first muscular movement and ends when the third step is completed. Two assistants mark the tip of the toe of the first, second and third steps and record these distances and the total distance covered to the nearest 1/4 inch.

Little data exist to evaluate test scores in this area. Comparisons are now being made using body weight, gender, age, sport and position. The times in Table 2.3 serve as a reference point for how fast male and female athletes usually move in the first three steps. Females are slower than males, mainly due to lower speed-strength and ground contact force.

Table 2.3 **The Speed, Length and Force of the First Three Steps in Track and Football**

	FIRST Male	STEP Female	SECOND Male	STEP Female	THIRD Male	STEP Female
Track*	10.50 to 13.89 fps	7.40 to 13.50 fps	12.54 to 16.33 fps	12:00 to 18.40 fps	16.57 to 20.00 fps	14.40 18.40 fps
Football**	8 to 15 8.7 40-yd.	9.5 40-yd.	13-16 fps 9.7 40-yd.	10.5 40-yd.	16 to 20 fps 6.7 40-yd.	7.3 40-yd.
Step Length	2.89 to 4.02"		3.00 to 4.6		3.74-5.10	
Force (lb.)	222 to 523	186 to 450				

** Gender estimations based on percent differences found in Adrian and Cooper, 1989.

*Ward, P. 1973. An analysis of kinetic and kinematic factors of the standup and the preferred crouch starting techniques with respect to sprint performance. Unpublished dissertation.

Is there a way to estimate how much improvement each athlete can expect in the 40-yard dash?

Complete the NASE future 40-yard dash test by having a coach or friend administer the test using a stationary position while being towed with surgical tubing. Connect the belt securely around the waist in front, with the other belt attached to a partner's waist at the back. With a partner standing 10 yards in front of the finish line, back up and stretch the tubing exactly 30 yards until reaching the starting line where a 3-point or 4-point stance is assumed. The timer at the finish line starts the watch on the first muscular movement and stops it at the finish line. After sprinting 5 yards, the partner sprints away in the same direction to provide additional pull throughout the test. Providing the sprint is completed without breaking form, this time, PLUS 3/10 of a second, is an estimate of what an athlete is capable of doing after several months of training when timed without assistance from surgical tubing.

POWER OUTPUT (SPEED STRENGTH)

(Ground contact force, Dead Lift, Double Leg Press, Single-leg kick back, Single and Double Leg Extension and Curl, Standing Triple Jump)

The most valuable tests of strength and power are those that measure ground contact force with each stride in sprinting. Although not as accurate as computer force plate technology, the speed-strength tests in this section provide valuable information about an athletes strength-weight ratios and ability to exert force against the ground, overcome the force of gravity and propel the body upward and forward in sprinting. In the near future it is anticipated that special sensors placed in shoes will record and store this information.

What are the most important speed-strength tests?

The two most critical tests are the Dead Lift and the Single Leg Kickback. Both tests measure ground contact force. Leg curls and leg extensions serve to identify muscle imbalance problems between the right and left leg and the hamstrings and quadriceps muscles.

For each exercise, scores are determined using 1RM testing. Athletes who have been involved in an ongoing free weight training program either know their 1RM (amount of weight they can lift for one repetition) or can provide a close estimate for each exercise. On the first trial after proper warm-up, use a low estimate of the amount of weight you can lift just one time and complete several repetitions. Rest 3-4 minutes and add 5-10 pounds. Continue to add or remove weight until locating the amount, to the nearest 5-10 pounds, that can be lifted only one time.

The Dead Lift (see Chapter 8) may be the single most important measure of an athlete's ability to exert a high amount of ground contact force during all phases of sprinting from the start to maximum speed.

The right and left leg kickback test examines and compares the force exerted against an area similar to a starting block and the ground during the accelerating phase of sprinting. It also allows a comparison of the force exerted by each leg. Stand to the side of a leg press station facing away from the leg pad. Place one foot on the pad and bend the knee to right angles before exerting as much force as possible to reach a full leg extension. Repeat the procedure until the 1RM is found for each leg separately. If the right and left leg scores differ by more than 5 lb., a muscle imbalance is indicated.

The Single and Double Leg Press identifies a key strength-weight ratio that can be evaluated and altered to improve sprinting speed. The objective is to find the maximum amount of weight each athlete can leg press for one repetition. Adjust the seat on a Universal, Nautilus, or similar leg press station or free weight stand (squat) until the knees are bent at right angles. On the first attempt, try an amount of weight equal to two times body weight. If that amount is too little or too much, rest 3-4 minutes and add or remove weight before trying again. Continue to add or remove 10 pounds until identifying the amount, to the nearest 5-10 pounds, that can be leg pressed only one time. Divide body weight into the total pounds lifted to find the leg strength/body weight ratio. This ratio indicates how easily one can get and keep the body moving at high speeds. A good ratio is 2.5:1, or a leg press score two and one-half times your body weight. If you weigh 150 pounds, for example, the leg press score should be at least 375 pounds (150 X 2.5 = 375). At college and professional levels of competition, ratios of 3:1 and 4:1 (three or four times body weight) are desirable.

For both the leg extension and leg curl test, find the 1RM in the same manner described above. The *Leg Extension* test measures quadriceps strength and is completed by sitting with the back straight while grasping both sides of the Universal or Nautilus bench. Hook both feet under the leg press pad and extend the legs. *The Leg Curl* measures hamstring strength and is also completed on a Universal Gym, Nautilus or similar equipment that has a leg curl station. To complete the Leg Curl test, lie on the stomach and hook both heels under the leg curl pad. Grasp the sides of the seat or the handles with both hands and flex the legs to the buttocks. Divide leg extension scores, in pounds, into leg curls to find the ratio. For example, if the double leg extension score is 100 pounds and double leg curl score is 50 pounds, the ratio is 50 divided by 100 or 50 percent (ratio of 2: 1). A score of less than 75 percent (ratio of 2: 1.33) is low and indicates the need to strengthen the hamstrings.

Ideally, leg extension scores (quadriceps) and leg curl scores (hamstrings) would be the same. In most athletes, however, the quadriceps are much stronger than the hamstrings. The average leg curl score of 1,625 middle school and high school football players tested was less than 50 percent of the leg extension score. Such an imbalance is associated with hamstring injuries and reduced sprinting performance. Experts also feel that the speed strength of the hamstring muscle group is the weakest link in most athletes and should be improved to 80-90 percent of the speed strength of the quadriceps group. A minimum of 75 percent is recommended for the prevention of injury.

Comparing the right single leg curl to the left and the right leg extension score to the left may also reveal a muscle imbalance that, when corrected, may improve speed in short sprints.

The Standing Triple Jump is also an excellent indicator of power output contributing to the start, acceleration and maximum speed phases of short sprints. Complete several standing triple jumps at slow speed until perfect form and technique are mastered. Now take the final maximum effort jump. The standing triple jump also provides a noninvasive technique (without resorting to muscle biopsy) of estimating the percent of fast-twitch muscle fiber in key areas. High scores are also associated with excellent starting and acceleration speed.

In the standing long jump position, jump forward as far as possible using a two-foot takeoff, landing on only one foot before immediately jumping to the opposite foot, taking one final jump, and landing on both feet. Practice the standing triple jump test at low speeds until the technique is mastered. The movement is identical to the triple jump in track and field, except for the use of a two-foot takeoff (standing broad jump). The test must begin with a jump off both feet for successful completion.

The Right and Left Leg Hops provide an excellent assessment of the speed-strength in each leg. High scores are associated with longer strides. After a 15-yard flying start, begin a one-legged hop at the start and continue hopping 20 yards to the finish line. Flags are used on the start and finish tapes. The test involves an all-out effort, first on the dominant leg, then on the non-dominant leg. Right and left leg hops allow a comparison of the power of the dominant and the recessive leg. Most athletes will show a difference and need to focus on the less explosive limb to correct the imbalance.

SUSTAINED POWER OUTPUT (SPEED ENDURANCE)

Speed endurance (anaerobic) tests are critical in sports that require athletes to make repeated short sprints after minimal rest intervals or long sprints during competition.

A high level of speed endurance allows athletes to sprint further before the onset of lactic acid buildup, recover more quickly between sprints, execute repeated sprints with minimum slowing due to fatigue, hold maximum speed longer, and exhibit less slowing at the end of a long sprint.

What is the best speed endurance test for team sports?

The part of the 120-yard dash test described previously (comparing the time required to cover 40 yards from the 40-80 mark with the time for the 80-120 yard mark) measures only one aspect of speed endurance--the amount of slowing that occurs during a long sprint. Equally important is the amount of slowing that occurs from one sprint to another during competition. Sports such as football, field hockey, basketball, soccer, rugby, lacrosse, and tennis, require repeated sprints throughout the contest. Athletes with a high level of speed endurance complete each sprint at nearly the same speed.

The *NASE Repeated 20-yard or 40-yard Sprint Test* is sport specific since the rest interval between sprints is determined from an athlete's sport and position. Ten consecutive sprints are completed using a predetermined distance and rest interval between each based on the information in Table 2.4. In football, ten 20-yard dashes are completed at 25-30 second rest intervals (huddle time) for offensive and defensive linemen, and ten 40-yard dashes for players in other positions. Scores are plotted in the order they are completed and analyzed for drop-off from the first repetition to the tenth. Ideally, there should be no more than a 2/10 second difference between the best and worst score. Basketball, soccer, lacrosse, rugby and field hockey use 10-40 yard distances and shorter rest intervals, depending upon player position. Shorter distances (5-10 yards) and rest intervals are used for tennis.

Table 2.4 Guidelines for Speed-Endurance Testing

Sport (Sec.)	Average Distance (Yds.)	Typical Interval Between Sprints (Sec.)
Baseball, Softball	30	30 to 60
Basketball	10 to 30	10 to 15
Football	10 to 40	25 to 30 (huddle time)
Soccer, Lacrosse, Rugby, Field Hockey	10 to 40	5 to 15
Tennis	5 to 10	3 to 5 (same point), 20 to 30 (between points), 60 (between games)

Does aerobic fitness improve speed endurance?

All sports have an aerobic component and attaining an optimal level of aerobic fitness expedites the removal of the lactic acid accumulated during repetitive anaerobic activity. This process allows athletes to recover faster after each sprint and minimizes slowing due to fatigue throughout the contest.

The *1.5 Mile Run* is an excellent test of aerobic fitness for team sports. Athletes should use a general walk-jog warm-up that produces perspiration, followed by a 5-8 minute dynamic flexibility stretching session before completing six laps around a track. Standards vary according to position in most sports, with large athletes 225-400 lb. permitted more time to complete the test (see the Standards column of your Speed Profile Form in Table 2.1).

QUICKNESS TESTS

What tests of quickness are used in team sports?

The Quick Feet Test provides information on the presence or absence of fast-twitch muscle fibers in the muscles involved in sprinting and indicates your potential to execute fast steps (stride rate) and quick movements.

Place 20 two-foot long sticks or a 20-rung rope on a grass or artificial turf field. A football field with each yard marked can also be used. Space sticks exactly 18 inches apart for a total distance of 10 yards. Pump the arms vigorously in a sprint-arm motion and use little knee lift while running the 10 yards without touching the sticks. The timer starts the watch when the foot first touches the ground between the first and second stick and stops the watch when contact is made with the ground beyond the last stick.

MUSCLE IMBALANCE TESTING

(Right and Left Leg Extension, Right and left Leg Curl, Right and Left Leg Hop)

What tests are used to identify muscle imbalance problems?

Numerous tests have now been completed that reveal muscle imbalances. Go to the Speed Profile Form (Table 2.1) and fill in the information requested under *Muscle Imbalance* for the following tests that have been presented previously: Right and left leg stride length scores, right and left leg kickback scores, right and left leg extension and curl scores, and right and left leg hops. These test scores should already be recorded and can now be used for muscle imbalance interpretations to obtain a more clear picture of how evenly speed-strength has been developed throughout the body. Since it is clear that muscle imbalances negatively affect speed of movement, more and more athletes and coaches take the time to compare dominant and recessive limb strength using various weight training exercises and other tests. Once a difference is noted, weight training programs can be altered until both sides of the body possess near equal strength.

The major focus on muscle imbalance in the past has been between joint agonists and antagonists such as the quadriceps (generally well developed in sprinters) and hamstrings (underdeveloped in most athletes). Numerous activities and exercises produce strength increases in agonistic muscle groups without a corresponding increase in the antagonistic muscle group. It is difficult to determine just how much a quadriceps-hamstrings imbalance and upper body imbalances of this nature affects speed in short sprints.

Although the type of imbalance discussed above needs to be corrected, there is an equally important imbalance in team sport athletes that is known to negatively affect starting, accelerating and sprinting speed (maximum velocity). *Contra lateral imbalances* or the speed-strength and power differences in the same muscle groups on the right and left side of the body do exist in many athletes. The dominant side (right arm for the right-handed athlete and left leg used for the one foot takeoff in right-handed basketball players), for example, gets more repetitions (jumps, throws), more use in daily chores, and is favored throughout life in all kinds of movements. These and other factors contribute to both the development of one side (upper and lower arm and leg) and to the underdevelopment of the other side. Although the prime movers in sprinting (knee extensors, hip extensors and ankle plantar flexors) tend to become well developed as a result of normal sprint training, the fact remains that these and other muscle groups may be much more developed on one side of the body than the other. Such imbalances affect every phase of sprinting and must be corrected if an athlete is to reach their speed potential.

It is relatively simple for coaches to identify the weaker side muscle groups and make the correction by improving the speed-strength of that limb through weight training exercises.

What is the correct procedure to find the 1RM for a speed-strength exercise?

After a 10-15 general warm-up period consisting of walking, light jogging (until perspiration occurs), and several minutes of dynamic stretching (upper and lower body), follow the six steps listed below as carefully as possible.

1. Complete two easy sets of 9-10 repetitions in the same exercise for which you are determining the 1RM (repetitions maximum).

2. Rest 4-5 minutes before placing an amount of weight on the bar equal to the closest estimate (not overestimate) of the maximum amount of weight that can be lifted for only one repetition.

3. Complete one repetition with that weight using proper form and a "spotter."

4. Rest 3-4 minutes and adjust the weight upward or downward and complete a second attempt with the new weight.

5. Rest 4-5 minutes to fully recover before adding or removing weight and making a final attempt to locate the 1RM.

6. Record the 1RM to the nearest 5-10 pounds.

FLEXIBILITY TESTS

To achieve maximum speed potential, an adequate range of motion in the shoulders, hips, and ankles must be present. Flexibility in these areas is affected by joint structure. Ball-and-socket joints (hip and shoulder) have the highest range of motion (ROM); the wrist is one of the least flexible joints with a ROM of 80 degrees, which is less than the 130 degrees of the knee joint. Excess muscle bulk (decreases ROM); age (decreases flexibility); gender (females are more flexible than males); connective tissue such as tendons, ligaments, fascia sheaths and joint capsules; injuries (restricts movement); and existing scar tissue (decreases ROM) are additional factors affecting range of motion.

Flexibility tests may also reveal excessive range of motion or joint laxity that can predispose athletes to injury. Once an optimum level of flexibility is developed, athletes should focus on other training areas while maintaining this flexibility. Because flexibility is joint-specific, a single test does not provide an accurate assessment of range of motion. It is also impractical to measure the ROM of every joint. In addition, the flexibility of some joints is not critical to sprinting speed.

The tests described in the following sections can be completed with little equipment and provide important information on ankle flexion and extension, shoulder flexibility, and hamstring flexibility.

Sit-and-Reach

What flexibility tests are recommended?

The Sit-and-Reach Test measures the flexibility of the lower back and the hamstring muscle group (the large group of muscles located on the back of the upper leg). An optimal level of flexibility in both areas is equally important.

After warming up to elevate body temperature, remove the shoes, and sit on the floor with the hips, back, and head against a wall, legs fully extended, and feet contacting a sit-and-reach box. Place one hand on top of the other so the middle fingers are together. Lean forward slowly as far as possible, without bouncing, slide the hands along the measuring scale on top of the box. The hands should reach at least slightly beyond the toes. Complete four trials and record the best score to the nearest one-fourth inch. If a sit-and-reach box is not available, one can be built by nailing a yardstick on top of a 12-inch by 12-inch square box. The yardstick extends exactly 9 inches from the front of the box where the feet are placed.

If your score does not merit at least a rating of "average" for your age (table 2.5), flexibility training is needed 5-6 times weekly.

Table 2.5 **Sit-and-Reach Scores (in Inches) and Ratings for Athletes in Middle School, High School, and College**

GENDER	MIDDLE SCHOOL	HIGH SCHOOL	COLLEGE	COMMENTS
Male	10.0 Average 11.0 Good 13.0 Excellent	13.0 Average 16.0 Good 17.0 Excellent	13.0 Average 16.0 Good 18.0 Excellent	A stretching session should follow each strength training workout.
Female	11.5 Average 12.5 Good 14.5 Excellent	13.0 Average 15.0 Good 18.0 Excellent	14.0 Average 16.0 Good 19.0 Excellent	Female athletes tend to be more flexible than males at all ages.

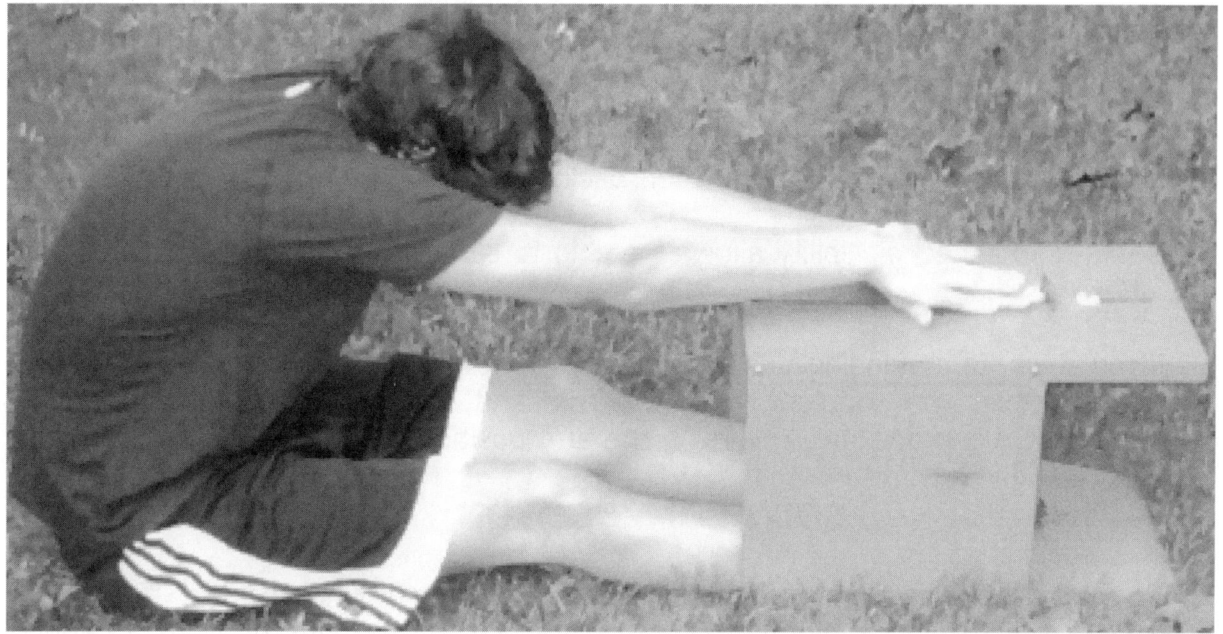

Figure 2.2 The Sit and Reach Test

What other tests can be used?

The range of motion in the ankle, neck, elbow and wrist, groin, trunk, hip, and shoulder can be quickly assessed in less than five minutes by self-administering the practical tests described below.

After completing the following tests, mark the space next to Practical ROM Tests on the Speed Profile Form.

Ankle. Lie on your back with both legs extended and the backs of the heels flat on the floor. Point the toes downward away from the shins and attempt to reach a minimum of 45 degrees (halfway to the floor). Now point the toes toward the shins to a minimum of right angles. Compare the flexion and extension of the right and left ankles.

Elbow and wrist. Athletes should be able to hold both arms straight with palms up and little fingers higher than the thumbs.

Groin. While standing on one leg, raise the other leg to the side as high as possible. A 90-degree angle should be achieved between the legs.

Hips. While standing, hold a yardstick or broom handle with both hands shoulder-width apart. Without losing or changing the grip, bend down and step over the stick (with both feet, one at a time) and then back again.

Neck. Normal neck flexibility allows the chin to sandwich a flattened hand against the chest.

Shoulders. In a standing position, attempt to clasp both hands behind the back by reaching over the shoulder with one arm and upward from behind with the other. Repeat this procedure, reversing the arm positions.

BODY COMPOSITION

The purpose of body composition tests is to determine whether the percent of body fat falls within an acceptable range. Excess fat and pounds provides an added burden that interferes with efficient movement and reduces speed.

What is the best way to measure an athlete's percent of body fat?

Unless underwater weighing equipment is available, the most accurate and practical method of determining the percent of body fat is through the skinfold technique. Because a major portion of fat storage lies just under the skin, measurements in millimeters can be used to predict total body fat.

The percent of body fat can be measured by determining the thickness of four skinfolds. The correct procedure is to grasp a fold of skin and subcutaneous fat (just under the skin) firmly with your thumb and forefinger, pulling it away and up from the underlying muscle tissue. Attach the jaws of the calipers one centimeter below the thumb and forefinger. All measurements should be taken on the right side of the body while the athlete is in a standing position. Working with a partner, practice taking each other's measurements in the four areas described until you consistently get a similar score on each attempt.

Triceps. With the arm resting at the side, take a vertical fold parallel to the long axis of the arm midway between the tip of the shoulder and the tip of the elbow.

Biceps. With the arm in the same position, take a vertical fold halfway between the elbow and top of the shoulder on the front of the upper arm.

Subscapula. Take a diagonal fold across the back, just below the shoulder blade.

Supra iliac. Take a diagonal fold following the natural line of the iliac crest, just above the hip bone.

Record the information on the Speed Profile Form to complete the evaluation. For example, Ted is a 17-year-old who weighs 185 pounds. His four skinfold measurements were 3, 4, 9, and 9 millimeters. Follow his evaluation to help you understand the procedure:

- Total the four skinfold measures in millimeters. Ted's total is 25 millimeters (3 + 4 + 9 + 9).

- Estimate the percent of body fat from Table 2.6. In this example,Ted possesses approximately 10 percent body fat. A reading of 25 millimeters for a female athlete places the estimate of body fat at about 17 percent.

- Determine the amount of weight that the athlete should lose, if any, to improve sprinting speed. Although the ideal percent of body fat may be somewhat lower for optimum sprinting speed, reasonable values fall between 10 and 15 percent for males and 15 and 20 percent for females. Growing athletes falling within these ranges do not need to diet. Ted is already at his ideal percent of body fat.

For a more accurate indication of body fat, *hydrostatic weighing* is recommended. In this test, the athlete sits on a scale in a tank of water, exhales as completely as possible, and is then submerged for 10 seconds while his or her weight is recorded. The proportion of lean mass and fat mass are determined from calculations that involve weight underwater, weight out of water, and known densities of lean and fatty tissues. *Electrical impedance* is a quicker, more practical method, but less accurate. Electrodes are attached to the wrist and ankle. In less than 2 minutes, a printout provides the percentage of fat and ideal body weight. Athletes must follow certain nutritional and exercise rules for 24 hours before the test. Ask your high school or university physical educator to help you find your percent of body fat with the skinfold test, or, if available, hydrostatic weighing or electrical impedance.

Table 2.6 Estimate of Percentage of Body Fat Using the Sum of Four Skinfolds for High School and University Athletes

Sum of Four Skinfolds (mm)	Percentage of Body Fat MALE	Percentage of Body Fat FEMALE
25 or less	10	17
35	15	21
55	20	27
85	25	34
120	30	39

How much fat should athletes possess?

The ideal percent of body fat for athletes depends upon age, sport, and position. For optimum sprinting speed, athletes should strive for 10 percent (males) and 15 percent (females). Although some body fat is essential to health (3 to 4 percent for men, and 10 to 12 percent for women), athletic performance (including speed and quickness) and health can be adversely affected by excess body fat.

How rapidly can body fat be reduced?

Dieting to lose body fat is dangerous and not recommended for growing athletes or anyone without careful supervision. The maximum rate of weight loss for athletes is 1 percent of body weight per week (1 to 2 pounds for those weighing 200 pounds or less). This rate requires a calorie deficit of 500 to 1,000 calories each day. Faster rates of weight loss, losing more than 5 percent of total weight, or weight loss programs exceeding four weeks may result in loss of lean muscle mass, dehydration, and overtraining and may cause changes in vitamin and mineral status that could hinder performance. A sound weight loss program requires careful supervision and a combination of caloric restriction, slow weight loss, and regular exercise, including strength training to avoid loss of lean muscle mass and to add muscle weight while losing fat weight. Make sure you consult your coach and physician (and parents, if you are under 18) before beginning any weight loss program.

ADVANCED TESTING

The advanced testing program is designed for athletes competing at the high school, college, and professional levels. The program requires more specialized equipment and coaches who are familiar with these procedures.

Strength Curve Testing

What is strength curve testing?

Dr. Stan Plagenhoef developed testing procedures to measure changes in leverage and muscle mass as a limb is moved through a range of motion. Anatomical strength curves reflect the body's ability to produce muscle contractile force at given points in the range of motion. These strength curves are used to determine how far above or below the strength potential an individual falls. Data collected on Olympic sprinters such as Carl Lewis, Leroy Burrell, Chris Jones, and Lamont Smith allow valuable comparisons to athletes in other sports who are striving to improve their sprinting speed. Strength curves can also be used to compare the right and left sides of the body (dominant to non-dominant side).

On-Field Analysis (Playing Speed)

How is On-field analysis used to evaluate performance?

On-field Game Analysis

New methods are rapidly evolving to help explain and evaluate performance more objectively. In the future, on-field analysis will uncover much of the information provided by a test battery with data obtained during actual competition. For sprinting analysis, this sophisticated system will use an Olympic champion sprinter as a basis for creating a digital athletic model of performance. Performances will be recorded in the computer with values assigned to points of movement. This information will then be compared to the database of the Olympic Champion Digital Model. The result will be graphically displayed through differences in performance characteristics such as leg lift, arm swing, stride length, and leg extension.

Radar Technology

How is radar used to test athletes?

Radar has been used in track and field to study sprinters by monitoring their progress on a daily basis without having to use a full distance race under meet conditions.

Radar technology can provide answers to questions such as: "Is your athlete running faster? Are they getting out of the blocks faster? Is each athlete accelerating to top speed too soon or too late? Is top speed improving? Are athletes keeping that top speed for a longer distance? Are they pushing harder on the ground with each step?" The answer to these and other questions allow coaches to focus their training on weakness areas that will have the greatest impact on speed.

Radar guns are also available to assist coaches with monitoring many components of a runner's form: Block speed (horizontal speed at first foot strike out of blocks), acceleration/deceleration ratio for the first step out of the blocks (this ratio should be as large as possible while maintaining good running form), step time (between two consecutive steps), step length (distance between two consecutive footprints on a track), step frequency (number of footprints per second hitting track), time and distance to maximum speed (relative to first step out of blocks), time and distance that maximum speed is maintained, presence of any left-right asymmetry in gait, and some details of the speed curve during the contact time of the foot with the track, indicating any gross abnormalities in running form.

If a coach has even a very modest budget ($350 for a month's rental) and access to a laptop computer and minimal skill at using it (or the willingness to learn!), all of the above parameters for any athlete can be discovered with processing times from a few seconds to a few minutes maximum and done immediately upon the finish of the run.

Overall, radar technology offers benefits that lasers do not. With a little patience until the user becomes familiar with the software, very useful information can be extracted for individual runners immediately after their run. Many times, for example, it is obvious to the coach that the novice runner's response to the command "run harder" is to take longer steps, and actually slow down their gait. The radar gun can make this painfully clear to the athlete and support the coach's visual analysis with some quantitative data. Radar has the ability to be a key component in the coaches' arsenal of weapons for training the elite or novice sprinter (Headly, 2003).

BUILDING YOUR PROGRAM

You now have enough information to design a personalized speed improvement program based on your test scores. For each score on the comprehensive test, check *Yes* in the weakness column on the Speed Profile Form if you failed to meet the standard specified. If you check *Yes* for a test, also check the programs listed at the bottom of Table 2.1 for that test area. These are the specific training programs you need to follow to eliminate the weakness areas.

TEAM SPORT COMBINES (NFL, MLB, MLS, NBA)

Pre-draft testing programs in team sports, such as the NFL Combine for pro football prospects, have become extremely important with scores having a dramatic effect on the draft round, signing bonus, salary, and other specifics in a contract. A poor combine 40-yard dash time, for example, can and has cost potential high round picks millions of dollars. So much emphasis is placed on the 40-yard dash and some other tests that prospects are forced to train for and practice specific tests for months before the scheduled combine. As a result, Combine Training Centers have sprung up throughout the USA. Specific player position tests are also important, and scores in these areas can be improved with training and practice.

The best way to achieve excellent scores in sports combine tests is to complete the comprehensive test battery described in this chapter and follow our sports-specific speed improvement program for 6-10 weeks to eliminate your weakness areas and improve your speed.

Practice and training for the specific tests used in a combine will also greatly increase the chance of achieving a higher rating for the draft. This section describes each test and scoring procedure in pro combines and tryout centers in baseball, basketball, football and soccer. Study the tables below carefully and master the techniques for each test prior to attending a combine or tryout.

NFL Combine

What physical tests are included in the NFL Combine?

Physical tests are offered in each of the areas described in table 2.7

Table 2.7 **NFL Combine Tests**

TEST	DESCRIPTION
PHYSICAL TESTS	
40 yard dash	Each player runs twice. The best time is recorded by pro scouts and the test is filmed.
225 lb. Bench Press	Each player, except kickers, completes as many repetitions as possible.
20 yard Short Shuttle	Each player, except kickers, is timed twice, once in the shuttle run left and once to the right. Both times are recorded and the drill is filmed.

Table 2.7 **(continued)**

TEST	DESCRIPTION
Vertical Jump	The test is conducted using the Vertec measuring device. Each player jumps twice. The highest jump is recorded.
Height & Weight	Height is measured to 1/8th of an inch and weight to the nearest pound.
FULL BODY VIDEO PORTRAIT	Provides a visual image of body type and build. Players are filmed from the front and back wearing shorts only.
PHASE II: SPECIFIC ONE-ON-ONE DRILLS (filmed, not part of grading system)	
QB	Filmed in isolation performing 3, 5 and 7 step drops and throws to WR's on one-on-one coverage against DB's.
RB/TE vs L	Running Backs and Tight Ends compete against Linebackers in man coverage during a one-on-one passing drill.
WR vs DB	Wide Receivers compete against Defensive Backs in man coverage during a one-on-one passing drill.
OL vs DL	Lineman are timed in the 10-yd and 20-yd dash before completing several cone drills to evaluate foot speed and quickness and compete in one-on-one competition during Run/ Block/React and Pass Rush/Block Drills. Helmets are worn during the blocking drills.
Punters	The Baseline Strength Test (hang time, distance and get-off time recorded on a total of six punts over two rounds) and Random Selection Scenario Test (ability to perform six different types of punts during two rounds - Direction Right, Direction Left, Deep Center, Deep Nose Over, Straight Pooch, and Float Pooch) is completed. Top punters in these tests may be asked to perform additional punts.
Kickers	Kick-offs (measured for hang time, location and distance on three consecutive kicks) and Field Goals (8 FG's over four rounds at randomly selected distances from 30 to 55 yards). The most successful kickers may be asked to perform additional FG's and KO's.
Long Snap	Seven snaps at each distance of 7 and 15 yards are graded for time and accuracy.

A Preparation Video Manual is available to help players prepare for the NFL combine.

Table 2.7 **(continued)**

Grading System - 5-10 scale.

Grade	Description	Player Type
9.00-10	Player significantly exceeds minimum pro standard.	Pro Player
8.00-8.99	Player meets or exceeds minimum pro standard.	Pro Prospect
7.00-7.99	Player scores slightly below minimum pro standard.	Potential Pro Prospect
6.00-6.99	Player scores below minimum pro standard.	College Level Player
5.00-5.99	Player scores well below minimum pro standard.	Below College Level

Are separate physical standards applied to each position?

Yes. Height and weight measurements and the results of the four physical tests determine a player's score in each of the four test grades: Size (height/weight), Speed (40-yard dash), Quickness (both shuttle run times) and Strength (bench press and vertical jump test). The four athletic test grades are averaged to arrive at a player's Final Test Grade (FTG). Players with an FTG equal to or greater than 8.00 are Pro Rated.

Table 2.8 **Minimum Standards by Position**

Pos	Ht	Wt	40	Shuttle	Bench	VJ
QB	6' 1"	200	4.90	4.50	10	28
RB	5' 10"	185	4.65	4.35	12	30
FB	5' 11"	220	4.75	4.35	14	28
WR	5' 11"	180	4.65	4.29	8	30
TE	6' 2"	230	4.85	4.55	18	28
CB	5' 10"	180	4.60	4.29	10	30
S	5' 11"	190	4.70	4.29	10	30
OLB	6' 1"	220	4.80	4.50	18	28
ILB	6' 1"	230	4.85	4.50	18	28
DE	6' 2"	270	5.00	4.60	20	26
DT	6' 3"	275	5.20	4.75	24	24
NT	6' 2"	275	5.20	4.79	24	24
OG	6' 2"	275	5.15	4.79	24	24
OT	6' 3"	275	5.25	4.79	24	24
C	6' 1"	275	5.20	4.79	24	24

The minimum pro standard equals a grade of 8.00. Higher than the minimum pro standard scores receive a score between 8.01 and 10.00, scores below the minimum fall between 7.99 and 5.00.

How are punters graded?

Averages are determined for touch-to-toe, hang time and distance during open-field punting.

Table 2.9 **Pro standard minimum by category and % in calculating the FTG**

Category	Pro Minimum	% of FTG
Touch-to-Toe	4.0 sec.	20%
Hang Time	4.25 sec.	40%
Distance	42 yd.	40%

How are place kickers graded?

Place kickers are scored based on field goals made and average kickoff KO) hang time and distance. The KO Grade is based 50% on distance and 50% on hang time. The Field Goal Grade is based on a starting grade of 5.00, with each successful kick increasing the grade by the point values listed below. The final grade (FTG) is based on 70% Field Goal Grade and 30% KO Grade.

Table 2.10 **Evaluating kickers**

Kickoff Category	Pro Minimum	Distance	Point Value
KO Hang Time	3.85 sec.	30 yd.	0.25
KO Distance	62 yd.	35 yd.	0.35
Field Goals		40 yd.	0.45
		45 yd. (left hash)	0,75
		45 yd. (right hash)	0,75
		50 yd. (left hash).	0,80
		50 yd. (right hash)	0,80
		55 yd.	0.85

How are long snappers graded?

Long snappers are graded based on the average time and accuracy for 7 snaps at each distance.

Table 2.11 **Long Snappers: Minimum Pro Standard (8.00 grade) For Time and Accuracy**

7 yd. Snap Time	**Pro Minimum**
Accuracy	0.28 sec. 1.29 sec.
15-yd. Snap Time	**Pro Minimum**
	0.75 sec.
Accuracy	1.57 sec.
Accuracy Scale: Grade	**Accuracy Scale: Description**
1 2 3 4	Excellent - Holder makes no adjustment Good - Holder makes minor adjustment Poor - Holder makes major adjustment Uncatchable - Snap is wild or short

What is the fastest 40-yard time ever recorded by a football player?

This is a difficult question since most 40-yard tests are hand-timed with the timer beginning the stop watch on the athlete's first muscular movement as opposed to a track event where the athlete is doing the reacting to a starting stimuli (sound of the gun). Even electronic timing used at combines allows the athlete to begin the 40-yard dash when they want to rather than having to react to a starting stimuli. As a result, hand-timed 40's and Combine electronic 40's are usually 2/10 to 3/10 faster than the same athlete could perform in a track meet. Coaches have also been known to use the hand-timed test to motivate athletes and inflate their times for encouragement. As a result, it is not unusual to hear of 40-yard times as low as 3.9; which is way out of reach even for the world's fastest 60-meter dash record holder.

In 1988, Ben Johnson of Canada set a world record in the 100-m dash (later annulled due to steroid use) by posting a 9.79 second time. Although one of the fastest starters of all times (he was two meters ahead of Carl Lewis at the 5-meter mark), his 40-meter time was said to be 4.69 and his 40-yard time was 4.38. This is still considered the fastest 40-yard dash ever run by an athlete in any sport. Claims of Michael Vick's 4.15, Stallworth's 4.26, and Deon Sander's 4.29 are inaccurate, although cornerback Tye Hill did post an electronic 40 time of 4.30 in a 2006 NFL Combine. If we add back the advantage of 0.2 - 0.3 tenths of a second gained by not reacting to a stimuli, Hill's time would be 4.5-4.6. Few believe that any football player can match the 40-yard times of a world class sprinter on a track in modern-day spikes.

The NFL's fastest official 40-yard dash time was 4.25 seconds by cornerback Fabian Washington. Prior to electronic timing, Deion Sanders held the official record at 4.29 seconds.

"Bullet" Bob Hayes may have been the fastest human of all times (mph speed) based on a 1.60 second 20-meter segment timing at an Olympic 100-meter race. If it's true that Hayes covered the 20 meters in 1.60 seconds, this is equivalent to a speed of 27.9 miles per hour.

While the 40-yard dash is an excellent test in a battery to evaluate NFL potential, the First Three Steps Test, and the 10 and 20-yard dash may be better indicators of success for most offensive and defensive positions in football. Times in a 20-yard dash correlate highly with times in the 40 and only players such as wide receivers, running backs and defensive backs routinely sprint distances as far as 40-yards.

How effective is the NFL Combine in predicting NFL success?

Few pre-season events receive as much attention in as the NFL Combine conducted each year during the 3rd week of February. Over 300 of the best college football players are invited to Indianapolis to participate. Top executives, coaches, player personnel and medical staffs from all 32 NFL teams are represented to evaluate draft-eligible players in an intense, 4-day physical and psychological testing period. Athletes are eager to display their skills to achieve their dreams of playing in the NFL. Potential NFL prospects attend combine preparation camps and clinics throughout the United States for months prior to the event. *Physical tests* include the 40-yard dash, 225 lb. bench press, pro agility shuttle, vertical jump, height, weight, and a full body video portrait. Minimum standards exists for each offensive and defensive position. In addition, specific *one-on-one drills* are filmed for various positions and punter, place kicker, and long snapper scores are recorded.

A poor 40-yard dash can keep a player from being drafted or cost him millions in signing bonuses. Other physical tests are also factored in to determine the potential of each NFL prospect. The tests are carefully administered and assumed to be highly reliable. But, are the physical tests valid? What is the predictive validity of each test and the validity of combined scores on all physical tests? Do high scores on the physical tests predict success in the NFL? Several studies have been conducted to answer these and other questions. Results provide valuable insight of the true value of the NFL Combine.

A study by Kuzmits and Adams (The NFL Combine: Does it Predict Performance in the National Football League, *J Strength Cond Res.* 2008 Nov;22(6):1721-7.) is perhaps the most negative about the true value of the Combine. Researchers concluded that, with the exception of the sprint tests for running backs, there is no consistent statistical relationship between combine tests and professional football performance. A more detailed account of how the study was conducted is described in the abstract below:

> The authors investigated the correlation between National Football League (NFL) combine test results and NFL success for players drafted at three different offensive positions (quarterback, running back, and wide receiver) during a 6-year period, 1999-2004. The combine consists of a series of drills, exercises, interviews, aptitude tests, and physical exams designed to assess the skills of promising college football players and to predict their performance in the NFL. Combine measures examined in this study include 10-, 20-, and 40-yard dashes, bench press, vertical jump, broad jump, 20- and 60-yard shuttles, three-cone drill, and the Wonderlic Personnel Test. Performance criteria include 10 variables: draft order; 3 years each of salary received and games played; and position-specific data. Using correlation analysis, we found no consistent statistical relationship between combine tests and professional football performance, with the notable exception of sprint tests for running backs. We put forth possible explanations for the general lack of statistical relations detected, and, consequently, we question the overall usefulness of the combine. We also offer suggestions for improving the prediction of success in the NFL, primarily the use of more rigorous psychological tests and the examination of collegiate performance as a job sample test. Finally, from a practical standpoint, the results of the study should encourage NFL team personnel to reevaluate the usefulness of the combine's physical tests and exercises as predictors of player performance. This study should encourage team personnel to consider the weighting and importance of various combine measures and the potential benefits of overhauling the combine process, with the goal of creating a more valid system for predicting player success.

A study reported in the *International Journal of Forecasting* by Bryan L. Boulier, H.O. Stekler, Jason Coburn and Timothy Rankins, Evaluating National Football League Draft Choices: The Passing Game, used a data base from NFL drafts between 1974 and 2005 and a range of measures to determine the success of players selected in the draft. The study *examined the success of drafting quarterbacks and wide receivers and also found combine test scores to be only slightly helpful in predicting NFL success at these positions.*

Another study compared the Combine performance differences between drafted and non drafted players entering the 2004-2005 drafts (Sierer, S, et.

Al. *Journal of Strength & Conditioning Research:* January 2008 - Volume 22 - Issue 1 - pp 6-12). The abstract below summarizes the study and reveals a slightly more positive view. Although drafted athletes were found to perform better than non-drafted athletes, the success of each athlete in the NFL was not used as a criterion measure and predictive validity was not established.

> The purpose of this study was to examine performance differences between drafted and non drafted athletes (N = 321) during the 2004 and 2005 National Football League (NFL) Combines. We categorized players into one of 3 groups: Skill, Big skill, and Linemen. Skill players (SP) consisted of wide receivers, cornerbacks, free safeties, strong safeties, and running backs. Big skill players (BSP) included fullbacks, linebackers, tight ends, and defensive ends. Linemen (LM) consisted of centers, offensive guards, offensive tackles, and defensive tackles. We analyzed player height and mass, as well as performance on the following combine drills: 40-yard dash, 225-lb bench press test, vertical jump, broad jump, pro-agility shuttle, and the 3-cone drill. Student t-tests compared performance on each of these measures between drafted and non drafted players. Statistical significance was found between drafted and non drafted SP for the 40-yard dash ($P < 0.001$), vertical jump ($P = 0.003$), pro-agility shuttle ($P < 0.001$), and 3-cone drill ($P < 0.001$). Drafted and non drafted BSP performed differently on the 40-yard dash ($P = 0.002$) and 3-cone drill ($P = 0.005$). Finally, drafted LM performed significantly better than non drafted LM on the 40-yard dash ($P = 0.016$), 225-lb bench press ($P = 0.003$), and 3-cone drill ($P = 0.005$). Certified strength and conditioning specialists will be able to utilize the significant findings to help better prepare athletes as they ready themselves for the NFL Combine.

It is understandable why it is so difficult to statistically determine success from a field test since football is skill specific and physical tests just cannot mimic the many key situations for each player position (NFL Combine One-on-one, kickers, punters, and long snapper tests DO simulate competitive game conditions fairly well). Conditions are also affected by the behavior and cooperation of teammates. In addition, very little quantitative test data is even obtained from linemen.

Although sport-specific and player-specific tests are more difficult to develop and substantiate, there is room for improvement even in the area of speed where researchers found some predictive value. Football is a game of quickness, starting, stopping and acceleration. An analysis of game play would reveal that it is a rare occasion when players in most positions sprint a distance of 40 yards. The First 3-step test and the 10-yard dash are much more sport specific for interior linemen (blocking, pass and run rushing) than the 40-yard dash. If the 40-yard dash is deemed necessary, the test should be changed to include split times at 5, 10, and 20 yards. Also, a plant, cut, and 10-yard acceleration test is also more football-appropriate for linebackers, defensive backs, and linemen.

The speed of the start and acceleration (drive phase) can easily be improved with the correct kind of training that focuses on increasing ground contact force and form and technique. At present, the best test indicator of ground contact force is obtained from Dead Lift/Body Weight ratio scores. A maximum Dead Lift (1RM) test should be added to the physical tests until a more accurate indicator of ground contact force is validated.

Soccer Combines

What tests are used in major league soccer?

Soccer combines are less common and not nearly as refined as NFL combines. Major league soccer teams use of a combination of the tests shown in Table 2-12.

Table 2.12 **Pro Soccer Combine Tests**

TEST	DESCRIPTION
Aerobic	12-minute run or Beep Test
Anaerobic (speed endurance)	Tall Cone at start and 30 yards. Players use a standing start and sprint up and back (60 yards) five times touching the top of the cone each time. Scoring: 57 to 58 - Excellent, Under 60-Good, 61-63 - weak
40-meter dash	Place two cones 40 meters apart. Time one 40-meter sprint.
MPH test	Radar gun
Muscular endurance	30-second Sit-ups (bent knee with spotter placing his palm on the knee (to be touched each repetition). Push-ups - lock out, chest to spotter's palm.
Sit-and-reach test	Same as the test described in this chapter.
Leg Power	Three consecutive bounds using a two-foot takeoff.
Strength	Bench and leg press (1RM)

Major League Baseball Combines

What tests are used in major league baseball?

Like major league soccer, MLB combines have not standardized their test battery and teams use a combination of the tests described below. Speed is critical for running the bases, scoring runs, and extending the defensive range at all positions. It is also receiving more attention by college and major league scouts. Although testing is not as sophisticated as the NFL combine, a similar trend is developing in college and professional baseball. MLB combines will be much more comprehensive in the future, especially in the area of speed.

Numerous speed tests are currently in use, although not all reflect the skills in the game of baseball. Baseball is a game of quickness and acceleration, not maximum speed, and tests should reflect this concept. Some of the recommended battery of tests discussed below are already in use; others are used by a few MLB teams, and still others have not been implemented.

Most MLB clubs use the stationary 60-yard dash as the measure of linear speed even though no base runner sprints more than 30 yards before making a left turn toward second or third base and no infielder or outfielder ever sprints 60 yards during a game. A 30-yard dash with splits at the 10 and 20-yard marks would be a more practical test.

Sixty yards is about the distance needed for a world class sprinter to reach maximum speed, so even this long sprint measures acceleration, and baseball is 98% acceleration. Although some teams use electronic timing, most testing is done with a stopwatch and standards are based on manual scores.

Typical standards and ratings for the 60-yard dash for baseball are listed below.

Minimum - Acceptable	Under 7.0 seconds
Good	6.5 - 6.9
Excellent	6.3 - 6.49
Superior	under 6.3

A sub 7.0 second 60-yard dash is expected of players in most positions. Justin Upton posted an impressive 6.23 seconds in his first year. Few players are as fast as Upton. To put times in perspective, a world class sprinter runs 60-meters (about 9% further in distance) in 6.39 seconds which is a rate of 10.27 yards per second (1 yard = 0.914 meters; 1 meter = 1.094 yards). Although unlikely, at this rate the sprinter would complete the 60 yards in 5.84. seconds.

What baseball-specific tests are used?

Most scouts start the stopwatch as the ball hits the bat, slightly anticipating the swing to get an accurate time. Some click their watch as the ball crosses home plate. The watch is stopped when the hitter's foot touches first base. Since left-handed hitters are a step closer to first base, their times are graded 1/10th of a second quicker. The same procedure is followed to test the crack of the bat to second, third, or home (inside the park home run).

A better way to record times from the crack of the bat is to time the action during an actual game. Results would also reveal situations where less than maximum performance was evident and allow coaches to compare times at all levels of competition to evaluate prospects and determine when an injured athlete is fully recovered and ready to return to the lineup.

An excellent study was conducted by Gene Coleman (2004) of the Houston Astros to determine how often and how hard professional baseball players run to first base during the season and whether or not they are able to maintain peak speed throughout the season. Ten MLB players participated in the study and 2,683 times were recorded during 162 games as players ran from home plate to first base (30 yards) in game situations. The study concluded that players do not run all-out on every play. There was also no significant change in speed from month to month during the 6-month season.

The main finding of this study was that running speed to first base in a subset of Major League Baseball players is maintained throughout the season.

Although unsubstantiated, one of the best times ever recorded was Mickey Mantel, who is said to have run from home-to-first base from the left side in 3.4 on a hit and 3.1 on a bunt.

Table 2.13 **Baseball Combine Tests and Standards**

CRACK OF THE BAT TO FIRST: STANDARDS AND RATINGS

	Right Handed Hitter	Left Handed Hitter
Average	4.3 seconds	4.2 seconds
Good	4.2 seconds	4.1 seconds
Exceptional	4.1 and under	4.0 and under

CRACK OF THE BAT TO THIRD: STANDARDS AND RATINGS

Average	11.3 - 11.7 seconds
Good	10.8 - 11.2 seconds
Exceptional	10.4 - 10.7 seconds

CRACK OF THE BAT TO SECOND - Not available

CRACK OF THE BAT TO HOME: STANDARDS AND RATINGS

Average	15.5 seconds
Good	14.1 - 15.0 seconds
Exceptional	14.0 seconds or less

BASE RUNNING: FIRST BASE TO SECOND, SECOND TO THIRD, THIRD TO HOME (EACH WITH A PRE-MEASURED LEAD)

Most teams have players assume the base running position with a pre-measured lead and begin timing when the beam is broken or muscular movement is noted and stop when the base is touched.

Table 2.13 **(continued)**

FIRST TO SECOND (BASE RUNNING)

Players must be below 3.2 seconds to steal second against the average time of major league catchers and pitchers.

TIME (Base runner to second)	Predicted Outcome
3.3 seconds or more	Will be thrown out
3.2 - 3.3 seconds	50/50 chances of stealing second
3.1 seconds or less	Stolen base

SECOND TO THIRD (BASE RUNNING) - Not available

FIRST TO THIRD (BASE RUNNING)

7.0 seconds	Average
6.8 - 6.9 seconds	Good
6.7 seconds or less	Exceptional

There are players in all positions in the Major Leagues who fall below the lowest standards in one or more speed tests. Some players survive on their hitting, fielding, arm strength and accuracy and lack of speed is overlooked, depending on their position. The *First 3-Step* Test is more important for players at all positions in base running, and for infielders, 10-30 yard speed and longer distances for outfielders. Obviously, the more players with enough speed to steal bases and run down balls, the better overall team performance. Faster athletes do get a closer look by scouts and coaches in Combines and other tryouts and it can be the difference between a contract, visit to camp, and a goodbye.

How can home-to-first base times be improved?

Achieving a GOOD to EXCELLENT crack-of-the-bat to first base time requires a combination of sound base running technique and use of the correct speed improvement training programs to aid the start and acceleration phases of sprinting.

The first objective is to get out of the box as fast as possible with absolutely no hesitation or time expiring after bat contact is made to watch the ball. One method is to avoid moving the feet after completing the swing and making bat contact, lean into the sprint, apply force first off both feet, then only off the lead foot as the rear foot leaves the ground. This approach is faster than dropping the front foot back (taking a negative step) before pushing off toward first base. At this point, regular arm, leg, and body lean sprint mechanics prevail as forward lean slowly decreases with the bend occurring from the feet through the hips and head (total body lean) after the first few steps; eliminating bending at the waist. For the first 3 steps, ground contact is made first with the ball of the foot and no heel-ground contact is made. The remaining steps involve the foot hitting almost flat with the outside ball of the foot contacting the ground first, followed by the heel. This movement allows the hip flexors and extensors to work efficiently to maximize ground contact forces in the right direction.

Work with a baseball coach to make certain the feet are in the proper position after the swing of the bat. Once that habit is established, the concepts of the standing sprint start can be applied to efficiently initiate and complete movements to first base. Care must be taken to avoid any type of excess emphasis that may interfere with the more important skill of "hitting" the ball.

NBA COMBINE

What tests are used in the NBA?

Tests in professional basketball (NBA) vary from team to team and lack the standardization and comprehensiveness of the NFL. Table 2-14 lists the various tests in use.

Speed tests for Young Athletes

What speed tests are used with young athletes?

The tests listed in Table 12.15 are helpful for the particular sport and provide baseline data for future comparison and improvement. The list does not include some key strength and power tests that are critical to some sports for older athletes.

TABLE 2.14 **NBA Combine Tests***

TEST	DESCRIPTION
No Step Vertical Jump	Using the Vertec device, two trials are made with no foot movement permitted (a shuffle step, side step, drop step, or gather step is disallowed); only a straight down and straight up movement. If an athlete reaches a new height on the second attempt, a third attempt is granted.
Maximum Vertical Jump	A maximum approach distance is measured from the free throw line extended in a 15' arch to the baseline. Athletes take as many steps toward the Vertec device as necessary to attain their maximum vertical jump, providing they start within the 15' arch. A one or two-foot takeoff is used. The best of two trial is recorded.
Pro Lane Agility	Cones are placed at each of the four corners of the pro foul lane (16' wide X 19' baseline to foul line). Athletes begin in the lower left-hand corner of the lane by sprinting toward the top of the lane, going around the cone in a right defensive slide to the edge of the lane and around the cone, back pedaling to the foul line, around the cone and defensive slide to the left and touch the floor with the feet even with the cone at the starting position. Changing direction back to the athlete's right, defensive slide around the cone and sprint to the top of the lane and defensive slide to the left around the cone and back pedal past the original starting position. The fastest time of two attempts is recorded. One false start (including knocking over a cone, cutting the corner of the drill, sprinting sideways instead of defensive sliding, not touching the line at the change of direction point at the start/finish line, or simply falling down) is permitted without penalty. Timing begins on the athlete's first movement by two coaches who average their readings to get the official time for that trial.
3/4 Court Sprint	Using a standing start, a baseline to opposite foul line sprint is made. Timing begins on the first movement. Four coaches time each of two sprints, eliminating high and low scores, averaging and recording the middle two as the official time. One false start is permitted.
Sit-and-Reach	The Acuflex Sit and Reach Box is used to used to administer this standard test described on page 2-23.
Bench Press 185 lb. Maximum Repetition	Following a warm-up (10 push-ups, 60-sec. rest, 5 repetitions of the bench press with 135 lb., and a 9-second rest) athletes complete as many repetitions of the bench press with 185 lb. (84 kg.) as possible. One spotter provides a lift off, counts the repetitions and verifies the lock at the top. The second spotter makes certain that the athlete's glutes stay in contact with the bench (no arching).

Source: The National Basketball Conditioning Coaches Association (NBCCA).

Table 2.15 **Sport and Recommended Tests**

Sport	Recommended Tests
Baseball, Softball	Crack of the bat to first base Crack of the bat to second Crack of the bat to third Base stealing: First to second base, Second to third base during a game
Basketball	First 3-step test, Speed Endurance test - 6-10 repeated 20 yard dashes at 15 second intervals
Football, Rugby	First 3-step test 10, 20, 40, 80, 120 yard dash (all in one sprint) Speed Endurance (10 repeated 20-40 yard sprints at 25-30 second intervals)
Soccer, Lacrosse, Field Hockey	First 3-step test from a standing position and a jog 10 and 20 yard sprint Speed endurance (anaerobic) - 6-10 20-yard dashes at 15 second intervals, 1 1/2 mile run
Tennis	First 3-step test, Speed Endurance Ten, 10-yard sprints (each timed separately with no rest between any of the runs); repeat the set after a 60-90 second rest period.

THE ACCURACY OF HAND-TIMED 40-YARD DASH TESTS

How accurate is a hand-timed 40-yard dash test?

The 40-yard dash is still the most widely used and misused test in modern-day sports. Although most team sport athletes rarely sprint this far during competition, the test remains tremendously popular. Even fans are well enough informed to interpret and evaluate 40-yard dash times by player position in football. Since the test is generally measured by two hand-held timers, rather than through the use of expensive electronic equipment, questions about its accuracy have surfaced on a regular basis throughout the years. Inflated times are often used as motivational tools by coaches to develop confidence and inspire athletes to speed train harder in the off season. This may be the source of much of the controversy.

In our early speed camps at Virginia Commonwealth University, we used both electronic and hand-timing. Athletes were constantly disappointed in their electronic times which consistently yielded a poorer performance than hand-timed 40s. Nesteor and Thobe conducted a very interesting study to compare the accuracy (reliability of timers) and validity of handheld times from two timers (Nesteor W. Sherfman and Mark A Thobe, The objectivity of timers for the 40-yard dash. *Research Quarterly*, March, 2001). Both an electronic and handheld test were administered to 235 collegiate football players at all different positions participating in a camp where they were being evaluated by pro scouts. Timers were trained and experienced in 40-yard dash testing. Most players completed two trials with the best time recorded for this study.

The findings of this study indicated the tendency for hand-held times to be slightly slower than electronic times by an average of 0.023 seconds. In the handheld test, the timers began their watches after observing the first muscular movement of the athlete, rather than the athlete reacting to a stimuli such as the sound of the gun in the sport of track and field. This difference between electronic timing and hand timing in the initial starting of the watches is most of the reason for the slower times. Findings also revealed that the 40-yard times of timer 1 and 2 were NOT significantly different and were, in fact, nearly identical and very reliable (.995).

Trained timers actually do accurately measure the 40-yard dash. The fact that these times yield a performance of about 2/10 of a second better than the readings of an electronic device is not a problem, and scores are not compromised and can be compared in football or other sports as long as all coaches are using the same method. Obviously, athletes prefer a timing system that yields the fastest time.

Is anyone capable of running a sub 4.0 40-yard dash?

A close estimate of 6′ 5″ Usain Bolt's 40-yard time can be calculated from his recent world record performance (9.58) and 10-meter split times in the 100-meter dash. When comparing this estimate to reported 40-yard times of football and other team sport athletes, it is important to keep several factors in mind:

1. Usain Bolt would not run a 40-yard dash the same way he ran the world record 100-meter dash. In a 100-meter dash, sprinters accelerate over a longer distance to reduce slowing at the end of the race and do not reach maximum speed for 60 meters or more. In Bolt's 100-meter performance, maximum speed was obtained at 65.03 meters (70.8 yards). In a 40-yard sprint, elite sprinters would alter their starting form and technique, take shorter steps out of the blocks, and reach maximum speed as early as possible since there is no concern over anaerobic fitness and slowing at the end of such a short race.

2. Training for the 40-yard dash takes on a different focus than training for a 100-meter sprint since the emphasis now involves approximately 50 percent horizontal force (first 20-yards) and 50 percent vertical force (second 20 yards). The early acceleration phase of a 40-yard sprint requires a tremendous amount of strength and power.

3. Hand-timed 40-yard dash scores are inflated. Since a team sport athlete begins the sprint whenever he or she is ready and the timer reacts to the first muscular movement of the sprinter, reaction time (RT) is eliminated. Usain Bolt's RT during his world record run was 0.146. Team sport athletes would take much longer to react to the sound of a gun shot. With hand timing, errors occur both at the start of the race (timer's reaction to the first movement of the athlete) and at the finish (timers reaction to the athlete crossing the finish line). The result is often 40-yard times that are grossly inflated and actually an impossibility for any human being.

4. An electronically timed 40-yard dash also eliminates RT and provides an advantage of 0.200 seconds or more for each athlete.

To estimate Bolt's time at the 40-yard mark during this record setting race, we used his 30-meter time of 3.78, determined the yards per second covered during the next 10-meter split (12.57) and used that figure to find his time for the final 7.192 yards of a 40-yard dash. Based on that information, Usain Bolt reached the 40-yard mark in 4.277 seconds. This estimated time by the fastest man in the world demonstrates how inflated 40-yard times are in football. If Usain Bolt did not have to react to the sound of the gun (0.146), his estimated 40-yard time time would still only be 4.131; considerably slower than reported times of some football players.

It is clear that had Usain Bolt trained for a 40-yard dash and used 40-yard dash strategy to complete the race, his time would be significantly better, perhaps as low as 4.0. It is doubtful that any athlete can legitimately run 3.9 or better when bound by the start and timing techniques used in track and field.

Table 2.16 Analysis of Usain Bolt's World record 100-meter Dash (9.58)

DISTANCE	SPLIT TIMES	CUMULATIVE TIME
Reaction Time = 0.146		
0-10m	1,89	1.80
10-20m	0.99	2.88
20-30m	0,90	3.78
30-40m	0,86	4.64
40-50m	0.83	5.47
50-60m	0.82	6.29
60-70m	0.81	7.10
70-80m	0.82	7.92
80-90m	0.83	8.75
90-100m	0.83	9.58

Maximum mph speed was obtained at the 65 meter mark (Maximum Velocity = 12.27 meters per second)

99% of maximum velocity was reached at 48.18 meters (1.094 X 48.18 = 52.7 yards).

Very little slowing took place after reaching maximum speed. A drop off of only 2/100th of a second occurred from the 70 meter mark to the 100-meter mark.

** Table above Courtesy of SpeedEndurance.com*

PART II

COMPONENTS OF PLAYING SPEED

Chapter 3

STARTING, STOPPING, ACCELERATION, FAKING AND CUTTING

Improving the ability to start, stop, accelerate, fake and cut requires athletes to master the correct form and technique for their sport. It also involves special training programs to increase ground contact forces and improve neuromuscular action. Proper starting technique, for example, depends upon the sport and position and may involve a stationary 3-point, 4-point, or standing stance, or acceleration from a walk, jog or three-quarter stride. Although there are numerous common factors, stopping, acceleration, faking and cutting varies from one sport to another. This chapter focuses on the basic techniques common to team sports to help athletes develop these important skills for their sport. The actual training programs and drills used to develop the techniques are presented in Part III: The 5-Step Model.

THE START

What is starting strength?

Starting strength is a key aspect of speed-strength and refers to the power required to begin a movement, such as the push off the ground to initiate a sprint or the foot plant cutting action commonly used in team sports. Starting strength can be improved by using exercises with weights and resistance of 60 to 80 percent of maximum strength at high speed (Tellez). Plyometrics, and sprint-resisted training (see Chapter 8) also develop starting strength.

What type of start should athletes learn?

Although not all athletes use a 3-point or 4-point stationary start during competition, timed 5, 10, 20, 40, and 60-yard dashes are a key part of the evaluation process when selecting players for university scholarships or the pro draft and for making the team in the high school, university and professional ranks. Unfortunately, team sport athletes rarely take the time to work on an effective start and the proper way to sprint a short distance even though this is critical for achieving their best times in these tests. During competition, only football uses a three point or four-point stationary start to begin a play. Athletes in baseball, basketball, field hockey, lacrosse, rugby and soccer accelerate to maximum speed from a standing position, slow walk, or jog and need to develop proper preparatory posture to perform this action as effectively as possible. However, speed tests from a stationary position are used in practically every sport, therefore, almost every athlete is forced to master the techniques of the 3-point or 4-point stance.

What is the proper technique for the 3-point stance?

For the 3-point stance, the stronger leg, usually the leg you jump with, is placed in the front position. For right-handed athletes, the left leg is generally the stronger leg. From a kneeling position, place the stronger foot forward so that the edges of the toes are approximately 16 to 20 inches behind the starting line. With the knee of the back leg on the ground, position it even with the ball of the front foot. Extend the right arm just behind the line, and raise the body to a position where the angle of the front leg is about 90 degrees and the angle of the rear leg is close to 135 degrees.

Extend the right hand on the fingertips with the index finger and thumb far apart to provide more stability. The left arm should rest on the thigh of the left leg or behind the body as if in a running position. Assume a relaxed posture with most of the body weight on the legs and a small amount of weight on the extended front arm.

The power of the start comes from the legs, not the arms, so don't lean so far forward that too much weight is on the arm. If most of the body weight is on the arm, there will not be enough pressure on the legs to drive and push out properly. If there is too much pressure on the arm, you will stumble out and catch yourself before regaining balance. Drive and push out with both legs and avoid trying to throw the arms out and forward. The arms are just working to create proper stride length and frequency, they do not replace the power of the legs.

After the initial thrust off both feet, the rear leg leaves the ground first, followed by the drive off the front leg with body lean occurring nearly in a straight line from the foot through the top of the head. A good start includes a balanced and stable position followed by correct driving and pushing with the legs backward and downward to set the body in motion.

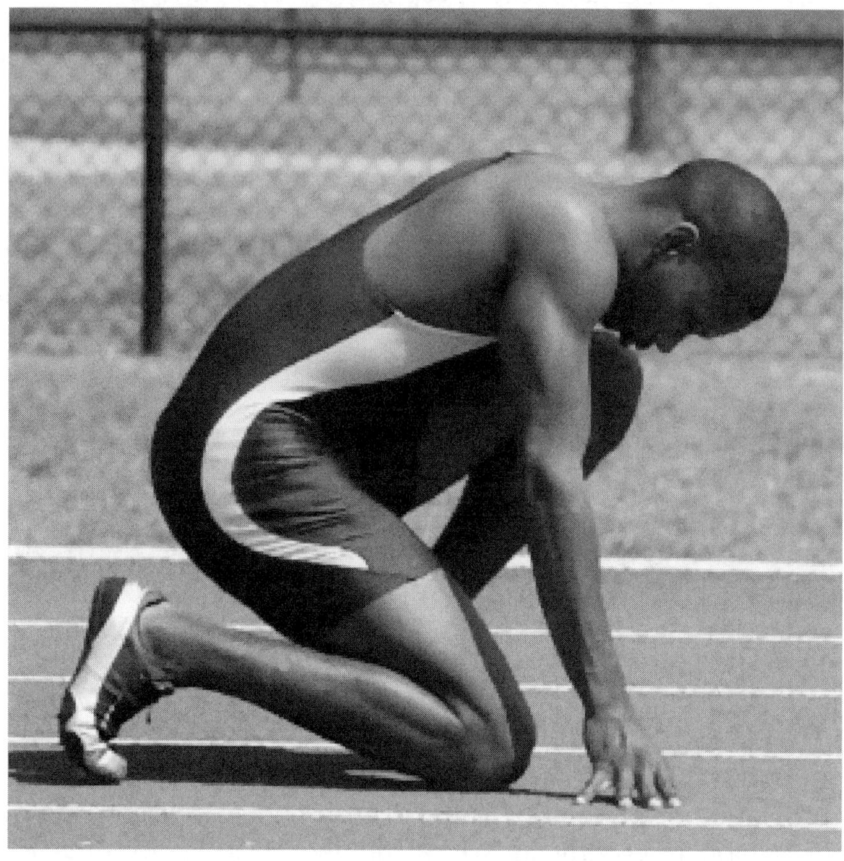

Figure 3.1a. Proper position for the 3-point stance using the medium start, with the knee on the ground. The stronger leg is in the forward position.

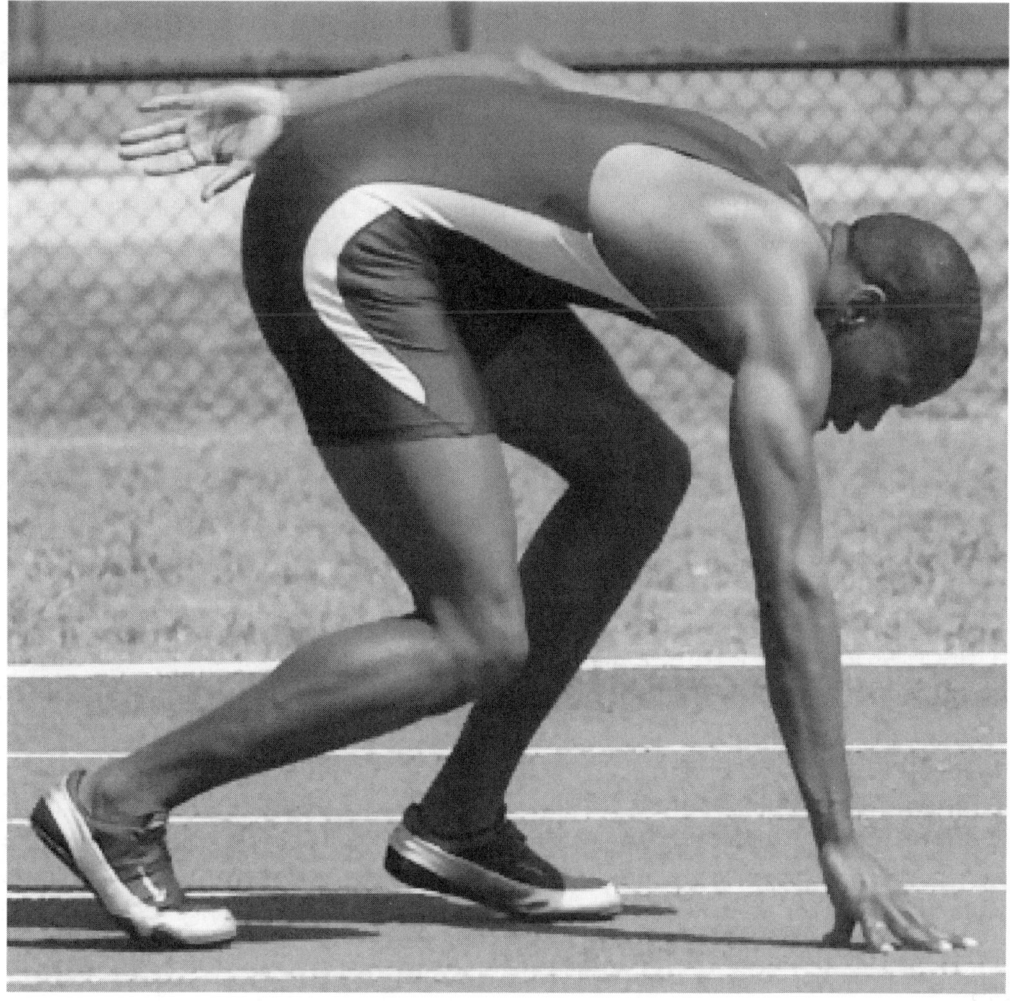

Figure 3.1b. Final set position with some weight forward. A powerful push-off occurs by applying the initial force to both legs to begin the starting action.

What is the proper technique for the 4-point track stance?

The 4-point stance is similar to the three-point stance except both arms are extended to the ground. From a kneeling position, place the stronger leg forward with toes approximately 16 to 20 inches behind the starting line. With the knee of the back leg on the ground, position it even with the ball of the front foot. Extend and spread out both arms behind the starting line about shoulder-width apart. Keep the fingers spread and arms straight. Rise to a set position where the front leg is at a 90-degree angle and the back leg is at a 135-degree angle.

Keep most of the weight on the legs so that you are comfortable and balanced. The driving action will come from the legs. Do not bend the elbows. The two key factors when starting in the 40-yard dash or other short sprint are balance and the driving and pushing action. As in the three-point stance, forward momentum is created by an initial thrust off both legs (see Figures 3.2a and 3.2b)

What is the most efficient way to run a 20- to 60-yard dash?

When racing the 20-, 40- or 60-yard dash, it is important to accelerate from start to finish. Although this sounds simple or even obvious, athletes who fail to understand acceleration are cheating themselves of their best times. The scientific analysis of sprinting has proven that athletes cannot sprint at top speed for much more than 1-2 seconds. In the 20-, 40-, or 60-yard dash, most athletes believe they have to run at maximum speed over the entire distance. They also believe that if they focus on increasing their stride frequency, they will run a fast time. The more efficient approach to sprinting a 40 - 60-yard dash is to accelerate over the entire distance and through the finish in order to reach top speed toward the end of the race. The fastest times will be recorded when you feel yourself accelerating through the finish line.

In the first 20 yards of a short sprint, stride length increases are easily handled by most team sport athletes. As the sprint continues beyond 60 yards, sprinters shift their efforts from stride rate to stride length.

How does foot spacing for a 40-yard dash test differ from spacing for a 100-meter sprint?

Several slightly different approaches should be tried by team sport athletes to determine which method produces the fastest 40-yard dash time or fastest 5-20 yard time for interior linemen in football and players in other sports where very short sprints are critical. In the 40-yard dash, the key factor is to find the technique that allows you to reach maximum speed as quickly as possible.

The *Medium* start described on pages 4 and 5 is used by most team sport athletes being tested in the 40-yard dash. Ralph Mann, outstanding researcher and former Olympic athlete provides several key suggestions in his book, *The Mechanics of Sprinting and Hurdling,* ©2007 for sprinters that also are sound for team sport athletes in short sprints. Although there are individual preferences, elite sprinters set their blocks in a similar fashion. The front block distance is set to allow the lead knee to be positioned at or slightly behind the starting line. Measuring from the front block, the back block is set back about 2/3 of the front block distance. Team sport athletes can experiment with these measurements to find the most effective position.

The *Bunch* Start is still another choice for athletes to consider. The main difference lies in the longitudinal distance between the toes of the front foot and the toes of the rear foot when the athlete is in the "On your marks" position. When using the Bunch start, the feet are closer together with the toe of the back foot approximately 11" behind the heel of the front foot. The Bunch start is not commonly used by elite sprinters who strive to reach maximum speed at approximately the 60-meter mark. The high hip elevation and forward lean may allow athletes to clear the ground (first two steps) faster and complete a faster short sprint of 5-10 yards. Early research indicated that this advantage may be lost and slower times may occur if used in longer sprints. The use of the 11 inch (28 cm) bunch stance resulted in clearing the blocks sooner but with less velocity than secured from medium stances, resulting in significantly slower time at 10 and 50 yards. In addition, the highest proportion of best runs and the smallest proportion of poorest runs resulted from starting with a 16-inch stance (41 cm). A 21 inch (53 cm) is nearly as good. Both of these are medium stances.

Regardless of the method used, both legs contribute to block or ground contact force with the greatest amount of force placed on the rear leg although the lead leg is in contact with the block or ground for a longer period and contributes more to block velocity. Once form and technique are mastered, athletes focus on training techniques to maximize force production--increasing the force of the pushing action away from the ground with each step.

Are there other tips to help improve times in the stationary 40-yard dash?

Some of the training tips have been mentioned previously, others have not. So much emphasis is placed on the timed 40-yard and 60-yard dash in team sports that it is important to acquire every small fraction of advantage possible. The *National Association of Speed and Explosion* 40-yard dash clinics stresses the following factors:

• The stronger leg should be placed in the front position since the lead leg is responsible for about two-thirds of the velocity at the start. To identify the stronger leg, compare the scores of the right and left leg in three tests: (1) right and left leg kick back, (2) right and left leg press, and (3) right and left leg stride length scores (see Chapter 2 for a description of these tests).

• Athletes should master the medium 4-point track start described previously and adapt it to the 3-point stance if they feel more comfortable in that position although the 4-point track start is more desirable since it makes it easier to support forward weight.

• A common error is to step forward with the back foot as the front foot pushes off. No track athlete would ever make this mistake. Near equal thrust off the front and back foot must be exerted to initiate the "drive" phase of the start and get out of the starting stance. The force exerted by the rear foot is about 75% of the force applied by the lead foot. This thrust off both feet occurs before the rear foot steps forward. To form the habit of pushing off both the lead and rear feet requires hours of concentrated practice. Have a workout partner block both feet with his feet and "tell" you about the thrust applied on each start.

• Take 4-5 "falling form" starts in each form training workout in Chapter 11 with just enough weight forward to allow a forceful push-off both feet.

• Lean forward until the shoulders are over the line while the right knee is still on the ground. This makes it easier to hold the weight over the line until moving to the "get set" position.

• Rise up slowly and maintain the "hold" or "set" position (keeping the shoulders over the starting line) only a very short time to reduce the strain on the hands and possibly surprise the timer who is reacting to the first muscular movement. Eyes should be fixed on the running surface as you maintain the "head down" position with the proper forward lean that will maximize your first two steps.

• Wear spiked shoes to improve push-off power.

• If you are being tested on natural turf, dig two small holes in the ground to increase traction during the push-off, or have a friend block both feet with their feet.

• The first movement is with the arms and involves an aggressive arm drive (one arm drives forward as the other moves backward).

• Use vigorous, smooth arm movement the first 10 yards and continue to work the arms hard throughout the sprint. To sprint fast, you must concentrate on sprinting fast. It does not occur automatically.

• Avoid straightening up too fast; stay low for the first 8 -12 yards with the head down.

• If you get a bad start, had a bad run or slipped, stop immediately and do not complete the run. Ask for another trial. If you complete the test, you may not get a second chance.

• Sprint 5-8 yards past the finish line rather than using the "lunge."

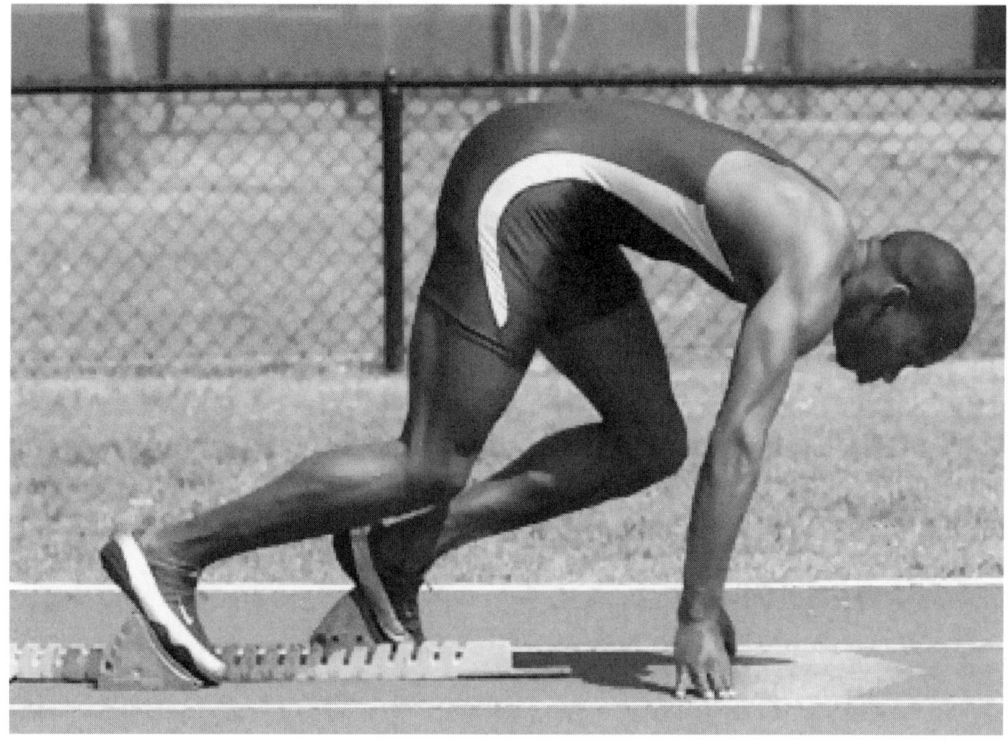

Figure 3.2a Track athlete in a 4-point stance

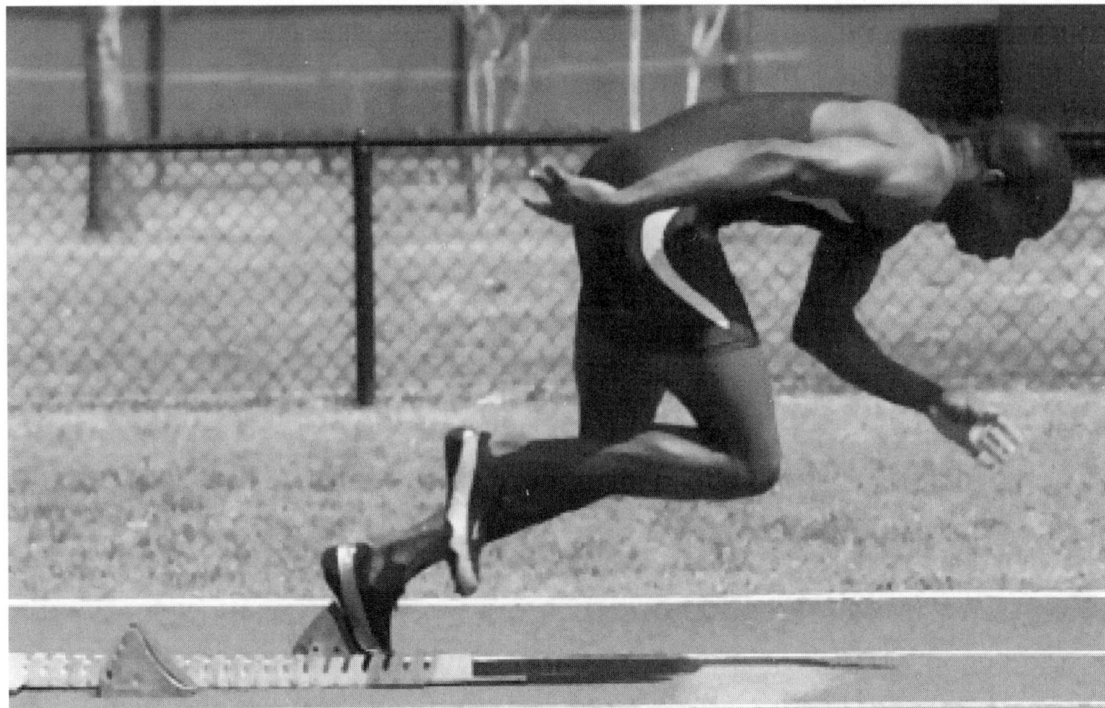

Figure 3.2 b First step after a two-foot push off the blocks.

• Drive out of the starting position and gradually come into full running position. Don't stay low or bent at the waist during the race because this will keep you from running with correct body position. In addition, you must stay relaxed. Speed over any distance requires the athlete to be disciplined enough to relax through the entire race.

Reaching maximum speed requires training. Many sports professionals believe that running is a natural act that needs no special focus. This belief has prevented athletes from improving performance. Concentrate on the principles of sprinting mechanics and your speed will improve.

Check List for the Stationary 3-pt and 4-pt Start

In the Preparatory Position

- Relaxed position with proper foot and arm spacing
- Weight evenly distributed between hands, knees and feet
- Straight arms are shoulder-width apart
- Head aligned with the back, relaxed neck

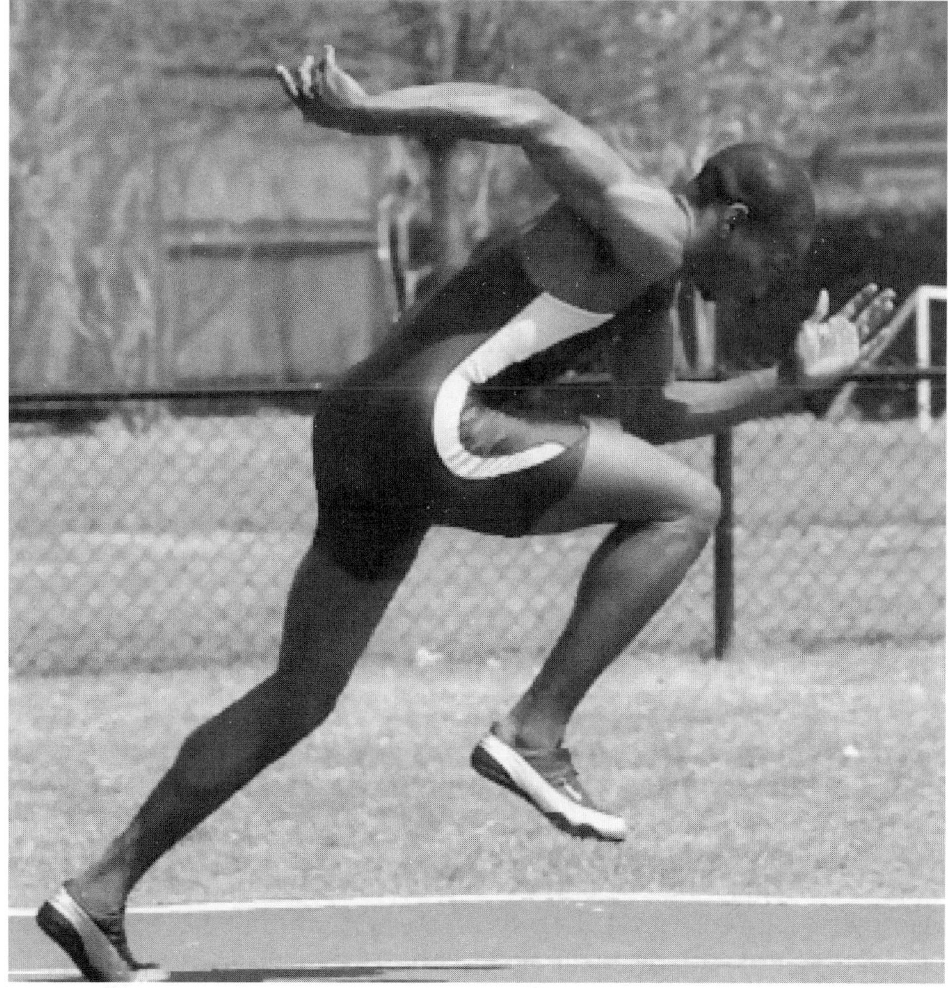

Figure 3.3c The drive phase after the start

Use the following list to evaluate the 3-point or 4-point start:

In the "Set" position

- Movement of the center of gravity above the front foot
- Front leg bent at 90-degree angle
- Hips slightly higher than the shoulders
- Both feet apply pressure to the ground
- Straight arms shoulder-width apart and in front of the hands

Takeoff (starting action)

- Explosive thrust exerted off both the lead and rear foot
- Rear foot leaves the ground first
- Fast, flat forward swing of the rear leg
- Active alternate sidearm motion

The "Drive" or acceleration phase

- Gradual straightening of the body and lengthening of stride
- Landing on the balls of feet and limited lowering of heels
- Head down position looking at the ground
- Straight line forward drive; no sideway placement of the feet

STARTING FROM A STANDING POSITION

How do athletes decide whether to use a standing or crouched start?

The standing start may be more suitable for younger athletes who do not possess the necessary strength and power to produce the forceful push off both feet and the powerful leg action and force against the ground required to accelerate from a crouched position. It also may be the best choice when taking a field test such as a 60-yard dash for athletes in sports such as baseball, basketball, soccer, lacrosse, and field hockey who are forced to use a type of standing start during competition. Other athletes who are unaccustomed to a crouched 3-point or 4-point start or have not taken the time to master the technique will also benefit from the standing start.

Improper form in the crouched start results in poor times. The standing start is easier to learn, places the lead foot closer to the starting line, is more forgiving if executed improperly, and is likely to result in a better time than what is recorded after an incorrect crouched start. However, high school and college athletes should not use the standing start for a 40-yard dash or other speed test. The fastest time will result from a perfected crouched start.

What is the proper stance and technique when starting from a standing position?

Assume a standing position with the strongest leg and foot as close to the starting line as possible. Kneel and place the knee of the rear leg even with the toe of the lead leg. Stand up, keep the rear foot in the same spot, feet shoulder-width apart. This is the proper foot spacing. Bend the knees, lower the head slightly and lean forward with approximately two-thirds of your weight on the front foot. Experiment with straight arms or with bending both elbows to 90-degrees to see which way works best. The arm opposite the lead leg is in front and the arm opposite the rear leg is back.

Push-off begins with both feet to get the body moving forward before the rear foot is lifted and the remaining push-off is performed by the lead leg. As described in the 3-point and 4-point stance, drive out of the start and gradually come into full running position. Do not stay bent at the waist during the race because this will keep you from running with correct body position. Body lean occurs from the feet through the head in a straight line during the sprinting action. The rear arm is thrust forward and the lead arm backward as you push off and begin the sprinting cycle.

Use the check list below for the standing start to correct your form.

Check List for the Standing Stationary Start

In the Preparatory Position

- Relaxed position with proper foot spacing
- Body weight evenly distributed on both feet
- Arms bent at right angles and shoulder-width apart

In the "Set" position

- Movement of the center of gravity above the front foot
- Front leg bent at a 90 degree angle
- Opposite arm of lead leg back, other arm forward
- Arms bent at 90-degrees
- About 2/3 of weight on the lead foot
- Both feet apply pressure to the ground

Takeoff/starting action

- Explosive thrust exerted off both the lead and rear foot
- Rear foot leaves the ground first
- Fast, flat forward swing of the rear leg
- Forward thrust of the rear arm

The "Drive" or acceleration phase

- Gradual straightening of the body and lengthening of stride
- Landing on the balls of feet and limited lowering of heels
- Head down position looking at the ground
- Limited bending at the waist

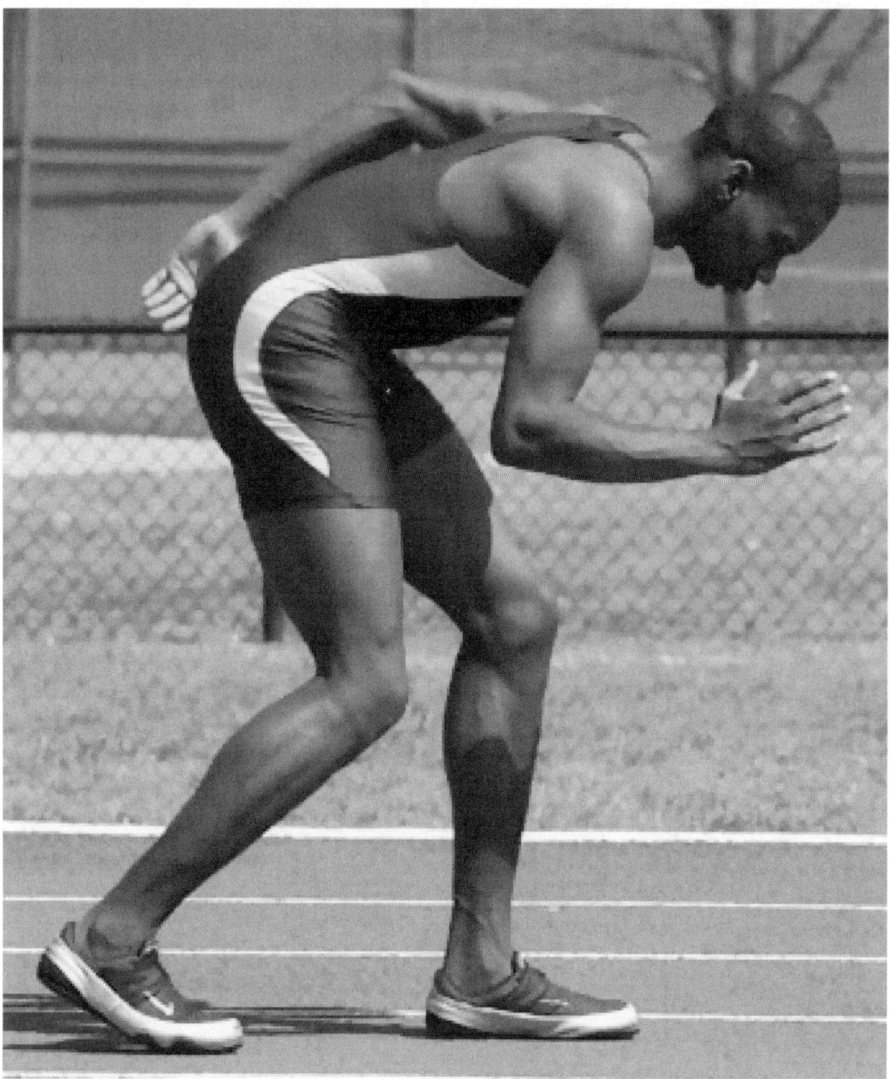

Figure 3.4 Standing Start. Ready Position with Knees and Elbows Bent. The push off involves both the rear and front foot.

STARTING FROM AN UPRIGHT MOVING POSITION

What is the correct technique when starting from an upright moving position?

In team sports such as basketball, soccer, rugby, field hockey, and lacrosse, athletes are in a pattern of continuous movement and need to develop efficient techniques of making the transition from a slow walk or jog to an all-out sprint. The transition requires a quick shift in the center of gravity, slight forward lean with little bend at the trunk, and vigorous arm and push-back action at ground contact off both legs. The pushing action of the legs comes from the ball of the foot, not the toes, which causes loss of power, stability, and speed.

Ask your coach or training partner to analyze your moving start using the following check lists:

Check List for the Moving Start

In the Preparatory Position

- Relaxed walking or jogging form
- Proper arm use during walking or jogging
- Only a slight, natural forward lean is evident

The "Drive" or acceleration phase:

- Explosive thrust exerted off both the lead and rear foot
- Gradual straightening of the body and lengthening of stride
- Landing on the balls of feet and limited lowering of heels
- Slight head down position looking at the ground
- Strong use of arms in synch with legs

HIGH SPEED STOPPING

Do athletes need to work on the "stopping" action?

Proper starting and stopping form is a major part of quickness in team sports and must be taught through the use of sport-specific drills that closely resemble the actual movements during competition. These techniques do not develop naturally. Most athletes of all ages have some faulty traits that need to be corrected or relearned. No two athletes sprint exactly the same; nor do two athletes start and stop exactly the same. There is also no perfect style that fits all body types. The key is to improve basic techniques without trying to mimic the exact form of others. You are an individual and must learn the concepts of starting, stopping and sprinting form in theory and adapt them to your personal traits. Unless your "start" and "stop and cut" form is "flawless," take the time to master the techniques and drills described in Chapter 11 and eliminate the major errors in each area.

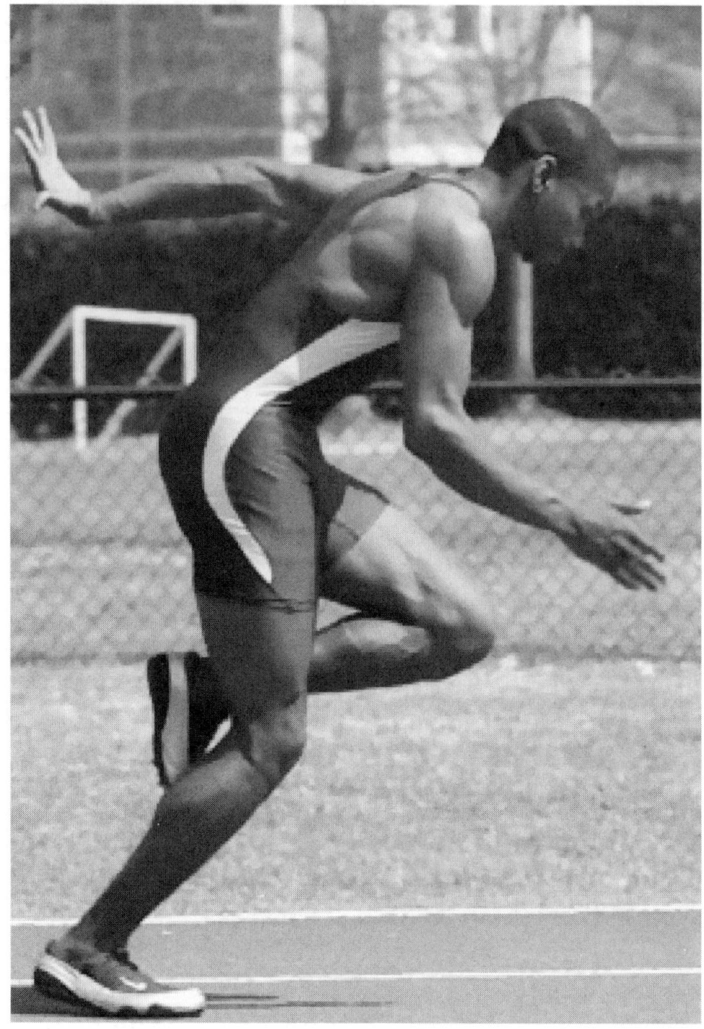

Figure 3.5a and 3.5b (a) The moving start from a slow jog or walk.

High speed stopping in team sports produces extremely high forces on the body that must be countered by the muscular system to prevent injury and bring a moving body to a complete stop or pause before executing a rapid change in direction. A football, basketball, or soccer player who is sprinting at high speed often must come to a rapid stop to change direction, execute a tackle, or secure the ball. The reactive forces of the ground or floor hit the athlete's body with the same force that hits the ground and must be rapidly absorbed to counter the shock and stress. Even with proper technique, it may be difficult to extend the time to soften the impact. The aid of special equipment and padding in football, soccer, field hockey, and lacrosse provide additional assistance; however, proper technique produces most of the needed delay in extending the time force is absorbed and spreading the force to allow explosive stopping and starting action in team sports.

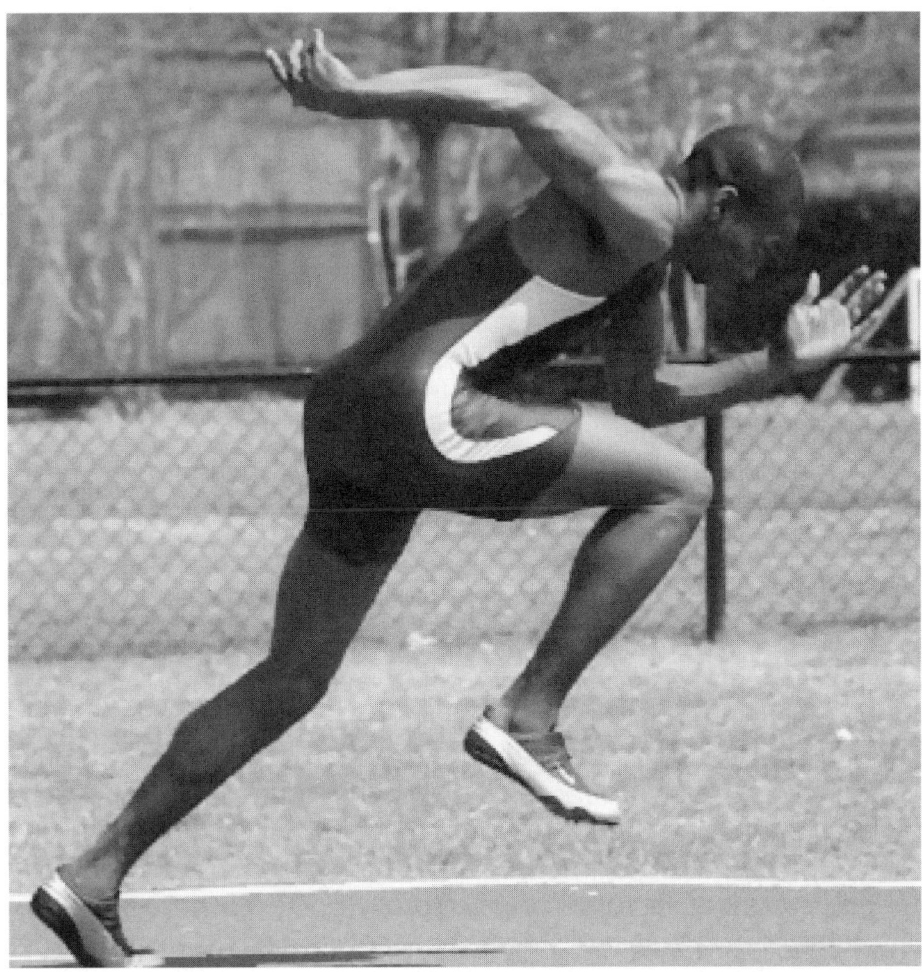

Figure 3.5b. A powerful "push" off the balls of both feet and proper body lean (from the ankle through the head with little bending at the waist) is needed for maximum acceleration.

The technique to produce an injury-free, high speed stop after a rebound or after reaching maximum sprinting speed involves proper flexing of the ankles, hips, and knees at landing or during the first one or two steps of the stopping action to extend the time the force is absorbed and spread the force throughout the body. Most athletes bend their knees as they land following a jump and during the stopping action while sprinting. The stopping action loads the legs with elastic energy as muscles stretch (lengthen) to absorb and control the high speed stop. The counter movement must now take place as quickly as possible to avoid losing this elastic energy to heat. The faster the counter movement is made after stopping, the more explosive the concentric contraction and the quicker the counter movement in another direction. During a rapid stop in team sports, the quadriceps are stretched and loaded eccentrically to produce stored elastic energy. If the stretch (stop) is too slow, no energy is stored and the counter movement will be slow. To improve quickness, an athlete must possess sufficient strength in the muscles involved to decelerate and stop rapidly.

Explosive stopping is the key to quickness in team sports and paves the way to executing rapid changes in direction under all types of conditions during competition. The object is to train the neuromuscular system and teach the muscles to fire more quickly. The nervous system will eventually increase the firing rate of motor neurons, cause maximum recruitment of fast-twitch fibers, quicker reaction, and improve the explosive force of the stop and start. A neuromuscular training program is described in Step V of the 5-step model in Chapter 10.

Drills to practice and speed up the stopping action are presented in Chapter 11.

ACCELERATION

In most sports, athletes accelerate to full speed from either a "dead stop" or a slow jog most of the game. It is no surprise that the average speed players reach during competition are well below their maximum. On only a few occasions will you accelerate for 60 meters, the approximate distance it takes a world class sprinter to reach maximum speed. A home run in baseball, a 100-meter or 200-meter sprint in track, and a long run in football, rugby, soccer, field hockey or lacrosse could approach or exceed 60 meters. What is generally referred to as *speed* is actually *acceleration* to maximum speed, and it is this quality that demands the most attention in sports.

Do all athletes reach maximum speed at about the same distance?

Rates of acceleration vary among athletes in various sports, including track and field. In some 100-meter races, Carl Lewis was still accelerating at the 70-meter mark. Although his accelerating rate was slower than his competitors in the early phase of the race, he continued to increase his speed longer which allowed him to pass athletes in the final 20 meters. Other athletes also accelerate more slowly only to reach higher speeds later in the sprint.

How important is the start in improving the rate of acceleration?

Tom Tellez, coach of numerous Olympic sprinters, indicates that the acceleration phase of a 100-meter dash completed in 10.0 seconds represents approximately 64% of the race and that efficient acceleration over the longest possible distance depends upon the position of the body as the athlete leaves the blocks. In other words, poor starting form in the first 2-3 steps in sports will affect the entire acceleration phase of the sprint.

Do team sport athletes have different acceleration needs than sprinters?

In sports such as football, baseball and softball, basketball, soccer, rugby, lacrosse, field hockey, and tennis it is important to accelerate faster, rather than later in the sprint, since it is unlikely there will be a later. Emmitt Smith and Walter Payton did not possess the blazing speed of Tony Dorsett or Herschel Walker; however, their acceleration speed was excellent and they became two of the best NFL running backs of all times. Using somewhat shorter strides the first 5-7 yards in team sports should help athletes reach maximum speed sooner.

How do athletes know if their acceleration speed is sub par?

Other than the numerous on-field indicators such as arriving to the ball late in soccer, field hockey, lacrosse, rugby; poor crack of the bat to first base times; slow in hitting the holes, rushing the passer, staying with a receiver in football; and getting beaten early in man-to-man coverage in basketball, several items in the test battery presented in Chapter 2 reveal inferior performance in this area.

If there is more than 7/10 of a second difference between your Flying 40-yard score and the Stationary 40-yard score and/or your First 3-step test scores are low, you need to improve your acceleration. Every athlete can improve their current acceleration time by increasing their power output. One of the most important tests to measure power output associated with a forceful push off the ground with each step during the acceleration phase of sprinting is the *dead lift.* This weight room exercise is also a key part of training to improve ground contact force. Your leg press test scores, standing long jump, standing triple jump, and kickback scores are also used to evaluate power output (explosive power or speed-strength) Speed strength plays a major role in early (first 20 meters) and late (20-60 meters) acceleration to maximum speed.

Training to Improve Acceleration

What training programs are used to improve acceleration?

The key program designed to improve acceleration is power output training to increase ground contract force; the power of the pushing action with each step. During the first 20 meters of a sprint, the most important factor is the production of horizontal ground force. Improvement requires the use of exercises performed in the weight room, plyometrics, and sprint-resisted training. These training programs are described in Step II of the 5-step model in Chapter 8.

Form training is also a key aspect of acceleration and proper technique is needed for optimal performance. The sprinting form techniques during acceleration (the leg drive phase of the sprint after clearing the ground and completing the initial two or three steps), also apply to the walk or jog-to-sprint transition. As in the 100-meter sprint, it is important to master proper form to ensure a fast acceleration since the start and ground clearance sets up the acceleration phase of a sprint. A series of acceleration or transition drills are described in Chapter 11: Form and Technique Training.

FAKING, FEINTING AND CUTTING

Not all athletes possess the natural faking and cutting instincts needed to become a great running back, basketball, rugby, soccer, field hockey, or lacrosse player. Although few athletes and coaches ever attack this area with a regular, organized program, these skills can be improved. The task is to identify the basic fakes needed for various sports and player positions, then practice and master these techniques until they become automatic during competition. Adding a new fake to one's repertoire requires an athlete to complete the maneuver hundreds of times, perhaps several thousand, in practice if the skill is to be used automatically at the right time during competition.

How do athletes in football and other sports improve faking and cutting skills?

Although it is beyond the scope of this book, we are in the process of preparing a manual entitled, *The Road to the NFL*, that presents a multiple year program for running backs to develop the fakes and cuts needed for the highest level of performance in football. The manual first presents the basic tactics that must be mastered prior to executing any type of faking maneuver. Athletes are taught to establish dominance, to display sufficient force, to neutralize the defender, and to draw the defender into the danger zone.

The 10 basic (Beginning Level) fakes and feints used by a running back are then described and a learning and practice plan to master these movements is presented. A similar procedure is followed for the Intermediate and advanced level fakes.

A summary of the three year plan is described in table 3.1.

Table 3.1 **The Road to the NFL**

LEVEL	CRITERIA	ESTIMATED TIME NEEDED
Beginning (High School)	Execute each basic cut correctly 10 times using a dummy, 10 times in a practice scrimmage, and 10 times in an actual game.	6-12 months
Intermediate	Meet the above criteria with the basic and intermediate cuts and fakes.	One Year
Advanced (NFL Level)	Meet the above criteria with the basic, intermediate, and advanced cuts and fakes.	Two Years

• You must complete hundreds of correct practice repetitions of each fake and feint before you will even begin to utilize that newly learned skill automatically in a competitive game.

• You should use every opportunity to fake backyard trees, living room furniture, parked cars, and imaginary defensive players to increase your weekly repetitions.

• Use mental practice daily for 10-15 minutes during leisure time to visualize each action.

• Complete 50 repetitions of walking fakes, 50 repetitions of jogging fakes, 50 repetitions of 3/4 speed fakes and 150 repetitions of maximum speed fakes. If you feel you are becoming obsessed with the mastery of these fakes and feints, congratulate yourself and continue with the same behavior. That's what it takes.

Are there common techniques that apply to all types of faking and cutting maneuvers?

Yes. Consider the following concepts below and how they can be applied to every maneuver.

• *Neutralize the Defender* by slowing his movement, breaking his concentration, altering his center of gravity, delaying his total commitment, and placing doubt in his mind. Keep in mind that you fake or feint, first to neutralize and second to go by untouched. Any fake will help neutralize, and any fake is better than no fake at all.

• *Draw the Defender into the "Danger Zone."* This allows you to manipulate the situation. For instance, if a move is to be effective, cutting must occur 2 –3 yards from the defender, therefore, a fake "Straight-ahead" break will draw him into the effective range.

• *Establish Dominance* by adding "Uncertainty" and "Discouragement" to the woes of the opposition. Use your playing skills, speed, power, and strength to get the job done. For example, if you are known to possess outstanding speed, defenders are more likely to go for an early cut that suggests you plan to outrun the opponent. A quick cut in the other direction as the defender commits would then do the trick. Power runners known to "run over" opponents can fake this straight ahead power move, then cut at the last second as defenders brace for the collision.

What types of fakes and feints should be mastered?

A partial list of the basic, intermediate, and advanced maneuvers recommended for running backs in football are listed below.

• *Single plant right and cut left.* Sprint directly at the defender in this and most other maneuvers. When you are within several feet and still out of the defenders grasp, convince the opponent you are breaking to the right with a committed upper and lower body movement in that direction; before planting the right foot, accelerating and breaking left. Although this is obviously one of the most basic moves, athletes often perform the task incorrectly, failing to "sell" the fake, beginning the move too far from the defender, and slowing down rather than accelerating with the cut.

• *Single plant left and cut right.* Opposite cut of above.

• *Double plant and cut left.* Run at the opponent before planting the left foot and breaking right, only to plant that foot also and return left to go by the defender. The first cut will neutralize, the second cut will draw, and the third will be one he'll only be able to watch.

• *Double plant and cut right.* Same as above with a right foot plant.

• *Open-field banana right.* With one defender to get by, execute a move early when you are as far away as ten yards by immediately committing at an angle to outrun the opponent. As the opponent reaches full speed, cut back to the left for 2-3 steps, then quickly accelerate again to the right to outrun the opponent.

• *Open-field banana left.* Opposite of above cut.

• *Ball Change*. Practice switching the football to the opposite arm and back at full speed. When you possess enough skill and confidence, you can use the ball change to make your opponent think you will be going a certain direction.

• *Triple Sideline Plant and Cut Right.* Fast feet are required to execute sideline cuts and spins when runners are trapped and have only a small amount of room to maneuver. These moves serve several purposes: additional yardage is acquired with the possibility of scoring a touchdown and the chance of injury is reduced. Quick movements of any kind help prevent opponents from "zeroing in" on you with maximum force. The movements add uncertainty and force the defender to use a bit of cautiousness. In the triple plants, the runner plants left, then immediately plants right, repeating this action with short steps and fast feet two more times before delivering the blow to the defender.

• *Triple sideline plants and cut left.* Opposite of triple cut above.

• *Dancing in Your Shoes.* Runners shift their weight back and forth without moving to force the defender to slow his movements and focus.

• *Overpower maneuver.* Although this tactic may seem out of place as a faking maneuver, it is an excellent example of how to establish uncertainty and actually condition an opponent to expecting the same action later in the competition. The idea is to execute a basic plant to the left or right before accelerating into the opponent to deliver the blow and become the "hitter" rather than the "hitee."

• *Shoulder drive, contact and spin left.* In conjunction with the overpower move, the runner delivers the blow with shoulder contact that prevents an opponent from "wrapping" the arms, then spins to the left and accelerates away from the defender.

• *Shoulder drive, contact and spin right.* Opposite drive, contact and spin of above.

• *Full Spin.* A pre-contact spin is especially good for moving around a clutter of players or changing directions.

• *Hit and side-step.* The hit and side-step is based on making good solid contact first and then using the energy the opponent gives you to initiate the sidestep. Walter Payton was a "brilliant" runner and is a good example of a player that was so advanced he dictated all aspects of play, even the use of contact.

• *Stop and back, cut at 10 and catch at 8.* One of the best stop and start actions used by receivers in football is to sprint directly at the defender, selling a "fly" pattern, then stopping quickly after a 10-yard sprint as the defender commits to a long sprint, and sprinting back 2-3 yards to catch the pass.

• *Stop, back and go.* At the end of the stop and back movement above, receivers can then accelerate into the fly pattern as a close defender approaches.

A series of faking and cutting drills are described in Chapter 11.

Chapter 4

MECHANICS OF SPRINTING

Although no two individuals run precisely the same way, basic sprinting mechanics are similar for all team sport athletes. Form is an important part of a holistic speed improvement program and athletes need to take the time to develop the proper mechanics of sprinting and eliminate all faulty actions that do not contribute to forward movement. This chapter describes sound mechanics of sprinting, including body position, proper lean, leg and arm action, eye focus, and relaxation. Proper starting techniques for team sports such as football, soccer, baseball, basketball, field hockey, rugby, and lacrosse were presented in Chapter 3.

An analysis of correct sprinting form has allowed researchers to identify key factors contributing to efficient movement. It has also revealed a diversity of styles and techniques among champion athletes. This diversity suggests the need for athletes to improve their basic style without trying to mimic the exact techniques of others.

Is correct sprinting form important for team sport athletes?

Proper mechanics in the start, acceleration and maximum speed phase reduces strength and energy requirements, delays fatigue and improves performance. It is also an area of training that cannot be done properly without adequate speed-strength to accelerate rapidly and speed-endurance to maintain performance with limited negative influence from fatigue. In general, the amount of horizontal force an athlete can generate depends on how much vertical force is applied during ground contact. This force is increased by gains in both strength and mechanical efficiency. Athletes who exhibit sound mechanics apply all available force in the proper direction during ground contact.

The preadolescent period is the ideal time to focus on sprinting mechanics. Developing these skills early provides a solid advantage when young athletes begin their holistic speed training program.

According to leading researcher, Ralph Mann, mastering correct form is often obstructed by the limitations that athletes develop during the formative years or through training practices. Observation of young elementary school children sprinting on the playground or athletic field makes it clear that poor sprinting mechanics are common. By the time athletes reach adolescence, these habits are deeply imbedded and difficult to change.

Body Position

What is the correct body position and proper lean in sprinting?

The ideal body position is perpendicular to the ground with the neck and head naturally in line. Depending upon the impulse (foot-ground contact), the body may lean from the ground, as in the drive phase of sprinting, or remain almost vertical, as in the maximum speed phase.

Running is instinctive, but the misinterpretation of the fundamental phases of sprinting sometimes interferes with natural and correct form. As an athlete, you must be aware of what is natural and what is unnatural or your efforts can make you sprint slower. Often athletes feel that they have to "bear down" and "stay low and pull" in order to run fast. The scientific analysis of sprinting suggests just the opposite. Reaching maximum speed depends greatly upon how relaxed you can keep your body in a naturally upright position. The human machine is much better at pushing than pulling, partly because the formation of the leg is unsuited as a pulling force. Therefore, the suggestion to "stay low and pull" prevents maximum speed. If you want to run faster, remember that sprinting is primarily a pushing action against the ground.

Leg Action and The Stride Cycle

What is the correct form during the stride cycle?

During any running stride, the leg cycles through three different phases: the *drive* phase, when the foot is in contact with the ground; the *recovery* phase, when the leg swings from the hip while the foot clears the ground; and the *support* phase, when the runner's weight is on the entire foot.

During the drive phase, the power comes from a pushing action off the ball of the foot (figure 4.1). Stride length, and therefore sprinting speed, is the result of a pushing action. The goal of the drive phase is to create the maximum push off the ground. The ball of the foot is the only part of the foot capable of creating an efficient and powerful push. Some misinformed sport professionals believe that the pushing action comes from the toes.

However, pushing from the toes reduces both power and stability and slows the runner. The drive phase contributes to overall speed only when the runner pushes off the ground using the ball of the foot.

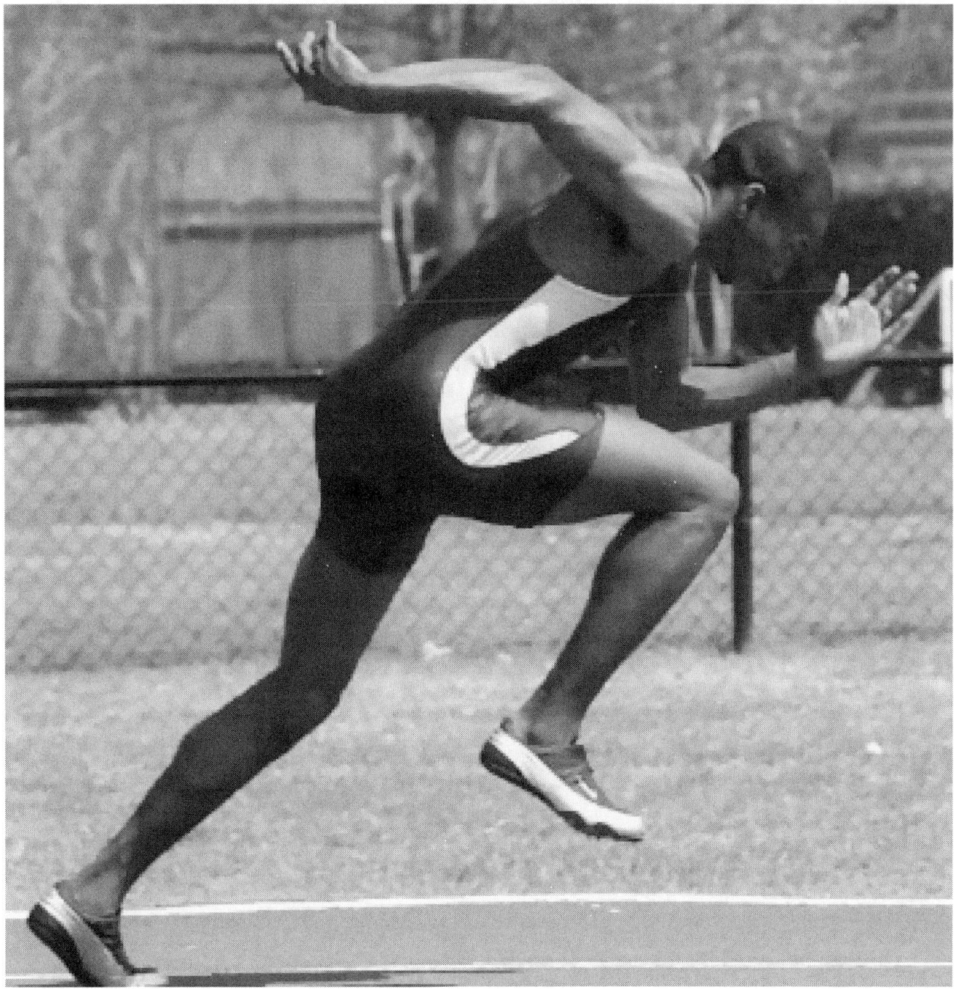

Figure 4.1 Natural lengthening of the stride by driving the center of mass forward.

The drive of the supporting leg during the sprinting action takes approximately 0.09 to 0.11 second though maximum strength in contracted muscles can occur after only 0.7 to 0.9 second. Obviously, maximum strength is not reached during the sprinting action. Fast training that improves speed strength, therefore, has the best chance of decreasing supporting leg time and thus improving sprinting speed. After an adequate strength foundation has been acquired, athletes should direct their attention toward the improvement of power output (speed-strength).

During the recovery phase, the knee joint closes and the foot cycles through as it comes close to the body. As the knee joint opens and the leg begins to straighten, the foot comes closer to the ground in preparation for the support phase. An important point to remember about the recovery phase is that the runner does not reach for the ground or force a stamping action. The leg should remain relaxed and allow the foot to naturally strike the ground.

During the support phase, the foot makes initial contact with the ground on the outside edge of the ball of the foot. The weight of the body is then supported at a point that varies according to the speed of the athlete. The faster the speed, the higher the contact point on the ball of the foot. Striking the ground first with this part of the foot serves to maximize speed but takes great energy. At slower speeds (jogging, for example), the contact point moves toward the rear of the foot between the arch and heel.

During longer and slower runs, energy is saved by using a flat foot plant. At all running speeds, the support phase begins with a slight load on the support foot that then rides onto the full sole. Even during sprinting, the heel makes a brief but definite contact with the ground. This analysis of the support phase shows how it is impossible to reach maximum speed by running on the toes.

Initial ground contact does vary depending upon the distance of the race or sprint:

RACE	INITIAL GROUND CONTACT
100-200-meter sprinters	Ball of the foot (inside top)
400-800-meter sprinters	In the arch
1500 meter runners	Almost the entire foot is in contact

How does an athlete avoid losing horizontal speed each time the foot hits the ground?

According to world renowned researcher, Dr. Ralph Mann (2007), "the only way to avoid slowing down with each stride as the foot hits the ground is to have the foot moving backward as fast as possible at ground contact. The quicker the foot moves, the faster the movement of the athlete. Applying the needed pushing force away from the ground is a real challenge when an athlete is sprinting at a high rate of 12 meters per second. At this rate of speed, the foot itself must be moving more than 10 meters per second backward with respect to the sprinter.

To help understand this concept, Dr. Mann uses the following analogy. If you are traveling 30 mph in a car with your hand out the window and your hand strikes a telephone pole, contact is made at 30 mph because that is how fast the vehicle is moving. If you are moving the hand forward 10 mph just before reaching the pole, the hand is traveling 40 mph as it hits the pole. Conversely, if you are moving the hand backward 10 miles per hour just before contact, the hand is moving only 20 mph when it hits the pole; moving the hand backward at 30 mph prior to contact would result in the hand contacting the pole at 0 mph causing no physical damage. The sprinter faces the same problem. To avoid hitting the ground with the foot moving forward at 10m per second, leg motion must allow the foot to move backward (in relation to the sprinter) at less than 10m per second.

As in the example of the hand striking the pole, if an athlete is incapable of producing a backward foot speed equal to the forward velocity of the body, a braking force occurs and forward speed decreases. In actuality, it is not possible to completely avoid producing some braking force. Although the horizontal foot speed at touchdown of elite sprinters comes close, foot speed still does not equal the horizontal velocity.

As shown in Table 4.1, even elite male and female sprinters are unable to reach "0" (equivalent to the hand moving backward at 30 mph as it strikes the pole with the car moving at 30 mph) and are striking the ground with the foot moving forward at 3.52-3.53 meters per second.

This concept is still another example demonstrating how the correct mechanical application of speed strength produces a high stride rate as a result of exact timing of force application.

Table 4.1 Horizontal Foot Speed, Speed of Forward Movement, and Forward Movement of the Foot at Ground Contact

CALIBER OF SPRINTER	HORIZONTAL FOOT SPEED AT TOUCHDOWN (mps)*		SPEED OF FORWARD MOVEMENT (mps)		FORWARD FOOT MOVEMENT AT GROUND CONTACT (mps)	
	Men	Women	Men	Women	Men	Women
POOR	6.71	5.55				
AVERAGE	7.59	6.46				
GOOD	8.47	7.38	12.0	10.9	3.53	3.52

* mps = meters per second *Source*: Mann, Ralph, Mechanics of Sprinting and Hurdling, 200

How do horizontal and vertical forces interact?

The two key aspects in understanding the factors limiting speed of movement in humans is *horizontal* and *vertical* force production. The discussion below includes numerous findings by Dr. Ralph Mann and his research team that are rarely examined and discussed. Few researchers have the resources and the capability of analyzing the act of sprinting as Dr. Mann whose findings provide further insight into training to improve speed of movement in team sport athletes.

Since the objective is to cover a distance of 5 to 100 yards as fast as possible in sports, all coaches assume that athletes need to generate as much horizontal force as possible while in contact with the ground. Dr. Mann points out that although the production of horizontal velocity is important, it is NOT the critical mechanical factor in achieving maximum sprinting speed. What is important for team sport coaches to remember is that it is only during the start and early acceleration phase of a sprint (first 20 yards) that producing horizontal ground force is the major factor. During this stage, large amounts of horizontal force are needed to move an athlete from a stationary position to a high velocity position as quickly as possible. *As an athlete approaches maximum velocity, force demands in a horizontal direction decrease and eventually approach zero since no additional mph speed can be obtained.* After maximum horizontal velocity is achieved, a shift from horizontal to a vertical or up and down direction occurs. The mystery for researchers has been to find out why athletes cannot produce additional horizontal force. In the past, it was assumed that the human body segments simply could not move fast enough to further increase speed of movement. Studies have revealed that this is untrue. The body can and does produce even greater forces at maximum horizontal velocity. This evidence has made it clear that the limiting factor is not in the horizontal direction.

Unlike the demands of horizontal force, there is no decrease in the requirements in a vertical direction. Ground contact time and air time are needed to produce vertical velocity and overcome the force of gravity. Dr. Mann describes these requirements:

> The sprinter must increase the vertical velocity of the body to a value of approximately 0.5 meters per second (1.6 feet) upward at the point where the foot leaves the ground. Then, during the air phase, gravitational pull rapidly reverses the sprinter's upward velocity and, as touchdown once again occurs, the performer's vertical velocity has been altered to approximately 0.5 meters per second downward. During the ensuing ground phase, the sprinter must reverse this downward velocity to again produce the 0.5 meters per second upward velocity as the next takeoff position is achieved. Thus, at maximum sprint velocity, although the horizontal

velocity is not changing, the vertical velocity is changing at the rate of 1.0 meters per second (from 0.5 meters per second downward to 0.5 meters per second upward) during each ground contact phase.

Vertical forces must project the body into the air throughout the sprinting action. The simple act of standing requires a vertical force equal to body weight to merely support an athlete. To stop downward velocity and produce enough upward velocity to propel the body into the air, the vertical force must also include body weight and amounts to approximately 2.15 pounds per pound of weight.

A 230 pound football player must generate an average vertical force of about 495 pounds with each step. During ground contact, a 230 pound athlete cannot produce a steady vertical force of 495 pounds and therefore must exert much higher than average forces at certain stages of foot/ground contact to counteract the lower values caused by changing body position at other stages. Since foot placement occurs directly in front of the body's center of gravity, a braking effect occurs during the first half of ground contact. The force generated during the second half of ground contact must regain the horizontal force lost during the first half and also propel the body into the air. THIS VERTICAL FORCE DEMAND IS THE LIMITING FACTOR IN SPRINTING PERFORMANCE.

The key for team sport athletes, after the initial 20 yards, is to increase vertical force production. This is the emphasis elite sprinters have successfully used to improve sprinting speed for decades.

How is flight distance (air time) and landing (touch time) balanced for optimum sprinting speed?

Flight distance refers to air time and the distance traveled in the non-support phase of each stride when both feet are off the ground. It is determined by the angle of impulse, the velocity at take off produced from the pushing action against the ground, relative height of the center of gravity (COG) at takeoff, air resistance, and acceleration due to gravity (natural body lean). Landing distance is the distance the center of gravity (COG) is away from the landing foot. This distance must be relatively short to reduce braking forces which decelerate the body. The correct landing spot is slightly in front of the COG before the body moves directly under the COG for push off.

Placement behind the COG results in stumbling; placement too far in front forces a reaching step, increases ground contact time, utilizes too much force, and results in loss of momentum as the body regains proper position to push off for the next stride.

Mastering proper sprinting form guarantees that the COG is in the correct position and that all forces are moving in the right direction with minimum resistance.

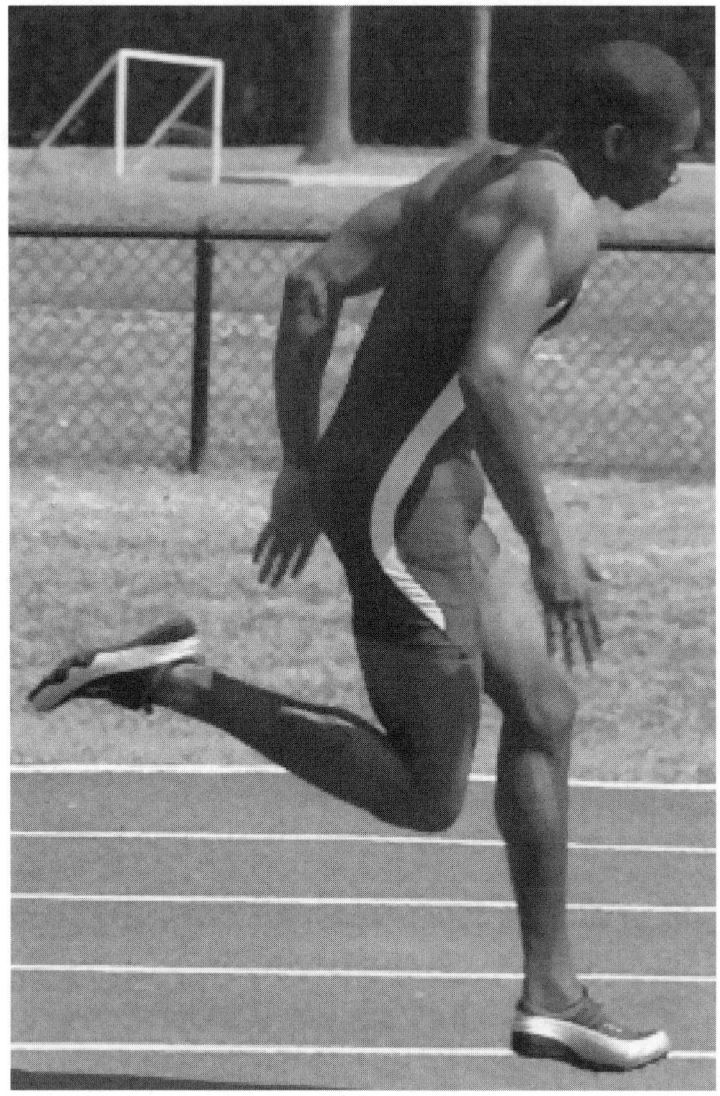

Figure 4.2. The foot strikes the ground directly under the center of gravity.

Is a high kick-up of the back leg (butt kick) important or just a waste of energy in sprinting?

A high kick up of the rear leg occurs during the recovery and support phase. In general, the harder the drive, the greater the fold up and closer to the buttocks the heel reaches. This is a natural reaction to the drive phase of sprinting. British sprint coach, Bill Marlow (1972), indicates that this allows the leg to come through as a short lever and, in the time available, permits a greater range of movement. As athletes learn to execute a powerful drive phase, the height of the back leg kick up will increase and actually come close to the buttocks. Butt kicking drills are an exaggerated form of the movement but do help some athletes develop the "feel" for the proper action of the leg and heel in the recovery and support phase. From a side view, observe a good sprinter or fast running back as they pass you at full speed. You will immediately notice the natural high kick up of the rear leg.

What do coaches mean when they tell athletes to run "in front" of the body rather than "in back?"

According to Ralph Mann and other researchers, "the more sprinters can shift ground contact efforts to the front of the body, the more successful the performance." Back side mechanics dominate the start and acceleration phase as athletes begin at a pace of about 4-meters per second with powerful thrusts against the blocks or ground. As the athlete moves past 20-meters, the switch to front side mechanics begins during ground contact. Mann's research indicates that if athletes do not make the transition after the start, they will complete the race poorly with back side dominance.

The theory is that the path taken by the recovering leg enhances front side landing mechanics. A foot lagging behind the butt would be counterproductive since the heel should come up under the butt with the hip flexors lifting the leg to prevent the heel from moving behind the midline of the body. With the upper leg vertical, back side mechanics are in play if the foot is recovered behind the butt. To apply the concept of front side mechanics, athletes must make certain the foot lands under the center of mass.

The amount of force an athlete can generate at the ankle, knee and hip determine speed of movement. Adopting the technique of front side mechanics is not a natural movement and takes time to master. Techniques to minimize backside action and maximize front side mechanics involve developing the correct muscular action at the ankle, the knee and the hip during ground contact. The goal is to help athletes develop a feel for active recovery of the upper leg during ground contact. Front side mechanics is practiced by all elite sprinters.

Is the common verbal cue, "drive the knees," helpful in getting athletes to sprint faster.

According to Latif Thomas, 2006 Massachusetts State Track Coach of the Year, coaches are telling athletes to lift the knees when they should be telling them to drive the thigh down and apply more force to the ground.

Thomas indicates that if coaches would have told him that the key is to "step over the opposite knee and drive down" instead of "knees, knees, lift your knees," he would have been a better sprinter. The object is to help athletes apply the concept of stepping over and driving down. Coaches need to make certain that verbal cues are clearly understood and are accurately communicating what is to be done.

Arm Action

What is the proper movement of the arms during the sprinting action?

Coordinated arm and leg movement results in efficient sprinting. The arms work in opposition to the legs, with the right arm and left leg coming forward as the left arm and right leg go backward and vice versa. The shoulders should stay square (perpendicular) to the direction of the run. The swing should be strong but relaxed. The hands are also relaxed and positioned about shoulder-high, not exceeding the chin, slightly in front of the chest. On the upswing, the hand should rise naturally to a point just in front of the chin and just inside the shoulder. During the upswing, the arm angle is about 90 degrees or less, coordinating with the quick recovery of the forward swing of the leg. During the downswing, a natural straightening of the elbow corresponds with the longer leverage of the driving leg on the opposite side of the body to allow horizontal drive. As the arm swings down, the elbow extends slightly. At the bottom of the swing, the hand is next to the thigh. However, toward the end of its backward movement, the arm bends and speeds up again to match the final fast stage of the leg drive. The elbows should stay close to the body. Attempts to keep the elbows away from the body will prevent relaxation of the shoulders and limit efficient running mechanics. Arm action is never forced or tense.

The shoulder is the axis of arm rotation and the elbow acts to shorten the lever when needed. Closing the elbow angle reduces the movement of arm inertia, increases angular velocity, to create quicker turnover. Arm movement without the elbow joint results in a straight-arm, penduum-like swing that moves too slow for leg coordination.

Should a 90-degree angle between the lower and upper arm be maintained at all times when sprinting?

Although this advice is commonly given to sprinters, no athlete keeps that angle throughout a sprinting cycle. As stated previously, when the arm is lowered, a straightening at the elbow occurs. The exact angles vary from sprinter-to-sprinter and with each individual depending on the length of the stride and the phase of a sprinting cycle. The key is to maintain relaxed shoulders, arms and hands with the swing coming from the shoulder joint.

On the upswing, the hand should rise naturally to a point in front of the chin and inside the shoulder with an arm angle of 90 degrees or less. During the downswing, a natural straightening at the elbow corresponds with the driving leg on the opposite side of the body to allow horizontal drive. At the bottom of the swing, the hand should be next to the thigh. Toward the end of the backward movement, the arm bends and speeds up again to match the final, fast stage of the leg drive.

Is it true that the faster one pumps the arms, the faster the legs will go."

This is only partially true, and the verbal cue to "overly pump the arms" is incorrect. Elite sprinters and athletes in other sports use their arms in a natural, relaxed manner and avoid any suggestion of "muscling" through the movement at any stage of sprinting. In addition, most athletes can move the arms at a faster rate than their legs. Researcher and coach, Ralph Mann, clarifies the issue in his book, *The Mechanics of Sprinting and Hurdling,*

> "Contrary to popular belief, superior arm action does not produce a superior sprint performance. In fact, regardless of the quality of the sprinter, there is no significant difference in the arm action. If a sprinter could improve the horizontal velocity simply by moving the arms faster, then even old, out of shape coaches could run faster than the elite sprinter since virtually everyone has the ability to move their arms fast enough to easily produce an elite stride rate of five steps per second. What the coaches and most other people cannot do, is produce the leg action required to produce an elite sprint performance. It is the legs that must not only move their own considerable bulk, but also contend with the large ground forces during each consecutive ground contact. In comparison, the arms must only move their own rather meager bulk, without any other external hindrance."

Eye Contact

Does where you focus your eyes during the sprinting action affect speed of movement?

According to Derek M. Hansen, author of the article "Where You Look Can Affect How Your Look: Running Mechanics and Gaze Control," (2009), eye focus is a key factor in sprinting. Coach Hansen became interested in the importance of eye focus after observing how team sport athletes pop their heads up after the first or second step from a stationary starting position which negatively impacts early and late acceleration. By making athletes look at a specific area on the ground 3-5 meters ahead, he was able to teach them to keep their head in the correct position - in line with their spine.

Research supports the value of "gaze-control" in sprinting. Elite athletes exhibit different eye movement, attention and decision making than non-elite athletes. Joan Vickers, author of *Perception, Cognition, and Decision Training: The Quiet Eye in Action* (2009) indicates that elite athletes:

> are faster to detect and recognize objects such as a ball within the visual field,
>
> posses superior recall and recognition of sport-specific patterns of play and an enhanced ability to effectively pick-up advance (pre-event) visual cues, particularly from an opponent's postural orientation,
>
> exhibit more efficient skill and use of visual-search behaviors, and
>
> have more accurate expectations of likely events based on the refined use of situational probabilities.

Researchers have been able to identify and record where an athlete's eyes are fixed when executing a sports skill in ice hockey goaltending, basketball shooting, baseball hitting, putting in golf, and speed skating. Vickers comments further on her experience with athletes:

> For long periods of time throughout the year, I will train sprint athletes in indoor environments to escape the cold and inclement weather. However, I find it is easier to get them to adopt proper posture in outdoor training situations. With indoor facilities, athletes will often see a wall in front of them when performing sprint repetitions. Even if they are not in danger of colliding with the wall, athletes will still change their posture and mechanics in anticipation of stopping prematurely. The body will tend to 'rear-up', impacting proper acceleration and/or maximum velocity mechanics. When training outdoors, I find that athletes do not feel the same confinement issues and tend to run more freely. I attribute this tendency to the power of vision and gaze. Almost innately, our bodies respond to not only 'where' we look, but also 'what' we see and take the necessary steps to change our posture and mechanics to anticipate a potential course of action. Some athletes are more sensitive to these environmental issues and coaches need to be aware of the impact of facilities on visual control and athletic performances.

Relaxation

How important is relaxation in Sprinting?

Coaches and athletes are well aware that the absence of efficient, tension-free muscular movement produces more rapid fatigue, poor performance, and increases the incidence of injuries. Executing short sprints in team sports also requires very efficient muscular coordination and relaxed movement patterns. During relaxed movement, less pliant tense muscles restrict range of motion and keep athletes from reaching their maximum mph speed. In addition, muscle involvement may occur that does not efficiently contribute to forward movement. Although the degree of "slowing" that occurs in all athletes at the end of a long sprint, or after repeated short sprints, is mainly determined by anaerobic fitness (speed endurance) and exhausted energy sources, it is also affected by muscular tension and an inhibiting processes that occurs in the central nervous system. According to Kehakultuur (1988), these inhibiting factors are not only caused by the reduced strength of nerve impulses but also by the frequency (sprinting) and duration (speed endurance) of the impulses. Successful sprinting that allows athletes to excel at their maximum potential will not occur without a relaxed running style free from tension.

To produce a relaxed style of sprinting in team sport athletes, some attention is needed on the developing the nervous process. The object is to sprint fast, but sprint effortlessly (relaxed) with a loose jaw, loose hands, and relaxed arm, shoulder and neck muscles. Team sport coaches and athletes need to incorporate sprinting relaxation techniques into their regular workout schedule until tension-free sprinting is automatic in all phases of their sport. The key is for athletes to avoid becoming too aware of the actual movement details of sprinting. As sprinting mechanics become automatic, emphasis is placed on relaxed movement patterns. Athletes are taught to relax their hands and eliminate tension from the shoulders to the finger tips. Since team sport athletes tend to make a tight fist as they accelerate and try to sprint faster, the thumb should make contact with the index finger as the remaining fingers stay relaxed.

Mike Smith, one of Britain's most successful sprint coaches, offers some key advice to improve relaxation during the start, acceleration, and maximum speed phases of the sprinting action. He points out that tension most often occurs when athletes "try too hard" and tighten the muscles of the hands, arms, shoulders, neck and jaw. The object is to avoid overdoing things and concentrate on remaining relaxed."

Muscle Involvement

What muscle groups are involved in propelling the body forward during the sprinting action?

Numerous studies have been conducted to identify the involvement and importance of various muscle groups during the acceleration and maximum speed phase of sprinting. One elaborate study by Klaus Wiemann and Gunter Tidlow (1995) summarizes the findings and answers this question very well. When looking for those muscles of the knees and hips which are responsible for the acceleration and horizontal velocity of the body during full-speed sprinting, the gluteus maximus, the adductor magnus, the hamstrings and the knee extensors have been identified as most important. Electromyographic results concerning the degree of muscle activity (ROA) in 12 elite sprinters show that the hamstrings are active during the whole phase of hip extension (back-swing and support phase) while the gluteus maximus, like the knee extensors, "fire" only during the back-swing phase and the first half of the support phase. However, the adductor magnus has already ceased to be active at the beginning of the support phase. The peak ROA of the muscles examined are clearly above 100% of MVC activity. The adductor magnus shows a conspicuously high peak ROA of 200%. These findings, together with biomechanical considerations, lead to the suggestion that the hamstrings in particular, together with a muscle rein consisting of gluteus maximus and adductor magnus, supply the energy needed for forward propulsion, by providing a high back-swing velocity of the support leg. In this context the adductor magnus seems to be loaded to an especially high degree. The vastus medialis in general and the gluteus maximus, to some extent during the support phase, fulfill only anti-gravitation functions. This leads to corresponding implications for sprint training.

How important are the Hip Extensor and Hip Flexor Muscles in Sprinting

The hip extensors and the hip flexors are the strongest muscle groups within the lower extremity. The extensors are the primary movers, by acceleration, of the body's center of gravity. The prime movers of the hips are also responsible for generating the most force during sprinting. Studies by Ralph Mann and others indicate that the bulk of forward propulsion and power generation in sprinting comes from the proximal musculature of the pelvis. The hip extensors are dominant in the back swing and the first half of the stance phase, and the hip flexors are dominant power generators in the second half of the stance and early swing phases. According to famed track coach, Tom Tellez, the athlete who can best utilize the hips joints will be more successful in sprinting. The most important phase in each stride for all athletes is the push-off the ground. The amount of ground contact force generated affects the length and rate of each stride, acceleration speed, and maximum mph speed. During this action, the body is stretched upward from the ground and the origin of the motion occurs at the hip joint. "The hip acts as a crank to deliver the force to the ground. This force is then returned to the center of the mass lifting it up off the ground." During foot placement, the hips continue to extend. The foot (ankle) is placed directly under the knee joint with the shin perpendicular (right angle) to the ground.

Research indicates that there is a strong relationship between hip flexion and hip extension strength relative to body weight when strength is assessed from an upright position. There also appears to be a cause-effect relationship between enhanced hip flexion/extension strength and sprinting speed (Guskiewicz, 1993). The hip musculature may be more important than knee musculature in evaluating sprinting speed.

In spite of the importance of the hip flexor muscles to sprinting and other movement patterns in sports, this muscle group is one of the most neglected in strength training. While exercises for the leg extensor muscles are common, hip flexor exercises are rare. The main muscles involved in hip flexion are the *psoas major* and the *iliacus* (the ilopsoas muscles). The *rectus femoris,* one of four quadriceps, crosses the hip joint and also operates as a hip flexor and knee extensor. The deep-seated ilopsoas muscles are difficult to strengthen with free weights and receive little attention in the weight room. The truth is that strong hip flexor muscles are critical for high performance in team sports and utilized anytime the thigh is brought up toward the abdomen or the abdomen is moved toward the thigh. Executing a powerful kick of the ball in football, rugby and soccer requires simultaneous knee extension and hip flexion. Strong hip flexors also play a role for ball carriers who are moving forward with opponents holding on. Hockey and lacrosse players also must skate and run through contact. The baseball player taking the first few steps out of the box or off a base will benefit from strong hip flexors. And, of course, sprinters who need extremely strong hip flexors.

The two most commonly used exercises to develop hip flexor strength are *incline sit-ups* and *hanging leg raises.* With body weight providing the resistance, strength gains are limited. *A multi-hip machine* is available that allows the athlete to push against a padded roller swinging on an arc with the thigh. If the position of the hip joint could be maintained, heavier weights could be used. The *MyoQuip HipneeFlex* is designed to strengthen both hip and knee flexors simultaneously from full extension to full flexion. Decreasing resistance occurs throughout the movement to provide the correct loading to both sets of flexors.

Kevin O'Neill, MS, CSCS provides a list of additional exercises to strengthen the hip flexor muscles:

Spread Eagle Sit-ups--Start by lying on your back. Spread your legs with locked knees and hook both feet on the vertical support beams of a power rack. Now complete a straight leg sit up. To add resistance, use a weight or dumbbell.

Hanging Knee/Leg Raises--While hanging from a pull-up bar, keep your upper body straight, bend your legs and bring both knees to your chest. You can also keep your legs straight and bring the toes to the ceiling with the legs parallel to the floor. For added resistance, hold a dumbbell with your feet.

Incline/Flat Bench Leg Raises--This exercise is similar to the one above, except, you adjust the angle to make it slightly easier. Lie supine while holding on to a bench behind your head. Complete either a straight or bent leg raise.

Cable/Band Knee Drive--Attach an ankle cuff cable to the low cable pulley. Place both hands on a a bench or box in front of you. Your body should resemble a sprinter leaving the blocks. Make sure you are far enough away to maintain tension on the cable. With a flat back, drive the knee forward and up in front of your chest. Stay in control of the weight on the negative phase so it doesn't jerk your leg at the end of the repetition. Focus on keeping the ankle cocked in dorsi-flexion. You can also use a band instead of the cable which forces you to accelerate through the movement.

Lying Cable Knee Drive--While lying on your back attach ankle cuffs to the low cable pulley and bring both knees to the chest.

Forward Sled Dragging--Using the sled strap attachment, place a loop around each foot. Proceed to walk straight ahead.

Muscle Hyperplasia and Hypertrophy

Is the increase in muscle size from weight training a result of hyperplasia or hypertrophy?

"Hyperplasia" refers to an increase in the number of new muscle fibers. This increase has been verified in birds and animals, however, there is currently no evidence of hyperplasia in humans as a result of various types of weight training. Even if some new muscle fibers were added, the effect on muscle size and body weight would be small, estimated at less than five percent of the gain. "Hypertrophy," the increase in the size of individual muscle fibers, accounts for muscle growth and additional muscle weight in humans as a result of weight training.

The number of human fat cells is generally set by the mid-20s and weight and fat changes occur from an increase in the size of these existing cells. There is some evidence that new fat cells can be added (hyperplasia) in adult individuals who become obese.

Does muscle fascicle length have anything to do with sprinting speed.

A fascicle is a bundle of skeletal muscle fibers surrounded by perimysium, a type of connective tissue. Kumagai (2001) and his colleagues investigated the relationship between muscle fascicle length and sprinting performance in 37 male 100-meter sprinters. The sample was divided into two performance groups according to their personal-best 100-meter times:

Group I: 10.00-10.90 seconds (Subjects = 22)
Group II: 11.00-11.70 seconds (Subjects = 15)

Muscle thickness and fascicle pennation angle of the vastus lateralis and gastrocnemius medialis and lateralis muscles were measured by B-mode ultrasonography, and fascicle length was estimated. Standing height, body weight, and leg length were similar between the two groups. Muscle thickness was also similar between groups for the vastus lateralis and gastrocnemius medialis, but Group I had a significantly greater gastrocnemius lateralis muscle thickness. Group I also had a greater muscle thickness in the upper portion of the thigh, which, given similar limb lengths, demonstrates an altered "muscle shape." Pennation angle was always less in Group I than in Group II. In all muscles, Group I had significantly greater fascicle length than did Group II, which significantly correlated with 100-m best performance (r values from 0.40 to 0.57). Researchers concluded that longer fascicle length is associated with greater sprinting performance. Longer muscle fascae length enhances the force generating capacity of the muscle which improves sprinting speed. Studies also indicate that there is no gender difference in the fascicle length of elite male and female sprinters.

Common Sprinting Form Errors

What sprinting form errors are commonly seen in team sport athletes?

The form errors most commonly seen in team sport athletes are listed in Table 4.2. The sooner flaws are corrected, the better. Developing proper sprinting technique in young boys and girls during the elementary school areas is the ideal approach.

Specific drills and techniques to correct faulty form are presented in Part III: The 5-Step Model, Chapter 11.

Table 4.2 Troubleshooting Sprinting Mechanics

Problem Area	Suggestion
Arm action	If you run with tense arms, practice loose, swinging movements from a standing position. Remember to swing from the shoulder and keep the arms relaxed at all times. Although the arms work in opposition to the legs, they must be coordinated with the action of the legs for maximum sprinting efficiency.
Body lean	Many athletes and some sport professionals suggest too much body lean. Your body should have a slight lean in the direction that you are running. It is important to note that the lean comes from the ground and not from the waist. The lean is only a result of displacing the center of gravity in the direction you are running. Leaning by bending at the waist interferes with the correct mechanics of sprinting.
Foot contact	Don't run up on your toes. The toes have no power or stability. If you run on your toes, you will not be able to run fast. Stay on the balls of your feet and push against the ground. Don't reach for and pull toward the ground; this strategy will develop injuries and result in poor sprinting mechanics and slow times. Allow the heel to make contact with the ground when running at any distance.
Overstriding	Over striding is the worst and most misunderstood element of sprinting. Don't reach and overstride to increase stride length. Push against the ground and let the foot land underneath your center of gravity. Any placement of the foot in front of the center of gravity will cause the body to slow down.
Understriding	Try not to be too quick. Too much turnover will cause you to run fast in one place, and you will not cover any ground. Quality sprint speed is a combination of both stride frequency and stride length. One does not replace the other.
Tension	Don't try to power your way through a race or sprint effort. You will not run fast if you are tight. To run fast, you must stay relaxed.

How do coaches correct the problem of feet crossing over the midline and turning outward?

This "out pointing" of the feet on ground contact is more common in preadolescent boys and girls who tend to have poor leg alignment in general possibly due to lack of strength and power. The problem seems to self-correct during the adolescent period in some athletes. It is also more common during the first 5-6 steps during the early acceleration phase.

One suggestion is to practice pointing the feet forward, inward and outward during a series of 10-15, three-quarter speed sprints for several training sessions to help develop a "feel" for foot placement and to gain control of these movements. Once you have control, breaking the habit of landing with the toes pointed outward will be easier.

Now, using line markers on a football field, sprint slightly to the left of the line concentrating on both the right forefoot and heel contacting the line with each step. Repeat coming back with the left toe and heel. Two lines at near shoulder width apart can also be used as you observe the foot placement at ground contact. The correction won't occur in one session but now that you are aware of and have control of the form error, change should occur in a few weeks.

The outside of the forefoot should make contact with the ground slightly in front of the body's center of gravity (except in the early acceleration phase during the first 5-15 meters when the foot strikes slightly behind the body's center of gravity) with the foot pointing directly forward. Avoid running up on your toes. The toes have no power or stability and will keep you from sprinting fast. Instead, make sure you stay on the balls of the feet, push against the ground and also allow the heel to make contact with the ground each step.

Chapter 5

STRIDE RATE AND STRIDE LENGTH

Sprinting speed is the product of stride length and stride rate. Maximum speed is reached only when these two components are in correct proportion. The rate of leg movement (sps--steps per second) is the time required to complete one stride and is limited by the length of each step. Stride rate is governed more by physiological function such as muscle fiber type, speed-strength, neuromuscular coordination, and flexibility than biomechanical function even though the path the legs take to create the speed is biomechanical. Both rate and length are limited by the length of the legs and the force applied against the ground during the pushing action of each step.

Which is more important, stride rate or stride length?

Stride length and rate are interdependent with the relationship based on the amount of resistance to be overcome. Power = Force X Velocity. The force and velocity generated by the muscles improves both stride length and rate. Research indicates that elite sprinters develop an optimal stride length, slightly above average, then concentrate their training on increasing stride rate.

STRIDE RATE

World class sprinters have a stride rate of about 4.5 (females) to 5 (males) steps per second. Women sprint the 100-meter dash 6/10 to 8/10 of a second slower than males mainly due to slower stride rates and shorter strides caused by differences in power output (speed-strength).

Children take faster steps than adults. As height and leg length increases, stride rate decreases. There is no advantage to having short or long legs. Long legs allow a longer stride, but slower stride rate. Short legs result in a faster stride rate and shorter strides. It also takes more strength, power, and energy to move long legs through a complete cycle than shorter legs.

Studies show that the ability to take fast steps is not common in young athletes. Among 13-14 year old students, only 15 had high stride rates.

Approximately 10 youngsters in 100 had a very short down time of 0.90 to 0.105 seconds (the support phase when one foot is contacting the ground).

The important thing to remember is that stride rate can be increased regardless of height or the length of the legs.

How is stride rate increased?

Stride rate can easily be increased by shortening air time. Unfortunately, this decreases the length of each stride. It is also a simple task to increase stride length by increasing air time. This decreases stride rate, and neither approach improves performance. The goal of elite sprinters and athletes in team sports is to find their natural, optimum stride length and develop an excellent stride rate. Maximum speed is achieved when stride length and stride frequency are in correct proportion. Forcing a stride frequency of more than 10% above the natural rate will only produce a shorter stride length and result in a loss in speed.

The first step in increasing stride rate is to master proper sprinting form (see Chapters 3 and 4) and develop a natural stride. Good sprinters then focus on two key training aspects; increasing power output or ground contact force through speed-strength training, plyometrics, and sprint-resisted training (see Chapter 8) and training the neuromuscular system to tolerate high rates of movement through the use of sprint-assisted training (see Chapter 11).

Does decreasing flight (air) time improve stride rate and speed in short sprints?

One study did show that air time (both feet off the ground) among elite and other sprinters varied only slightly by 2/100 to 3/100 of a second. From this study, some have erroneously concluded that this difference is insignificant. In reality, an improvement of 2/100th to 3/100th of a second each step is far from insignificant. In the 100-meter dash, races are lost by such a small margin. Decreasing air time 2-3 hundreds of a second each step for 50 steps (100 meters) is about a 2/10 second difference and places a sprinter 6-7 feet behind the winner. Try covering a fly pattern as a defensive back in football when you are 6′ behind, or covering Michael Jordan in basketball when only 1′ behind. Athletes arrive to the soccer, rugby, or field hockey ball and gain control a tenth of a second or so before an opponent dozens of times during competition Small improvements in speed translate into big improvements in performance in most sports.

Even if neuromuscular training reduces air time each step by a mere 1/100, the improved speed is significant for competition in any sport.

Does brain activity affect sprinting speed?

Brain activity affects the speed of all movements. Recent research indicates that how fast the brain cells fire determines how fast you run, throw a ball, or perform any rapid muscular movement pattern. How fast we move depends on the width of myelin (sheet of fat coating nerve fibers). Maintaining healthy myelin (thick and tightly bound insulation) allows quick conduction of electrical signals. These high frequency electrical charges speed muscular movement. Fast firing depends on good insulation for the brain's wiring. In addition, it appears that some athletes are born better myelinated (insulated) than others and have an edge in all types of speed of movement associated with sports.

As we age, some insulation in the motor control portion of the brain is lost along with a subsequent loss in speed. By age 40, the part of the brain affecting motion begins a gradual slowdown. According to Dr. George Bartzokis a neurosurgeon at UCLA, these changes make it difficult to remain a world-class athlete after the age of 40.

The good news for athletes and the exercising population is that the physically and mentally exercised brain identifies fraying insulation quicker and signals the body to make repairs. To maintain speed as the years pass, it is important to be physically and mentally active, maintain normal blood pressure, cholesterol, body weight and fat, prevent diabetes, and reduce stress. Physical activity appears to make myelin last longer since it causes the body to send the "repair" signal. As we age, the system that repairs myelin becomes less efficient and causes the gradual weakening and loss of speed.

Muscle Fiber Types

Is stride rate genetically determined by the amount and location of fast twitch muscle fiber?

Hereditary does determine how much each athlete can improve since improvement is somewhat based on the the preponderance of fast twitch fiber in the muscles involved in sprinting.

A considerable amount of conflicting evidence has been reported in the past. This is partially due to the advances in muscle fiber typing over the last several decades that now includes many different subcategories depending upon the study being reviewed.

What are the main types of muscle fiber?

The three main types of muscle fiber described below are present in various proportions throughout the body.

Slow-twitch red (type I). This type of muscle fiber develops force slowly, has a long twitch time, a low power output, is fatigue-resistant (high endurance), has high aerobic capacity for energy supply, but has limited potential for rapid force development and anaerobic power.

Fast-twitch red (type IIa). This intermediate fiber type can contribute to both anaerobic and aerobic activity. It develops force moderately fast and has moderate twitch time, power output, fatigability, aerobic power, force development, and anaerobic power.

Fast-twitch white (type IIb). This fiber type develops force rapidly and has a very short twitch time, a high power output, high anaerobic power, low endurance and low aerobic power.

Although we commonly speak of "types" of muscle fiber, the metabolic activity of muscle is really a continuum ranging from slow firing and long lasting to fast firing and quickly fatigued. This is illustrated more clearly in Table 5-1.

Table 5.1 **Characteristics of Primary Muscle Fiber Types**

CHARACTERISTICS	ST RED	FT RED	FT WHITE
Contraction Time	Slow	Fast	Very Fast
Aerobic Capacity	Very High	High	Low
Anaerobic Capacity	Low	High	High
Force Production	Low	High	Very High
Primary Fuel	Triglycerides	Creatine Phosphate, Glycogen	Creatine Phosphate, Glycogen
Resistance to Fatigue	High	Moderate	Low
Motor Neurons	Small	Larger	Largest
Activity of Use	Aerobic	Long term anaerobic	Short term anaerobic

Training to improve sprinting speed focuses on the FT white (type IIb) and the FT red (type IIa) fiber type. Specific training programs to accomplish this goal are presented in Chapters 8 and 11.

What do research findings reveal about fiber types and speed?

Unfortunately, the early research literature is inconsistent and often confusing. Many studies used animal subjects and/or small samples. This has been problematic for coaches who must develop complete training programs for power athletes in team sports and track and field. Recent studies utilizing improved technology and more precise measurement are providing better answers to many of the questions coaches have been asking about ST and FT fiber and speed-strength training.

The summary of findings in this section provides an overview of the basic concepts of ST and FT fiber, the characteristics of muscle fiber types, altering fiber type, and the effects of various training techniques on ST and FT muscle fiber in the form of a True/False concept test.

Take a few minutes to test your knowledge by placing a "T" (True) in front of each statement about muscle fiber type and training that is correct and an "F"(False) for incorrect statements. After completing the exercise, score and review your responses (answers are located at the end of the last question) and correct any misconceptions that may be reflected in your training techniques.

CONCEPTS OF ST AND FT MUSCLE FIBER

(True-False Knowledge Check)

• The three basic types of muscle fibers are Type I: Slow twitch (ST) and Type II: Fast twitch red (FTIIa) and Fast twitch white (FTIIb). Each type also has various subtypes.

• The percent of Type I and Type II fibers in the body varies for each person with most human muscle containing a mixture of ST and FT fibers.

• The percentages of fiber type in the human body depend mainly on hereditary factors and, to a small extent, on training adaptations.

• Different muscles in the body have different percentages of Type I and Type II fibers.

• Elite marathon runners have higher percentages of ST fibers in their legs.

• Elite power lifters and sprinters have higher percentages of FT fibers throughout the body.

• The dark meat of turkey or chicken legs is red or ST fiber. These slow muscles have more mitochondria (red pigmented cyctochrome complexes) and more myoglobin within the muscle cells, giving them the red color.

• The breast meat of chicken or turkey is white or FT fiber and has limited blood supply.

• ST and FT fibers are not that different in the amount of force produced, only in their rate of force production.

• Although training may cause small changes in fiber type composition, the changes occur mainly from one subgroup of muscular fiber to another.

• An athlete cannot change Slow Twitch Red muscle fiber (Type I) to Type IIa or Type IIb fibers.

• Some Type IIa fast-twitch glycoltic fibers are converted to Type IIb fast-twitch oxidative glycolytic fibers through resistance training.

• In order to recruit the Type II fibers and achieve a training effect, exercise must apply heavy loading or demands for higher power output.

• Regardless of the exercise intensity, ST motor units are recruited first, followed by fast-twitch IIa and fast-twitch IIb as intensity becomes high.

• Depending on the type of training, FT IIb fibers may take on some of the endurance characteristics of FT IIa fibers, and FT IIa fibers may take on some of the strength and power qualities of FT IIb fibers.

• Training to improve speed in short sprints produces selective hypertrophy of the fibers involved in the sprinting action.

• Muscular endurance training, in the absence of speed and power training, can cause FT fibers to atrophy and ST fibers to increase in size.

• While aerobic fitness is important to speed and power athletes, elaborate aerobic training is not recommended.

• Strength training with low or moderate intensity (high repetitions, low weight) does not train FT-IIb fibers.

• To increase the neuromuscular component of strength for sprinters with weight training, heavy weight that approaches the 1RM and low repetitions (1-3) are recommended.

Each of the preceding statements about ST and FT muscle fiber are correct.

Read each question you missed or were not sure of again. Briefly review the topic of muscle fiber types in an Exercise or Human Physiology Text or a recent (2006 or later) strength training book in areas that are unclear.

Estimating the prevalence of FT muscle fiber

Can the presence of fast twitch fiber be determined without a muscle biopsy analysis?

At the present time, there is no method available that is more accurate than muscle biopsy and fiber typing. Adding to the problem is the fact that typing is now much more sophisticated and categorizes types into more than just Slow Twitch, Fast Twitch White (FTIIb) for explosive short duration activity and Fast Twitch Red (FTIIa) for somewhat longer high intensity work.

To determine the predominant fiber type in a particular muscle in the weight room, follow the steps listed below:

Find your 1RM (amount of weight for a particular exercise that allows the completion of only one full repetition using correct form) for various muscle groups such as the quadriceps, hamstrings, and hip flexors.

For example, John was able to complete only one repetition of the dead lift with 400 pounds.

Using 80 percent of 400 or 320 pounds, he was asked to complete as many repetitions as possible. John completed a total of 6 repetitions.

4-7 repetitions in any exercise, indicates a preponderance of FT fiber in that muscle or muscle group. John has a preponderance of FT fiber.

Approximately 10 repetitions indicates a mix of ST and FT fiber.

15-20 or more repetitions indicates that the muscle group contains predominantly ST fiber.

Over the past 40+ years, we have collected data from our speed camps to determine the correlation between standing triple jump scores using the same movement as the triple jump in track and field, except the athlete begins with a two foot takeoff (see Chapter 2 for a detailed description of how to complete the standing triple jump). Athletes with the longest standing triple jump scores also produced the fastest 40-yard dash times. Although the standing triple jump was a better predictor of 40-yard times, the relationship between vertical jump scores and 40-yard dash times was also quite significant. We were not able to convince the human subjects committee to allow a muscle biopsy study to verify the findings. The standing triple jump and the standing broad jump are also effective plyometric exercises in increasing the ground contact force of athletes during the start, acceleration, and maximum speed phases of sprinting.

Obviously, most coaches can observe athletes completing various drills and physical tests and make a fairly solid estimate of the prevalence or absence of FT muscle fiber. By the time athletes reach high school, coaches have had numerous looks in various settings and are aware of who is or is going to be quick and fast. Coaches rely on this method of observation to determine player position and to identify the areas to focus on in the off- season.

It is important to avoid judging athletes too quickly who have not yet reached puberty. It is easy to make a mistake, and nothing improves speed like the adolescent growth spurt and the hormonal changes that occur. The key also is to avoid giving up on "slow" athletes since this is a group that will show considerable improvement after following a holistic speed training program.

STRIDE LENGTH

As long as stride length changes occur naturally from improved form and technique and increases in ground contact force, and not over striding, changes are helpful and will improve speed in short sprints. Unnatural attempts to merely jump further with each stride result in the landing of the plant foot beyond the center of gravity and produce a slowing effect. Such efforts also have a negatively effect on proper sprint mechanics.

Does a small increase in the length of each stride make a difference?

In the example in table 5.2, the athlete increased stride length by 6" without altering the number of steps taken per second. As a result, the flying 40-yard dash time improved by 4/10 of a second. This is a dramatic change for athletes who already can run 5.0 or better and will occur only from proper training, not over striding.

How is stride length improved?

The first step to increasing stride length is to master proper sprinting form (see Chapters 4 and 11) and develop a natural stride based on your current power output or ground contact force. Training programs then focus on increasing ground contact forces by improving the speed-strength of the

Table 5.2 **Stride Length Changes and 40-yard Times**

Stride Length	Stride Rate	Feet per Second	40-yd. Time
Current 6' X	4.0 sps*	24	5.0
New 6'6" X	4.0 sps	26.4	4.6

* steps per second

muscles involved in the pushing action against the ground with each step (see Chapter 8). Power output training occurs through the use of speed-strength training in the weight room, plyometrics training, and sprint-resisted training. Speed endurance training allows athletes to maintain proper sprinting form and ideal stride rates and lengths for a longer period of time during a long sprint.

When the foot makes contact with the ground, it must be directly under the body's center of gravity. For example, if the foot lands too far out in front and ahead of the center of gravity (over striding), it will cause a braking effect resulting in a loss of speed. Great force (downward push) yields great stride length. Misapplication of this force translates to poor technique and loss of momentum. This slowing effect is seen in athletes who over exaggerate the natural sprinting stride.

It is only possible to improve performance by increasing the length of each stride, providing stride rate is not compromised. Once optimal stride length is reached for an athlete's leg length, only increases in ground contact forces can change the length of each stride.

Chapter 6

SPEED ENDURANCE

A successful performance in sport is determined by several factors. One key component for power-based athletes is the ability to execute rapid, powerful movements throughout the competition. A low level of sustained power output, known as *speed endurance,* occurs when energy requirements exceed the body's ability to deliver oxygen. It is important to note that speed endurance will not increase stride rate or length in short sprints, but it will help athletes maintain proper sprinting form, minimize fatigue during competition, and increase the anaerobic threshold. Every athlete is expected to execute repeated short sprints with each performed as close to maximum speed as possible throughout competition. The goal is for the athlete to be as fast in the fourth quarter as he or she was at the start of the game.

Those who have a high degree of speed endurance gain several advantages:

- Each sprint is performed at close to the same speed throughout competition,
- A longer distance is covered before the start of lactic acid buildup;, and
- Less slowing occurs at the end of a long sprint of 60 yards or more.

Many examples of poor speed endurance are evident in sports. In each case, a low level causes a reduction in speed due to fatigue:

Football/Lacrosse/Rugby: A ball carrier is caught from behind by a slower player after a long sprint,

Track: A sprinter is passed in the final 10 meters of a 100 or 200-meter dash.

Baseball: A player runs out of steam and is tagged out at third or home.

Basketball, soccer, field hockey, lacrosse: A player is beaten to the ball by a slower opponent.

These performance related factors make speed endurance training essential to athletes in power sports. Since training for a sport performance goal requires a careful analysis of the energy requirements associated with the sport, such an analysis provide the basis for a sound speed endurance training program. This chapter will familiarize the speed coach with the three major energy systems, help coaches understand the energy system demands of specific sports, and describe training to develop each energy system.

Does every athlete slow down at the end of a long sprint?

Although no athlete can maintain maximum speed for more than 2 seconds or 20 meters, the amount of "slowing" after a 60-80-meter sprint depends on a number of factors. For example, not all 100-meter sprinters follow the same race strategy. Carl Lewis accelerated more slowly than most sprinters, was still accelerating at 60-meters, and reached a higher mph speed later in the race. At times, he was accelerating while athletes he was passing were barely "holding" their current mph speed. Most elite sprinters cross the 40-meter mark at 4.72 to 4.84 seconds, reach maximum speed at 60 meters, hold maximum speed for 20 meters, and slow 1/10 of a second or less the final 20 meters. For team sport athletes, maximum speed may be reached sooner and slowing may be more dramatic.

In the 1992 Olympic 100-meter finals, Leroy Burrell (USA) finished second (Silver Medalist), crossing the finish line in 10.10 seconds. He reached the 40-meter mark in 4.82 seconds, the 60-meter mark in 6.58, the 80-meter mark in 8.32, and the finish line in 10.10. Analyzing the 20-yard segments (see Table 6.1), we find that Burrell covered the 20-40 meter segment in 1.83 seconds. This was only slightly less than 1/10 second (.09) off his maximum mph hour speed for the race. Burrell was at near-maximum speed at the 60-meter mark but did not reach his true maximum until somewhere between 60 and 80 meters. During the final 20 meters (80-100 meter segment), he slowed down only .04 second.

Burrell was about 1/10 second slower than winner, Christie of UK, at each of the 20-meter segments. His "estimated" 40-yard dash time was 4.374. Olympic sprinters are capable of slightly less than 4.3. The 4.1, 4.2, or lower 40-yard times reported by some athletes in football are often inaccurate.

Table 6.1 Analysis of Leroy Burrell's 20-meter Segments in the 1992 Olympic 100-meter dash Finals

20-meter Segment	Time to Cover (seconds)	Difference between previous 20-meters	Analysis
0-20 meters	2.99		
20-40 meters	4.82	1.83	Still accelerating at the 40-meter mark
40-60 meters	6.58	1.76	Almost at his maximum speed for the race; still accelerating slightly
60-80 meters	8.32	1.74	Maximum mph speed reached
80-100 meters	10.10	1.78	Slowed only .04 seconds the final 20 meters of the race.

For team sport athletes, the decline in speed from the 80-100-meter mark would be greater. Team sport athletes are also likely to be unable to hold that speed for a full 20-meters. Well controlled speed-endurance training programs can greatly improve the performance of team sport athletes, reduce the amount of slowing at the end of a long sprint, and improve recovery time between repeated sprints.

THE ANAEROBIC ENERGY SYSTEM

How does the anaerobic energy system work?

The anaerobic energy system consists of two energy pathways: the ATP/CP source (Creatine Phosphate) and the ATP Lactic Energy Source. The ATP/CP System requires no oxygen to supply 5-8 seconds of maximum effort energy. In fact, athletes could hold their breath for this short time period without affecting the energy supply or performance. Phosphate substances and amino acids in the muscles are metabolized to produce cellular energy. This system provides the fuel for the first 60-80 meters of an all-out sprint and compliments the ATP (adenosine triphosphate) energy already present in the muscles. The CP energy system can be fully recharged after 2-3 minutes of rest.

The ATP Lactic Acid System

This system also requires no oxygen. When anaerobic energy is needed beyond the supply of the CP system, working muscles release pyruvic acid that is converted to lactic acid. These two by-products are metabolized to produce ATP to allow energy output to continue without oxygen. Continued maximum effort exercise beyond this point will eventually produce more lactic acid than can be metabolized, resulting in fatigue until exercise cannot continue. At this point, approximately one hour is needed to fully remove lactic acid from the system. Light activity at 40-50% of maximum can slightly reduce recovery time.

Lactic acid energy is what allows continued exertion at near maximum effort once the CP energy is exhausted (after about 60-80 meters). This permits a sprinter to complete the powerful striding effort the final 20 meters of a 100-meter dash when athletes try to hold their current speed or gently build up if they are not at their maximum speed. It also allows team sport athletes to sprint longer distances, recover faster, and execute repeated sprints with little or no "slowing" due to fatigue.

The Anaerobic Threshold

The anaerobic threshold, also called the lactate threshold (LT) or lactate inflection point (LIP), refers to the point at which exercise intensity causes lactic acid to begin to accumulate in the blood stream. Lactic acid, per se really doe not exist at the pH levels found in the body; rather, *anion*, the lactate molecule is what accumulates in the blood. During high intensity anaerobic exercise, such as repeated 40 yard sprints with little rest between each repetition, high rates of ATP hydrolysis in the muscle releases hydrogen ions as they are transported from the muscle into the blood and bicarbonate blood stores are used up. This onset of blood lactate accumulation begins as soon as lactate is produced faster than it can be metabolized.

When athletes exercise at a lower intensity, below the anaerobic threshold, muscle lactate is metabolized and no buildup occurs. Blood analysis identifies the threshold as the point at which lactate reaches a concentration of 4 mM (at rest it is around 1 mM).

With speed endurance training, the anaerobic threshold increases and athletes are capable of sprinting longer distances before the onset of lactic acid buildup.

How do athletes prevent lactic acid buildup and avoid fatigue?

Lactic acid is actually a source of muscle fuel, rather than a waste product that brings muscle contraction to a halt. Muscles actually produce lactic acid from glucose and use it for energy so high intensity exercise can continue. "Glycolysis" is a process in which ATP (adenosine triphosphate) is produced through the breakdown of glycogen to glucose. This takes place both with oxygen (aerobic glycolysis) and without oxygen (anaerobic glycolysis). Aerobic glycolysis not only produces more ATP but does it without producing lactic acid. During high intensity exercise there is insufficient oxygen to meet energy demands and anaerobic glycolysis is the major way ATP is produced. The lactic acid buildup allows all-out activity for only a short period of time. For this reason, anaerobic glycolysis is also referred to as the lactic acid system.

As anaerobic conditioning improves, it takes longer for the buildup of lactic acid to produce fatigue that reduces maximum effort, and, the mitochondria mass increases and allows the muscles to more efficiently convert lactic acid back into fuel. It is best to view lactic acid as a form of stored energy that will be readily available as soon as sufficient oxygen enters the system. At this point, lactic acid is converted to pyruvic acid and used to produce ATP.

Lactic acid has also been suspected of causing muscle soreness and damage following exercise, specifically in the deconditioned or unconditioned athlete. Researchers have now discovered that a small portion of the muscle fibers reveal a distorted pattern (microtears) and that this is more likely the cause of post-exercise muscle soreness.

How do athletes train to improve the anaerobic energy system for power sports?

The maximum training effect to improve speed-endurance for power sports is determined by workout intensity, volume, and the length of the recovery or rest period. To improve anaerobic capacity, each repetition begins while an athlete is still in a state of reduced performance capacity and not fully recovered from the previous sprint. The number of repetitions and sets must also result in maximum oxygen debt and provide partial repayment of this debt. When the pulse drops to 110 to 120 beats per minute, this indicates a repayment of the alactacid part of oxygen debt (ATP-CP) and reduced actacid one. Korchemny (1985) points out that training regimes involving sub maximal (75-90% of maximal) and maximal intensity increase both glycolytic power and the capacity of FT muscle fiber. Power increases occur by using near maximum intensity (>90%); capacity improvement is achieved through use of sub maximal exercises (75-90%).

To develop anaerobic power, for example, all-out sprints of 30-60 meters (3-5 repetitions, 2-3 sets) would involve 2-3 minutes rest between each repetition, 4-6 between sets, and begin before resting heart rate reaches 110 beats per minute. Longer distances of 150 to 250 meters may involve 2-3 repetitions, 2-3 sets, 8-15 minutes rest between repetitions, 2-15 between sets, with each repetition beginning before resting heart rate reaches 120.

Four key principles of training are applied to develop a sport-specific program: progressive overload, specificity, reversibility, and individual differences.

- *Progressive Overload:* Duration, volume, rest intervals, specific movement patterns/distances/exercises, or combinations of each are prescribed at intensities above normal in order to produce adaptations which enable the athlete to function more efficiently. This overload principle is important for the speed coach to progressively increase the load in order for the athlete to function at an optimal level during competition.

- *Specificity:* Drills and exercises should mimic exact sport movements as closely as possible during speed endurance sessions. Adding resistance may create a different skill pattern and place undo stress on the body that could result in injury. Specificity also involves the manipulation of work and rest intervals to concentrate on the predominate energy system(s). Drills and activities should be functional for a specific skill in terms of the number of training days and evaluation(s) performed. A review of the SAID principle (*Specific Adaptations to Imposed Demands*) provides further help in designing training programs and improving conditioning levels. In general it means that "specific training adaptations utilizing specific training variables will create specific training effects."

- *Reversibility:* Training, if terminated, for a sufficient period of time (sometimes a week, sometimes slightly more or less) will result in significant reductions in physiologic function and exercise capacity. It is important to stay consistent with a good speed endurance program.

- *Individual Differences:* This principle refers to the understanding that all athletes (especially novice athletes) vary in their fitness state and will respond differently to a speed endurance program. Training is not optimized if individual differences are not considered.

To improve anaerobic capacity, distances of 60 meters (90-95% of maximum intensity) to 100 meters (80-90%) and 300 (80-90%) to 600 meters (75-85%) are used. Each repetition begins before the athletes heart rate returns to 120 beats per minute.

The training programs described in Chapter 9 are more sports-specific and attempt to regulate the intensity, duration, volume, and recovery phases without heart rate monitoring. It must be said, however, that track coaches who use heart rate as an indicator of when to begin the next repetition can secure better speed endurance results for team sport athletes.

THE AEROBIC ENERGY SYSTEM

Is the aerobic energy system important for athletes in power sports?

Although short sprints rely mainly on CP and lactic energy sources, athletes with high levels of aerobic endurance obtain a higher anaerobic threshold and experience the benefits discussed previously. Anaerobic work also produces pyruvic acid, which is later converted to lactic acid. Since these two by-products are eventually removed *aerobically* during the rest period, a high aerobic capacity expedites recovery between repeated short sprints both during competition and during speed endurance training sessions. In sports that have a higher aerobic component such as basketball, soccer, lacrosse, rugby, and field hockey, aerobic fitness is more critical than for athletes who compete in power sports such as baseball, softball, football, gymnastics, and wrestling.

It is important to remember that the anaerobic and aerobic processes function continuously and at the same time. Anaerobic energy is used at the beginning of any type of exercise and during exercise of high intensity such as all-out sprints. If exercise demands are beyond an athlete's maximum oxygen uptake capability, anaerobic metabolism must supply the additional energy.

When do the two systems come into play in team sports?

Table 6.2 displays the percent contribution of the anaerobic and aerobic systems based on the number of seconds of an all-out maximum effort. In an all-out sprint of 1-5 seconds, for example, 95% of the energy is provided by anaerobic metabolism. Sports such as football, baseball, and softball fall into the 1-5 second category. Soccer, basketball, field hockey, rugby, and lacrosse are more likely to be in the 5-10 second range and therefore require a slightly different training approach.

Study table 6.3 to determine the predominant energy system used and the approximate percent requirement of the anaerobic and aerobic energy sources used in your sport. These percentages are used to design sport specific speed endurance programs.

Should athletes in power sports engage in rigorous aerobic training during the off-season period?

A solid aerobic base is important for athletes in all sports; however, the energy requirements for each sport determines how much and how frequently aerobic work should be done. A good standard is the 1.5 mile run

Table 6.2 Approximate Percentage Involvement of the Anaerobic and Aerobic Energy Systems during Maximum Effort

	Duration of Effort (seconds) 1-5	30	60	90
Percent of maximum power (Intensity)	100	55	35	30
Percent of anaerobic mechanisms	95	75	50	35
Percent of aerobic mechanisms	5	25	50	65

described in Chapter 2. For players who weigh less than 220 pounds, this means completing the one and one-half mile distance in less than twelve minutes. For those weighing 226 to 300 pounds, a target time of under fourteen minutes is recommended. Finally, for those over 300 pounds, the recommended minimum time is less than thirteen and one-half minutes.

Heavy aerobic training, however, is not recommended for power athletes since some studies show hypertrophy of slow twitch fibers and atrophy of fast twitch fibers following such training programs. Atrophy in FTa and FTb fibers may be a result of limited anaerobic work both in the weight room and on the field. One to two days per week can involve some aerobic work to maintain current levels. Aerobic work is also very important in the fat burning process and in the regulation of body weight and fat among interior linemen.

TABLE 6.3 **Predominant Energy Systems Used in Sports**

Sport	ATP-CP and LA	LA-02	02
Baseball	80	20	0
Basketball	85	15	0
Field Hockey	60	20	20
Football	90	10	0
Ice Hockey			
Forwards	80	20	0
Defensemen	80	20	0
Goalies	95	5	0
Lacrosse			
Goal Keeper	80	20	0
Defensemen	80	20	0
Attackers	60	20	20
Midfielders, man down situation	60	20	20
Soccer			
goalies, wings, strikers	80	20	0
Halfbacks, linemen	60	20	20
Tennis (singles)	70	20	10
Track and Field			
40-220 Yards	99	1	0
400 Meters	80	15	5
Mile	20	55	25

Chapter 9 describes several speed endurance training programs and provides an 8-week workout program that can be adapted to any sport.

PART III

TRAINING PROGRAMS
THE 5-STEP MODEL

Chapter 7

FOUNDATION TRAINING

Foundation training is the root system that supports and sustains every play in any sport. Playing situations arise in every sport that reveal an athlete's weaknesses. A careful look at these situations will determine whether an identified weakness can be corrected.

How do athletes prepare for foundation training?

The first part of Foundation Training involves a period of general preparation. During this period, practical experience and research shows that muscle adaptation occurs slowly. It may take several months to years before change can be measured, depending on the intensity and amount of training. In contrast to general adaptation, muscle size chances are visible in a short period of time, changes in skill can happen in a few hours, and positive changes in maximum strength and power can occur in two weeks.

Practical experience with *Inertial Impulse Training* is a good example of how the nervous system can be trained in the art of delivering a blow or hitting. Using force transducer measurements to document the quality of a "hit", even trained Karate Black Belts have increased their hitting power in a few minutes. These short-term improvements in performance are based on neuronal changes brought about by recruitment of motor units and greater tolerance in activity levels of the motor neurons. The objective is to increase all of the body's resources to optimum levels before beginning a program to improve playing speed.

Each of the following resources is vital to sports performance: awareness, reactions, reflexes, quickness and control of body segments in all directions, quickness in close-range movements in all directions, basic movement elements of the body, basic movement elements required for sports (movement patterns, hand-eye and foot-eye coordination), sustained power output, speed in all directions, maximum strength, muscular endurance, anaerobic conditioning, and aerobic conditioning.

This chapter covers five key foundation areas that help prepare athletes for advanced speed improvement training in Steps II, III, IV. and V of the 5-step model: warm-up, stretching (before and after a workout) and flexibility; body composition and speed; combat breathing; training the brain; body control and power; and dominant and recessive movement patterns in sports.

WARM-UP, STRETCHING, AND FLEXIBILITY

Flexibility (stretching) exercises are often too closely linked with warm-up. As a result, athletes make the common mistake of stretching cold muscles rather than warming the body first with large muscle activity so joints can be safely stretched. Athletes warm up to prepare to stretch, they do not stretch to warm up. This section clarifies other misconceptions and covers all aspects of a sound warm-up, stretching, and flexibility training program for team sport athletes.

Who should stretch?

Although all athletes benefit from regular stretching, lean body types with a good range of motion may need very little stretching, whereas the stocky, more powerfully built athlete with limited range of motion may need a minimum of 15-30 minutes daily.

Why is stretching necessary?

Research shows that daily stretching increases range of motion, conserves energy, increases fluid motion, aids muscle relaxation, supports good sprinting form, and helps cool the body at the end of a workout. Increasing overall range of motion (ROM) may also improve speed by increasing stride rate and decreasing energy expenditure and resistance. Chu, (1999) identifies four specific areas where flexibility plays a key role in improving sprinting speed:

1. In sprinting, flexibility and elasticity in the gluteals and hamstrings can benefit the athlete during the knee lift and help to produce a longer stride.

2. Flexibility in the quadriceps is essential for maximizing the recovery of the leg during the swing phase.

3. After take-off, the further the legs can be separated, the more the elastic recoil can help in closing the angle at the point of landing to maximize stride length.

4. An optimal degree of shoulder flexion and extension is needed to match that required of the legs.

What stretching techniques should be used?

Dynamic stretching exercises are completed in the beginning of each workout immediately after a general warm-up period to prepare the body for vigorous activity. A second session involves the use of static exercises as part of a cool-down at the end of the workout and is designed to improve an athlete's range of motion. Static stretching can also be used whenever time permits to aid in the recovery from soft tissue injuries.

How is this approach used in a typical workout?

The first stretching session involves dynamic exercises and is completed immediately after a 12-15 minute general warm-up period that raises core body temperature several degrees and produces perspiration. The purpose of this session is to prepare athletes for a high intensity workout or competition and reduce the chance of soft tissue injury. This is not the time to concentrate on improving ROM.

Dynamic Stretching. Kapooka Health Center researchers (in New South Wales, Australia) studied 1,538 army recruits for three years. The conclusion was that static stretching, the most common type used in the beginning of a workout session in the past may harm muscles, ligaments and joints and decrease performance. Evidence also indicated that the force output potential of static-stretched muscles was reduced by 8-15% for as long as one hour. This reduction in muscle strength may also increase the chance of injury. Although the findings of one study do not merit a complete change of tactics, this is not the first time static techniques have been questioned. The NASE combines *dynamic stretching* and some sprinting form training in the beginning of a workout, immediately following the general warm-up period. Exercises move from slow movements to medium to near maximum speed in 2-3 sets of ten repetitions. Sprinting form drills are taught by a track coach the first week until athletes can perform each correctly. A 15-minute combination dynamic stretching/form training can be used.

- *Jog-stride-sprint in place*--Using proper arm movement, jog in place slowly for ten repetitions (left foot contacts the ground ten times) bringing the knees waist high.

- *Sprint-arm-movement*--Standing erect with only a slight forward lean with the arms and hands in a relaxed sprinting position, move the arms through one complete sprinting cycle at medium speed (forward hand rises to shoulder height, backward hand to the hip), repeat ten times.

- *Butt Kickers*--From a slow jog, the lower leg swings back and approaches the buttocks; the upper leg stays vertical as athletes move forward for 10-yards.

- *Shoulder Twirl*--Swing both arms slowly in a clockwise circular motion in front of the body with the hands moving below the waist 10 times; repeat with a counterclockwise circular motion above the shoulders 10 times.

Repeat #1 (jogging in place) at 3/4 speed.
Repeat #3 (butt kickers) at 1/2 speed
Repeat #2 (sprint-arm-movement) at 3/4 speed
Repeat #4 (shoulder twirls) at 1/2 speed.

• *Cycling*--Lean against a wall or bar, cycle one leg through a sprinting action. Keep the leg from extending behind the body, allow the foot to approach the buttocks during recovery, and "paw" the ground to complete one repetition. Ten repetitions are done with each leg.

• *Pull-throughs*--Extend the lead leg in front of the body like a hurdler, bring the leg down and paw at the ground for ten repetitions.

• *Down-and-Offs*--Jog in place using high knees, hit the ground with the balls of the foot and push off as quickly as possible; bouncing up into the high knee position for ten repetitions.

• *African Dance*--Run forward, raise each leg to the side of the body as in hurdling and tap the heel with the hand for ten repetitions.

Repeat #5 (Cycling) at 3/4 speed
Repeat #6 (Pull-throughs) at 3/4 speed
Repeat #7 (Down-and-offs) at 3/4 speed
Repeat #2 (sprint-arm exercise) at full speed - 2 sets, 10 repetitions
Repeat #8 (African dance) at 3/4 speed
Repeat #1 (Sprinting in place) at 3/4 to maximum speed - 2 sets of ten repetitions

Static Stretching. This technique is designed to increase ROM at the end of each workout. Two phases are emphasized: *easy stretching* for one repetition, moving slowly into the stretch and applying mild tension with a steady, light pressure, and 1-2 repetitions of *developmental stretching* that increases the intensity and movement for an inch or less. Slow, relaxed, controlled, and pain-free movement are made as athletes learn to judge each exercise by the "stretch and feel method," easing off if the pain and strain is too intense.

The position at the end of each exercise is held for a minimum of 30 seconds to allow stretch to progress from the middle of the muscle belly to the tendon. Athletes begin with a 15 second hold and add 2-3 seconds each workout until the hold position can be maintained in each exercise for 30 seconds. Exercises should use the major joints: neck, shoulders, back, hips, knees, wrists, and ankles, be as specific to the sport as possible with a goal of reaching equal range of motion on both sides of the body. Research indicates that when a joint on one side of the body is 15% more flexible than the same joint on the other side, an injury is 2 1/2 times more likely to to occur.

Proprioceptive neuromuscular facilitation (PNF)

This two-person stretching technique is based on a contract-and-relax principle. PNF stretching requires a partner to apply steady pressure to a body area at the extreme range of motion until the person being stretched feels a slight discomfort. When stretching the hamstring muscle group, for example, lie on your back with one leg extended to 90 degrees or a comfortable stretch. Have a partner apply steady pressure while attempting to raise the leg overhead further. As pressure is applied, begin to push against a partner's resistance by contracting the muscle being stretched. This isometric hamstring contraction produces no leg movement because a partner will resist whatever force is applied during the push phase. After a 10-second push, relax the hamstring muscles while a partner again applies pressure for five seconds to increase the stretch even further. Repeat two to three times. Many other stretches can be devised to meet the needs of each athlete. Some other common problem sites are lower back and shoulder girdle for all throwers.

The PNF method involves four phases: an initial easy stretch of the muscle, an isometric contraction with resistance provided by a partner, relaxation for five seconds, and a final passive stretch for five seconds. As a variation, a partner may allow the leg to move slightly downward during the push phase. PNF stretching relaxes the muscle group being stretched, which produces greater muscle length and improves flexibility. Disadvantages of this method include the presence of some discomfort, a longer workout time, and the inability to stretch without a partner.

How much Intensity should be used?

Regardless of the technique used, stretching should take the form of a slow, relaxed, controlled, and relatively pain-free movement. Too much pain and discomfort is a sign of overloading soft tissue and increases the risk of injury. After experiencing mild discomfort with each stretch, relax the muscles being stretched prior to the next repetition.

How long should athletes stretch?

Total workout time requirements for static stretching will increase from the beginning to the advanced stages as the length of the "hold" reaches 30 seconds. Static stretches that are longer than 30 seconds only slightly increase the benefits and may be impractical. After proper warm-up, complete each exercise gradually and slowly, beginning with a 15-second hold and adding two to three seconds to the hold time each workout until you can comfortably maintain the position at the extreme range of motion for 30 seconds.

If the main purpose of stretching is to prepare the body for exercise and to maintain the existing range of motion in the major joints, 6-9 minutes of dynamic stretching should be enough following a general warm-up period.

How often should athletes stretch?

As pointed out earlier, dynamic stretching always follows the general warm-up routine every workout prior to performing any phase of the 5-Step Model. Athletes who want to increase their ROM should shoot for 15-30 minutes of careful static stretching daily at the close of each workout. Several different stretching exercises may be performed for each joint.

How flexible should athletes become?

The gymnast, ballet dancer, and hurdler must be more flexible than sprinters and athletes in most team sports. The stretching routine described in this section is geared toward improvement in all major joints and emphasizes key areas for high-speed sprinting action.

Orthopedic surgeons are treating more injuries related to excessive stretching and attempts to reach a very high level of flexibility than injuries due to a failure to stretch. This increase may be partly due to a renewed interest in stretching and the popularity of yoga. In some cases, these methods emphasize over-stretching and extreme flexibility, a range of motion not needed in most sports.

What exercises should be avoided?

Decades ago, a group of Orthopedic surgeons developed a list of potentially dangerous stretching exercises that were commonly used by coaches and athletes. Since that time, each of the risky movements described below have been eliminated by most coaches and replaced with a similar, safe movement pattern that stretches the same muscle group. When a joint is bent beyond the body's ability to control it with muscle strength, there is a risk of tearing muscles, tendons, or ligaments that support the joint or damaging the joint surface.

The so-called "Orthopedic hit list" below includes outdated, potentially dangerous stretching exercises that should be avoided:

• Yoga Plow--Athletes lie on their back, arms to the side, and bring both legs straight overhead until touching the ground. Football players are often asked to dig the tips of the shoes into the ground with a running motion. This is one of the most dangerous exercises ever used that puts stress and strain on the blood vessels to the brain, the upper spinal cord, and spinal disks and ligaments.

• Hurdler's Stretch--Athletes sit on the ground with one leg extended in front and the other at right angles to the side in the hurdler's position and attempt to bend forward and lay the chest on the thigh of the lead leg. This exercise over stretches the muscles and ligaments in the groin and can cause chronic groin pull, injure the knees (meniscus cartilage and the medial collateral ligament) and irritate the sciatic nerve.

• Knee stretch--Athletes rest on their knees with the lower legs underneath, then lean back until their head is on the ground. This stretch exceeds the skeletal range of motion of the knees and over stretches the patellar and collateral knee ligaments, destabilizing the knee.

• Duck walk and deep knee bend--Walking like a duck in a deep knee bend position is very likely to damage the knees.

• Straight-leg toe touching--This exercise can over stretch the posterior longitudinal ligament, a main supporter ligament of the spine. Disks can also be damaged and the sciatic nerve is in danger of being pulled from its connection.

• Ballet stretches--Placing an extended leg in front of the body resting on a bar and bouncing forward is hazardous to the sciatic nerve, low back ligaments, muscles, joints and discs.

• Straight-leg raises--Raising a fully extended leg overhead while lying on the back stretches the sciatic nerve beyond its normal limits.

• Straight-leg sit-ups--This exercise is similar to the standing toe-touch except that one begins in a sitting position. After sitting up 30 degrees, a hip exercise, not an abdominal exercise, is being performed, Beyond that point, abdominal muscle strength is not improved. Bent-leg sit-ups and variations of the crunch are more effective and safer.

• Fast neck circles--May pinch discs and over stretch delicate ligaments.

• Straddle jumps--Jumping jacks that cause the feet to land further apart than shoulder-width can strain the knees.

What static stretching exercises are recommended for sprinting?

Table 7.1 describes some key static stretching exercises designed to increase ROM for sprinting. static exercises are completed at the end of the workout.

Table 7.1 Static Stretching Exercises for Sprinters

Body Part	Description
Achilles tendon and Soleus	*Gastroc*–Stand 2' from a wall in a stride position with the front knee slightly bent., back leg fully extended, both heels on the ground. Lean forward with a straight back until you feel the stretch in the calf of the rear leg. *Soleus*-- Assume a similar position as above with back straight and palms against the wall. Begin in a seated position with legs bent and buttocks dropped. Lean into the wall until you feel the stretch in the lower calf.
Lower Legs	From a push-up position, with the hands close to the feet, raise the hips and form a triangle. At the highest point, press the heels to the floor or alternate flexing one knee and extending the other.
Hamstrings	Lie on your back with eyes focused upward. Grasp the back of one bent thigh with both hands and pull to a 90 degree angle, then slowly straighten your knee.
Adductors	Stand with one foot on top of a chair, slide the rear leg backward while holding onto the chair. Exhale and lean forward and downward while bending the knee of the leg resting on the chair.
Quadriceps	From a standing position on the right leg, reach down to grasp the front of the left foot and pull the leg upward to the "butt kick" position. Keep the back straight and do not allow the knee to drift forward ahead of the stance leg.
Hips	Lie on your back, relax and straighten both legs. Pull the left foot toward the chest and hold. Repeat using the right foot.
Lower Torso	Kneel on the floor, legs slightly apart and parallel and the toes pointing backward. With both hands on the upper hips, arch the back, contract the buttocks, and push the hips forward. Exhale, continue to arch the back, drop the head backward and slide the hands onto the heels.
Upper Back	Stand with the feet together, 3' from a supporting surface about hip to shoulder height, arms overhead. With arms and legs straight, flex at the hips, flatten the back, grasp the supporting surface with both hands. Exhale and press down to arch the back.
Shoulders	Sit or stand with one arm raised to shoulder height, flex the arm across to the other shoulder. Grasp your raised elbow with the opposite hand, exhale, and pull your elbow backward.
Neck	Lie on the floor on your back with both knees flexed. Interlock the hands behind the head near the crown. Exhale and pull your head onto your chest while keeping the shoulder blades flat on the floor.
Groin	Assume a sitting position of the soles of your feet together. Place both hands around your feet and pull yourself forward.
Arms and Wrists	Sit with one arm behind your lower back as far up on the back as possible. Place the other arm overhead while holding a folded towel and flex your elbow. Grasp the towel with the lower hand and inhale while you pull the hands toward each other.

Does stretching improve sprinting speed?

Researchers from the Department of Kinesiology at Louisiana State University examined the effects of a variety of stretching protocols on 20 m sprint times. Eleven males and five females were recruited from the nationally ranked Louisiana State University track and field team to participate in the investigation. Subjects used the different stretching protocols in a randomized manner. Prior to each of the stretching protocols all athletes performed a series of warm-up exercises which included 1) an 800 m jog, 2) forward skips 4 x 30 m, 3) side shuffles 4 x 30 m, and 4) backwards skips 4 x 30 m. Four stretching protocols were then tested: 1) no stretching on either leg (NS), 2) both legs stretched (BS), 3) forward leg in the starting position stretched (FS), 4) rear leg in the starting position stretched (RS). Each stretching protocol was performed four times with each stretch being held for 30 seconds. Overall the data suggested that the NS condition produced the fastest 20-m sprint time (3.17 ± 0.04 s), while BS (3.21 ± 0.04 s), FS (3.21 ± 0.04 s), and RS (3.22 ± 0.04 s) produced the slowest sprint times. There were no statistical differences noted between the BS, FS, and RS groupings. Based upon the findings of this investigation the authors suggest that performing passive stretching exercises before sprinting activities can result in a significant decline in sprinting Speed. Therefore, it was recommended that the use of passive stretching techniques be avoided by athletes prior to the performance of sprinting activities. *Source:* Nelson AG, Driscoll NM, Landin DK, Young MA, and Scheznayder IC. (2005). Acute effects of passive muscle stretching on sprint performance. *Journal of Sports Sciences,* 23(5):449 – 454.

Other researchers have also examined the effects of an acute bout of stretching in 23 additional studies; 22 articles suggested that there was no benefit for the outcomes isometric force, isokinetic torque, or jumping height; one article suggested improved running economy. Of 4 articles examining running speed, 1 suggested that stretching was beneficial, 1 suggested that it was detrimental, and 2 had equivocal results.

How common is low back pain in athletes?

Pain in the lower back occurs as often in our society as the common cold. The disorder affects 8 to 10 million people in the United States alone. Informal surveys of middle and high school athletes suggests that as many as 40% have experienced back problems severe enough to miss practice. The prevalence of nonspecific lower back pain (LBP) in 14 to 16-year old adolescents occurs almost as often as with adults due to sedentary lifestyles, intensive sports, and participation in high impact leisure-time physical activity (Ebbehojl, et al. 2002). Injuries to the lower back are also common among amateur and professional athletes in sports such as golf and tennis (Grimshaw et al. 2002).

What causes lower back pain in athletics?

The exact cause of most lower back pain (LBP) in the general population remains a mystery. Blaming pressure against a spinal nerve caused by bulging spongy discs is incorrect when a normal back without some degree of bulging is the exception. Other theories suggests that lower back muscle spasms or arthritic spurs on bony overgrowth compress spinal nerves. Trauma of some type in athletes certainly contributes to the condition.

How can athletes protect their lower back and reduce the chance of injury and loss of practice time?

Everyone can lower the risk of developing LBP by changing the way they stand, bend, lift objects, sit, rest, sleep and exercise. In most cases, part of the treatment is the correction of faulty posture. A summary of key tips provided by Schering Corporation will help athletes keep their back healthy:

General:

- Avoiding strain must become a way of life as you protect the back while lying, sitting, standing, walking, working and exercising.

Standing:

- Lifting--bend the knees and hips, not the waist.
- Use a footrest when standing to avoid sway back; one foot rests on a stool a foot or two high.
- Hold heavy objects as close to the body as possible, not out in front.
- Always bend the knees when bending over.
- In correct standing posture, a line dropped from the ear goes through the tip of the shoulder, middle of hip, back of kneecaps, and front of the ankle bone. In correct posture, the chin is in, head is up, back is flattened, and the pelvis is held straight.

Sitting:

- Sit forward, flatten your back, tighten the abdominal muscles and cross the knees.
- Use a foot rest to elevate the knees higher than the hips to relieve swayback.
- Keep the neck and back in a straight line with the spine, bending forward at the hips.
- When driving, sit close to the pedals and use a hard back rest.

Sleeping:

- Use a firm mattress or 3/4-inch plywood.
- When lying on your back, knees should be supported with a pillow.
- If lying on your side, bend knees and use a flat pillow to support the neck.
- Avoid sleeping face down. This position strains the neck and shoulders.

What can be done to prevent a low back episode after feeling the common sharp pain or twinge that often precedes the condition?

Two key exercises suggested by Robin McKenzie (2006), a leading authority on lower back problems, and others, are tremendously effective in heading off lower back episodes that may last days and weeks and cause loss of valuable practice time. As soon as any symptoms appear, even mild pain and discomfort or a slight twinge, stop and complete the exercises described below and shown in Figures 7.1, 7.2, and 7.3.

Lying face down in elbow extension - Lie on the stomach flat on the floor. Place both elbows under the shoulders and lean on the forearms. Breathe deeply and relax the lower back and legs completely. Remain in this raised, extension position for five minutes. Emphasize complete relaxation of the lower back and lower extremities.

Extension in lying - Remain lying face down with the hands under the shoulders in the push-up position. Straighten both elbows to push the top half of the body up as far as pain permits. Strive to keep the pelvis, hips and legs completely relaxed and allow the low back to sag. Hold the "up" position for 3-5 seconds. On each of 10 repetitions, try to raise the body higher.

Extension in standing - If traveling in a vehicle and you cannot assume the lying position, this exercise, although not quite as effective, can be substituted for the previous two. Stand upright with the feet slightly apart, place the hands in the small of the back with the fingers pointing backwards. Bend the trunk backwards from the waist as far as possible, using the hands as the fulcrum while keeping the knees straight. On each of 10 repetitions, try to bend backwards slightly further.

These exercises provide a tremendous quick fix for most LBP among athletes and should be performed 5-6 times daily beginning with the onset of any pain or discomfort in the lower back. Once you have recovered, use the exercises as a preventive procedure, especially after working in a sitting, bent position for an extended period of time.

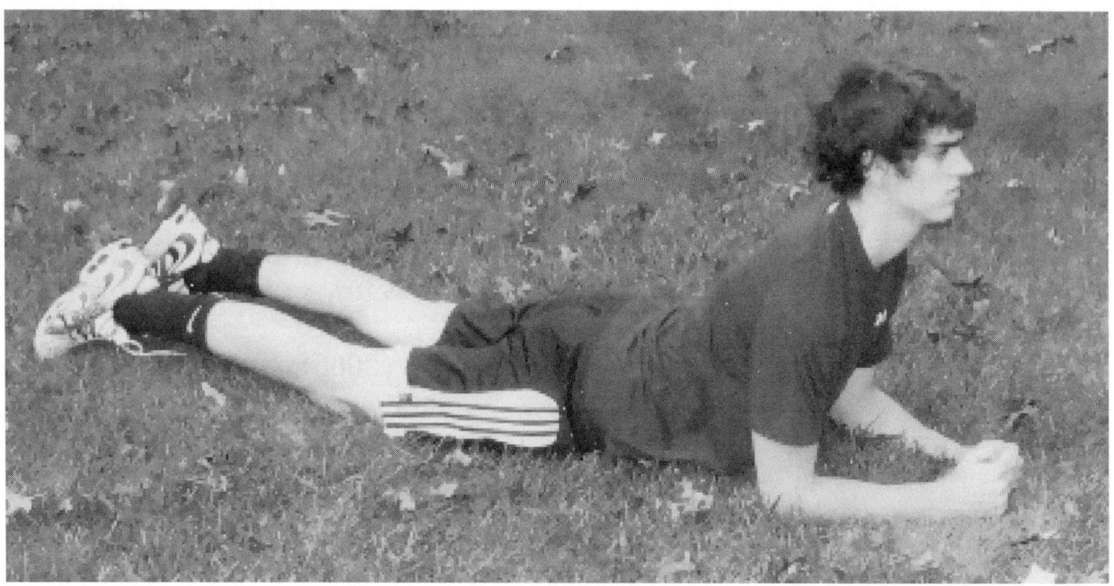

Figure 7.1 Lying face Down in elbow extension

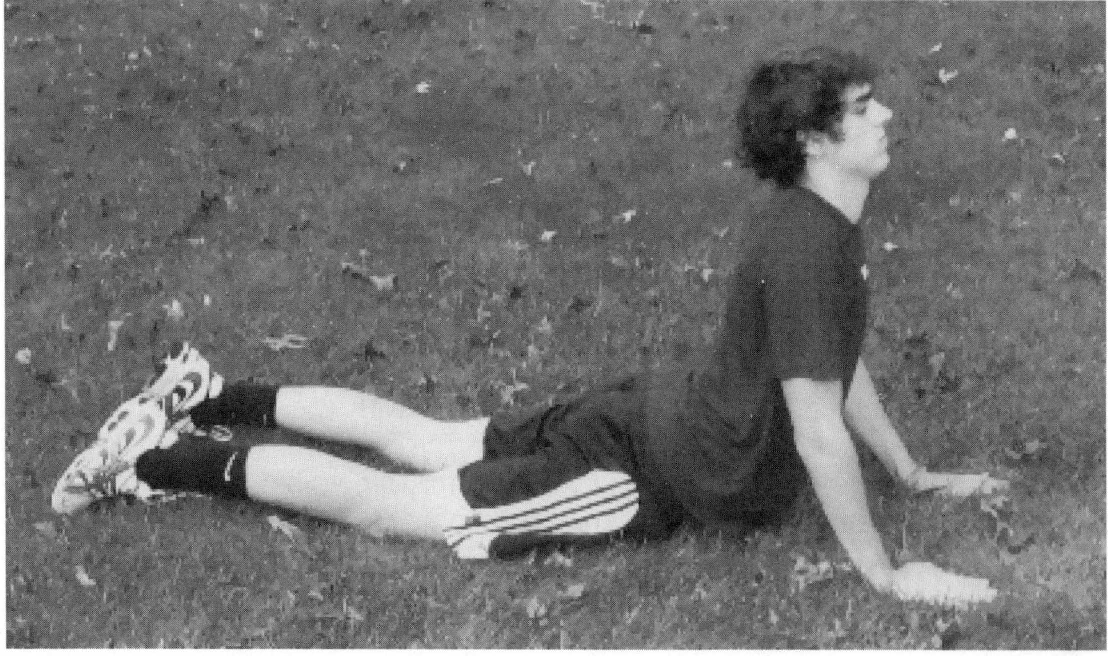

Figure 7.2 Full extension lying down

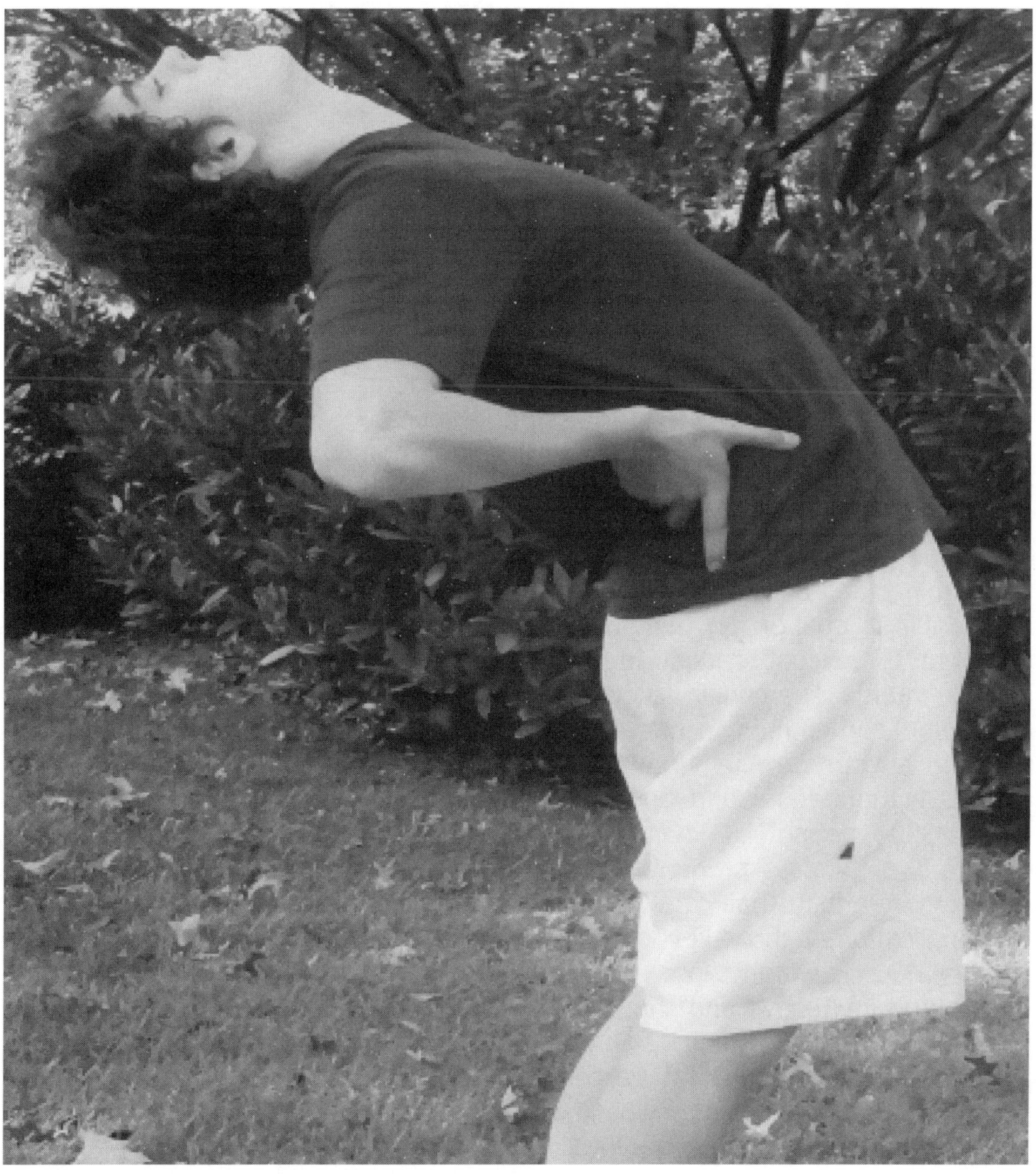

Figure 7.3 Extension in standing

BODY COMPOSITION AND SPEED

How much does excess body fat affect speed in short sprints?

Extra pounds of body fat on any athlete, regardless of their position in a sport, change strength/weight ratios and decrease speed in short sprints. For every pound of weight (fat and muscle) added, slightly more than two pounds of additional ground contract force is needed during the pushing action against the ground with each step in sprinting just to maintain the athlete's current speed. On the other hand, eliminating body weight in the form of fat decreases the ground contact force needed by *favorably* changing strength/weight ratios.

A 220-lb. athlete, for example, needs approximately 460 pounds of thrust or force against the ground each step to sprint at high speed. If 10 pounds, are added, approximately 481 pounds of ground contact thrust are now required to prevent a decrease in sprinting speed.

The ideal percent of body fat for optimum health in the general population, less than 15 percent for men and 20 percent for women, is considered high for athletes in some sports and positions. For male sprinters and athletes in speed positions in football (wide receiver, defensive backs, running backs), basketball (except centers) soccer, lacrosse, field hockey, and tennis, a goal of ten percent is ideal. For female athletes in most sports a goal of 15 percent is ideal. In positions where "push" weight and mass are critical (interior linemen in football, rugby players in the scrum, the center and some corner men in basketball), up to 20 percent is acceptable. The trend to encourage linemen in football to reach a body weight of 350 – 390 pounds without regulating body fat is unhealthy and dangerous as studies of retired 300+ pound NFL linemen have shown.

Safe weight loss programs require the involvement of a physician or registered dietitian that carefully monitors the rate of loss, caloric intake, and the application of three key principles of nutrition: variation, moderation and balance. Quick weight loss schemes presented in national magazines are unsafe and ineffective and should be avoided.

If hydrostatic weighing, skinfold measures, or other body composition tests reveal a high body fat percentage, a 220-lb. athlete with 20 percent body fat playing a position where speed is critical, for example, can safely lose 8-10 percent or 17-22 pounds. The new weight of 198 to 203 pounds would reduce the amount of ground contact force needed from 460 to a range of 426 to 415 pounds. Assuming that the weight loss would result in zero loss of ground contact force, keeping the athlete at 460 pounds of thrust per step, speed would improve at every distance as the athlete takes both a faster and longer step.

Adding muscle weight also increases the demand for ground contact force. Athletes involved in safe muscle weight gain programs need to make certain that their pushing force against the ground increases as muscle weight gain occurs to prevent a reduction in speed. Chapter 8: Power

Output Training, describes several speed-strength training programs designed to improve ground contact force with minimum gains in muscle mass and body weight.

How much abdominal work must be done to obtain a washboard" stomach?

If one believes all the "hype," you would think it can be done in a week or two. Unfortunately, this is far from true. Most of us will never again see the flat stomach and definition (muscle lines) we remember in our youth; nor is it necessary to do so unless you are a competing body builder.

The truth is that even athletes can do sit-ups until doomsday and still not achieve this goal. Dr. Dintiman once did a short TV piece to demonstrate this point.

> "On camera, Bob, a 25-year old male, walked toward me with a somewhat protruding stomach. When I punched him firmly in the abdominal area, he doubled up. I then said, 'We will take a short commercial break. When we return, you'll see Bob after having completed 1,000 sit-ups every day for six months.' After the break, Bob reappeared on camera and walked toward me. I again punched him in the midsection, but he did not double up this time. Unfortunately, he looked the same with his stomach fat protruding although the underlying muscle tissue was quite strong and firm."

Bob made one big mistake. Muscle and fat are two separate tissues; increasing muscle firmness and strength requires exercise. Bob did that and was successful. To decrease the size of the fat cells in the abdominal area, more calories must be expended than taken in. Since Bob failed to decrease the calories he took in, stomach fat remained the same and his appearance did not change.

Obtaining a flat stomach requires reduced calories, regular aerobic exercise, *and* abdominal work. With calorie restriction, fat cells will shrink, and the stomach will get smaller. A varied sit-up routine will strengthen the underlying muscle tissue and a very high number of repetitions on a regular basis may even produce some "definition," Both adipose (fat) tissue and muscle tissue need changing; you cannot convert fat tissue to muscle tissue; nor will muscle tissue change to fat when you become sedentary. It is possible to obtain a flat "washboard" stomach with a combination of calorie restriction, exercise in a sport, and high repetitions of at least 4-5 different exercises for the upper and lower abs, but it won't be easy.

Is it possible to change the shape of the entire body?

Changing the shape or the body or body sculpturing requires a 1-2 year commitment and use of the following steps and exercise programs:

- If you are "over fat," consult a physician and engage in a safe, sound, long-term nutritional program that results in no more than 1-2 pounds of fat loss per week to shrink fat cells in the back of the upper arms, stomach, hip, waist, and thighs.

- Begin an aerobic exercise program 3-4 times weekly to maintain health, improve cardiovascular fitness, and expend enough energy to enter into a calorie reduction of 500-750 per day (1 to 1 1/2 lb. of fat loss per week).

- Consult a personal trainer or physical educator to develop and master the proper form and techniques in each bodybuilding exercise to add muscle mass and definition throughout the body and to help the skin fit better in areas where fat cells shrink (back of upper arms, thighs, hips, stomach and buttocks). A serious approach involves daily strength training exercises alternating the upper body one day and the lower body the next, resting on Sunday.

- Although you cannot spot reduce (lose body fat only in areas exposed to exercise), you can concentrate on problem areas by completing multiple sets and 5-6 different exercises for each muscle group. Combining this approach with calorie restriction and shrinking of fat cells can also result in greater muscle definition.

- Plan to stay with the program for up to two years and remain patient the first 5-6 months until you see noticeable results. You did not get in this shape in six months and cannot expect to completely reach your goal in that short time period.

COMBAT BREATHING

What is Combat Breathing and why is it important in sports?

Breathing is an essential human function that plays a major role in the production of energy at sleep, rest, or playing a sport at top speed. However, very few of us have been trained to use the most efficient mechanics for meditation, relaxation, or executing the basic tasks of daily life. Most of us are walking around each day with limited breathing skills. Athletes cannot afford to lack skill in any aspect of breathing while engaging in their sports. Relaxation, starting and stopping, body contact, hitting or punching, blocking, running, sprinting, and throwing all require specific breathing skills.

Checklist for Proper Breathing Mechanics

NOSE: Breathe through the nose to warm and filter air.

MOUTH: Breathe through the nose and mouth during high oxygen demands. Regulate the release of air through the mouth during contact and high-output skills, such as body contact, hitting in baseball, punching in boxing, or throwing in all sports.

LUNGS: Use lower portions of the lungs to breathe when sleeping, meditating, relaxing, and during times of maximum oxygen transfer.

DIAPHRAGM: Put your hand on the stomach to check that it moves inward with each breath.

SHOULDERS: Raise and roll the shoulders back to provide additional volume for combat breathing.

RIB CAGE: Increase the chest volume by maximizing breathing during high oxygen demands, for protection from forces of contact, and for high force output. This added volume requires the use of the intercostal muscles of the rib cage.

TRAINING THE BRAIN

What is involved in what coaches refer to as "Training the Brain?"

In the past, training the brain to react quickly by using the latest technology has been overlooked. Amazing human feats have demonstrated that, through training, athletes can gain more control over their nervous systems than people ever dreamed possible. We have all seen the Yogi on the bed of nails. Some may also have observed a Yogi get into such a small box that it appeared to be an impossible fit. The box was lowered in "ice water" for 5 minutes. Then the box was pulled out of the water and the Yogi emerged slowly, unraveling himself in tact, with no signs of bodily harm.

Like the Yogi, athletes can learn to tap into this kind of performance-enhancing total body control to accelerate their speed to uncommon levels by keeping abreast of the latest information emerging from numerous laboratories around the world. The computer age has brought all forms of sophisticated devices to the laboratory and the field for sports scientists and coaches. Special software exists that can monitor most body functions. Heart rate monitors now include computer connections and software to collect and evaluate information for each individual heart beat and its relation to the next beat. Today's coaches are very lucky to have such immediate and powerful objective information for the training of athletes.

Some of the more important findings from these studies that will help athletes sprint faster and play at higher speeds are listed below:

• Technology has now given us immediate and precise information about all forms of sport. One example is the disqualification of Linford Christie in the 1996 Olympic 100-meter finals for a second false start. His gun-to-leaving-the-blocks time was below human capability. This time difference was used to confirm that he had jumped the gun. However, the time difference was so close to human capability that without today's timing devices it would have been impossible to determine. During the preparation meets for the 2000 Olympics, Michael Johnson was highlighted on TV and the internet as using science to evaluate how he was performing during the actual competition. Real time data was being collected for rapid evaluation and implementation.

There is little doubt that On-Field Analysis evaluations can offer immediate and objective information. This specific performance data about how players are moving on the field provides the necessary information for evaluation, selection, and training. Game action and sprinting takes place at such high speeds that thinking before acting interferes with performance. Players must react to the situation and ask questions later.

• Brain research and the practical playing experiences of elite athletes reveal that there is a state of high artistic and sports performance. Many have described it as being in an effortless state called "the Zone." Research reveals that the Zone, also known as the flow state, is associated with lower heart and breathing rates coupled with brain wave frequencies of 8 to 13 Hertz.

Too much or not enough stress can negatively affect performance. Athletes must be able to control stress levels for maximum performance. The best-known way to control stress is to get in the Zone. According to John Douillard in Body, Mind, and Sport, "The coexistence of opposites—rest and alertness, composure and vigorous exercise is the formula for the Zone."

One common fault of many athletes is trying too hard. Invariably, the harder one tries, the tighter one gets, which is just the opposite of what you want and what the Olympic motto, "Swifter, Higher, Stronger," is all about. If an athlete is in the Zone before performing, the proper muscle control or optimal coordination reaches exceptional heights. The Zone is one of the most critical performance principles for the beginner or elite athlete.

• Athletes can control visual awareness in such a way that they can see everything in the visual field. The running back who sees all defensive players as they are positioned and then runs to daylight is using a technique called *open focus*, a term coined by Dr. Les Fehmi. This technique is similar to the ultimate camera that takes a clear picture, without a shutter, of anything it wants, even at the same time another picture is being taken. Can you imagine the luxury of processing all incoming information and automatically sorting out what you need at any one moment in your sport? Obviously, your performance would improve dramatically.

One way to improve visual awareness is by doing turns or rolls while a coach throws you a ball as you recover body control. Another way is to juggle or use the mini-trampoline as a rebounder of two or more objects. With practice, you will be able to juggle more balls, increase the area of visual recognition, and be able to manage other sensory input with improving ability.

• We all have experienced the adaptation to high-speed travel. Driving at 70 miles per hour seems fast at first due to acceleration and the relative speeds and positions of other cars or objects in the field of vision. However, in a short period of time, this sensation is replaced by a sense that 70 miles per hour is not fast at all. This feeling describes the exact playing sensation you want to have on the field. The programs for speed of movement and speed of thought provide drills and exercises that will help improve this "flow" state condition on and off the field. The best way to develop this "slowing" sensation is to incorporate the skills of combat breathing and visual awareness. Once you have learned how to expand your field of focus, perception of motion tends to slow down.

• Training both sides of the body by developing near equal skill in both hands and feet assists in improving skill levels by producing higher levels of synchrony or coordination in the nervous system. It is not uncommon to find that sensory processing or skill dominance varies on left and right sides of the body. Differences can be found in every paired organ system in the body: the two sides of the brain, eyes, ears, hands, and feet. Research shows that hand preference affects the tissue (muscle, tendons, ligaments, capillaries, arteries, veins) and composition of the upper limbs in all age groups. A large amount of tissue changes occur in bone density and the fat-free soft tissues of exercised limbs. In addition to these changes, you can expect to improve the functional skills required for your sport.

Research also shows that sprinters and cyclists produce uneven amounts of power output with their legs. This is an example of dominant and recessive motor patterns that limit speed of movement. These imbalances in speed-strength, identified in Chapter 2, can be corrected through the use of the power output training programs presented in Chapter 8.

• Computers have created games that assess (measure, record, and evaluate) neuromuscular and brain function and train the neuromuscular system. Alternate hand and foot patterns, along with running patterns (for example, left arm and right leg), have been programmed into the game. These specific patterns, rhythms, and distractions are used to systematically guide players to higher levels of handwork and footwork. A powerful advantage of using the scientific game is its ability to record correct responses. There is evidence to specific benefits (structural and functional changes in the nervous system) gained by playing this game that may help athletes sprint and play faster.

BODY CONTROL AND POWER

Can your describe the Body Control Program?

The major objective of a body control program is to perfect a large number of movement patterns to the point where they occur automatically. As more movement patterns are developed, athletes increase their ability to move quicker and faster in a variety of directions. The ability to use all body parts, in all of their movement patterns and in a variety of game situations, when called upon to do so, is the ultimate goal of the body control program.

Can Sport Hitting Power be improved?

One of the most formidable defensive players to ever take the field in the NFL, Randy White, needed instruction on how to improve his ability to hit with his hands properly on and off the field. Randy came to the Dallas Cowboys as a highly recognized and decorated player. One would think that if he was asked him to hit a bag with his left hand, right hand, or both hands together, you'd better step back! Surprisingly, this was not the case. The results of a simple test to measure hitting power convinced the coaches and, more importantly, Randy, that he should begin a training program to improve the power of his hits. Randy did improve his hitting power. An NFL "Tough Man" boxing match in Las Vegas demonstrated the fact that a well learned skill...Hitting...can be retained for some time with a little work. Randy knocked out his opponent in the first few seconds of the 2nd round with a sizzling, short left hook.

Starting Power (Power Trainer Curve)

What is the Power Training Curve and how is it used?

Starting power is the ability to get moving in the appropriate direction in the most efficient way possible. A sprinter reacting to the starting gun, a linebacker reacting to a running play to fill the hole, or an NBA basketball player fast-breaking down the court for a two-point lay-up are all examples of actions that require a lot of starting power.

Some of the best advice for improving this ability comes from Bruce Lee, the famous martial artist. Bruce suggested that athletes use his quickness principle of a slow, phased, bent-knee position to move quickly into an attack, evasion, or retreat. In sports that allow movement, this position means that you keep the body in a slow movement pattern, which helps to overcome the inertia that makes it harder for you to get started from a still position. Some coaches call it "dancing in your shoes". In sports where the athlete must remain still, like the start in swimming and track or the offensive linemen in football prior to the snap, the slow, phased, bent knee position takes place in the mind.

Driving Power

What is driving power?

Driving power applies to contact sports such as football, rugby, soccer, or basketball where initial contact is made and then the player has to follow through to clear an area by moving the opponent out of the way. No matter how contact originates, the physical properties must be managed to minimize or avoid potential injury. Once contact is made, driving power is the ability of the player to maintain the contact and move the opponent in the appropriate direction. Repeated drills against a challenging opponent in many situations are the best way to develop driving power. This is why inter-squad scrimmages are so effective and are the preferred method for high-level development.

High-Speed Quickness

Do the speed and quickness drills coaches use in practice make athletes faster?

It is true that drills are becoming more sports- specific as coaches more closely simulate game conditions. Rather than just sprinting from point A to point B, a football drill may force a defensive player to first recognize a specific game situation such as a pass or run before executing a controlled sprint toward the quarterback. Rather than using a lateral shuffle in basketball to move from one cone to another, a drill may force the defensive player to recognize and anticipate the movement of the offensive player before rapidly shuffling to the left or right. These types of drills are attempts to improve "playing speed," which is the main objective of speed training in sports. Most improvement in speed from drills result from faster recognition, reaction, starting and accelerating in that sport-specific scenario. The mechanics of that movement are improved with this added efficiency contributing to improved playing speed.

If all that was needed to improve speed was drills and more drills, every athlete would be a speed demon. The typical on-field or on-court-drill is not the magic speed improvement bullet. Most drills do not overload the muscles involved in the various phases of sprinting, nor do they force athletes to take faster and longer steps than they are normally capable of taking, or improve speed-strength and change strength-weight ratios.

To achieve these goals, drills need to contain another element to make sure tissue changes occur that have implications for improving the start, acceleration, and maximum speed by increasing stride rate, stride length, and speed endurance. This involves combining known speed improvement techniques into the drill such as sprint-assisted training (towing), sport loading, and form and technique training.

Coaches are beginning to combine drills with speed training and focus on the primary goal of improving "playing speed." Defensive backs, for example, are connected to two sets of surgical tubing. As a wide receiver begins a sideline pattern, the DB is towed in a backward sprint with one set of tubing. As the receiver makes his cut, the DB is towed diagonally by a second set of tubing to complete the coverage at super high speed. These types of drills increase playing speed by improving recognition and reaction time in specific movements and by producing physiological changes in the body that increase raw power, strength, and speed.

DOMINANT AND RECESSIVE MOVEMENT PATTERNS

Athletes in practically every sport are quicker and faster when executing their favorite or dominant side movement pattern. Right-handed basketball players drive to the right faster than to the left, soccer and rugby players favor movement to one side depending upon their dominant leg, football players favor carrying the ball in a particular hand and move faster and more efficiently in one direction, and so on for athletes in every sport. This difference exists for two reasons--lack of skill in the recessive hand or foot and the underdevelopment of movement patterns toward the recessive side. Years of repetitive dominant movements produce muscle memory, additional speed-strength, and automatic, efficient, and fast action.

What is the so-called athlete's "forgotten side" in sports?

In this modern era of sports, it is almost unbelievable that only a select few athletes have mastered the skills in their sport with near equal ability on both sides (left and right hand and leg). Clearly, ambidexterity would enhance both the speed with which movement patterns are completed and overall performance in many sports, yet training to master such skills is almost nonexistent. The recessive (non-dominant), undeveloped limb is referred to as the forgotten side.

Why is this aspect neglected?

Decades ago, many misconceptions delayed this movement in sports; however, it is well known that these beliefs are outdated and unfounded. Research has shown that 1) left-handed individuals are not inferior and there is no need to try to convert a left dominant person to right dominance, 2) training to develop the recessive side will not cause mental confusion, 3) improved skill in the recessive side will not decrease the skills of the dominant side, and 4) recessive side skills can easily be improved with training. Even with this knowledge, little is being done in any sport.

If you took the time to watch every move of any athlete for a 24-hour period, you would observe that about 95% of daily routines, from grooming to carrying books, eating to standing and sitting, and all play and sports activity would be performed with the dominant side. Not only does the dominant hand and leg (the right in most athletes) get the majority of use, there is also a dominant standing, sitting, and walking posture. There is a side in most movements that is less involved and less developed in both skill and size. After decades of repeated behavior, it is no wonder the recessive side has atrophied, able to perform only simple gross motor movements, and nearly useless in modern day athletics. In some cases, overuse of the dominant side and underuse of the recessive side has also resulted in muscle imbalance differences that slow down athletes in short sprints due to the reduced ground contract force of the recessive leg.

Should coaches encourage athletes to develop equal skill in each limb?

"Handiness" refers to your consistent lateral (side) preference when completing a complex manual movement pattern. "Lateral dominance" and the "recessive hand" indicate the preference of one hand or leg over the other. There are also degrees of handiness in athletes:

Ambidexterity - The athlete uses both sides (arms, legs) with equal skill.

Approximate Ambidexterity - The athlete carries out large muscle group movements with the recessive side nearly as effective as the dominant side.

Slightly Handed - The athlete prefers one side over the other in detailed movements but can use the other side equally well for most activities.

"Approximate ambidexterity" should be the goal of every athlete in carrying out movement patterns and skills since both affect speed and quickness. Our present system of training fails to provide near equal exposure to both sides. As a result, adequate recessive limb skill at the high school, university and professional levels is uncommon. How many times do you see football players running with the ball in the wrong hand, basketball players who cannot control more than 1-2 high speed dribbles, shoot, pass, or rebound with their recessive hand, soccer and rugby players with inferior kicking skill in one leg, and volleyball players who favor one side for passing, blocking, spiking, and net retrieving? Switch hitting in baseball, quarterbacks throwing with both hands, tennis players serving right and left-handed, and players with near equal skill on both sides should be commonplace in modern day sports. Unfortunately, only a few athletes have mastered the use of their recessive side and most will never achieve this goal unless recessive side training becomes a part of regular off-season and in-season workouts.

Can the Recessive Side be Improved?

Striving for perfect ambidexterity with equal skill in both sides in all athletic movements is not practical and is nearly unattainable. We suggest that coaches, athletes, and parents strive for approximate ambidexterity. As a Head University basketball coach, Dr. Dintiman was quite upset with his starting guard who violated off-season rules, went skiing and broke his right wrist. With his wrist in a cast, he continued to play recreational basketball daily during the off season using his uninjured left hand. When he reported to opening day practice the following October, his ability to control the basketball and perform the key skills with his left hand, which was clearly now as good as his right hand, amazed everyone. This observation made recessive side training a priority for all his players in off-season work. Numerous studies have also shown that the recessive side is trainable and can be improved to a level nearly equal to or slightly less than the dominant side. Throwing accuracy in baseball and softball, soccer kicking accuracy, and basketball dribbling and shooting skill have all improved when athletes follow a 6-10 week training program.

Research has also revealed that recessive side training can help prevent lateral deviations of the spine such as pelvic tilt, compensatory curvatures and drop shoulder. Eliminating muscle imbalances on the recessive leg will also improve speed in short sprints.

Developing the recessive side in athletes will not occur from normal workouts, team and individual sport practice sessions, or free play where most athletes repeatedly execute their best dominant side moves. Just as improving speed requires sports-speed training, training for approximately ambidexterity requires a specialized approach. It also will not occur in a week or two.

How can coaches implement a program to reach the goal of approximate ambidexterity?

Although recessive side skills can be improved at any age, the most effective strategy is to begin this type of training before age 10 with emphasis by parents, elementary physical education teachers, and youth sports coaches. A few recommendations to help implement a program follow:

- Appoint an assistant, graduate student or helper friend as the official Recessive Side Coach.

- Assign off-season recessive side work in your sport that includes a minimum of 30 minutes daily.

- Use a minimum of 15 minutes of recessive hand or feet drills during each practice session.

- Occasionally run a 15-30 minute scrimmage that forces everyone to use only the recessive side during actual competition.

- Discourage athletes from only practicing their best shots and moves in pre-practice and free play. Devise a series of sport-specific recessive side warm-up drills for your sport.

- Test athletes every 6 months to determine their improvement in various skills.

- Make recessive side training a key aspect of your off-season training program.

- Use recessive limb exercises such as one-hand push-ups, pull-ups and half-squats.

- Devise drills to emphasize sport-specific recessive side training.

  Football - Carrying the ball in both hands, cutting and faking while moving to the right and left, lateral passing, tackling and blocking.

  Basketball - Dribbling, shooting, passing, rebounding, defensive stance.

  Baseball/Softball - Switch hitting, fielding, throwing, and moving to the left and right.

  Field Hockey and Lacrosse - All stick work and defense.

  Soccer - All kicks and traps from both side.

  Tennis - Movement to the right and left at the net and baseline.

  Volleyball - Passing, spiking, blocking, net retrieval.

Chapter 8

POWER OUTPUT TRAINING

A major objective of power output training (speed-strength) is to increase the force applied against the ground during the pushing action of each step during the starting, accelerating and maximum speed phases of sprinting. To improve playing speed, the force must also be applied at the right time and in the right direction. As power output increases, so will horsepower reserve, which allows athletes to play the game at a lower percent of capacity, with more available power for the demanding adjustments that arise during the game.

A second key objective of power output training is to develop the required force and tissue capacity for a sport, which includes the ability of body tissue to defend, build, repair, heal, regenerate, remodel, and self-regulate. Any builder knows that the materials used in construction must be able to sustain the loads within all stress ranges. The human body also has its limitations. These limitations are evident when players are seriously injured because functional demands are placed on body parts that exceed the physiological limits of bone and soft tissue. When forces exceed the tissue's capacity to protect the body, injuries occur. Although a high level of speed-strength does not guarantee a career free from injury, it does provide additional protection.

The ability to propel a stationary body into rapid movement and exert maximum force requires both strength and power (speed-strength). An athlete may be strong yet lack explosive power and be incapable of sprinting a fast 40-yard dash. Speed and power training also involves movements that are similar to those in the sport (the principle of specificity). The speed-strength programs described in this chapter apply sound concepts of training to prepare athletes for team sport competition by improving starting speed, acceleration, and maximum speed; improving the ability to deliver and receive force, and providing protection from injury. A complete program to maximize ground contact force and speed-strength is also presented in this chapter.

CONCEPTS OF POWER OUTPUT TRAINING

What is the principle of work hypertrophy and how is it applied?

Commonly referred to as *Progressive Resistance Exercise (PRE)* this principle, must be applied to every phase of training if speed-strength, speed endurance, and overall speed in short sprints are to improve.

The PRE is a simple concept that involves gradually overloading one of the body systems (muscular, circulatory, respiratory). The object is to perform more work (exercise) in terms of frequency (exercise more often), volume (exercise longer), or intensity (exercise faster with fewer and shorter rest periods) each session. When this occurs each workout, the body gets the message and repairs itself through elaborate cellular changes to prepare for even more difficult future exercise demands. Use of the PRE produces dramatic changes in the heart and circulatory system and the strength and endurance of muscles.

Each athlete begins a training program at their current level of conditioning, such as level A in Figure 8.1. During and immediately after the first workout, this fitness level temporarily declines to point B. During the next 24-48 hours of the recovery or resting phase, tissue rebuilds beyond the original level to point C. The athlete is now able to perform more work than before with no more effort and actually has slightly improved his or her conditioning level. As this process is repeated over and over, fitness continues to improve as indicated by A-2, A-3, A-4, and so on, *providing certain guidelines* are followed:

- Each workout must be strenuous enough to cause an initial decrease in conditioning levels. In fact, the amount of improvement during recovery depends on the intensity and length of a workout.

- A 18-24 hour recovery period is needed following an anaerobic (speed endurance) or aerobic workout, and approximately 48 hours between strength training workouts, to receive the full benefits.

- The next workout must occur within 24-48 hours to avoid a decline in fitness levels.

- Each week, training must be progressively more strenuous (more workouts, longer workouts and more intense workouts) than the previous week.

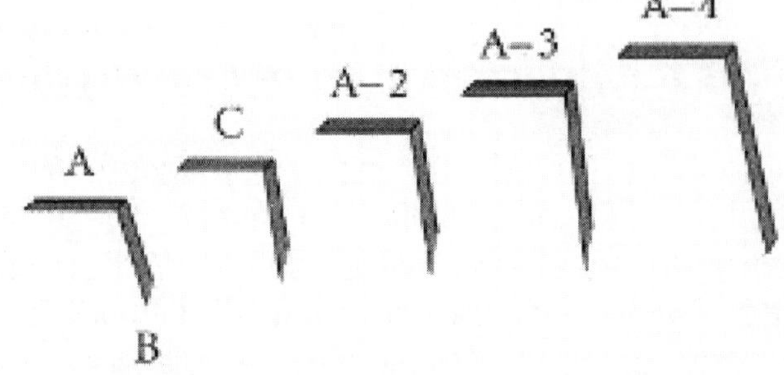

Figure 8.1 Progressive resistance exercise: how improvement occurs
A - Starting fitness level B - Lowered fitness level after the first workout
C - Elevated fitness level after recovery, and the proper time to begin the next workout, A-2, A-3, and A-4 - Elevated level after additional workouts and rest

Is it necessary to work or train fast to be fast?

The "work fast" principle is essential in all power sports and in the improvement of speed for any sport. There is a fine range of speeds and loads that must be adhered to in order to maximize transfer to a specific sport. Tissue strength will be gained over a wide range of high intensity explosive lifts. Several training programs have been used successfully to bridge the gap between strength and power to improve speed-strength and sprinting speed. Combinations of weight training, sprint-resisted training and plyometrics are used.

Are free weight exercises better than machines?

The actual muscle involvement of movements in specific sports can be simulated more closely using free weights, making exercises more sprint-specific. The three-phase response of the body to stressors (see Seyle's General Adaptation Syndrome) is also enhanced.

What is more important, acceleration or mass?

The amount of force generated is influenced by either a change in a player's mass (weight) or acceleration (speed of movement). Fast running backs may match the force output of 300-pound linemen due to rapid acceleration and high speed. Large and fast running backs like former all-pros Jim Brown and Earl Cambell create the most force. The most effective way to generate force is to increase both acceleration and mph speed.

What is the relationship of work and power to speed of movement?

Imagine yourself completing the simple task of moving 100-ten pound weights onto a one-foot high train in ten seconds. The train will depart in ten seconds; therefore you get credited only for weight placed on the train. In a similar manner, the foot of the sprinter has a window of time to apply force. This is why it is important that you train to meet the many specific power output requirements in your sport. Table 8-1 summarizes the power output of an athlete who moves 10 weights from the platform to the train in 10 seconds. Remember that in most explosive sports, there is about .1 to .3 second to apply additional force at the foot. The only way to increase speed of action is to increase the speed with which the 10-pound weights are moved.

This illustration helps us understand what must be done to sprint and play at faster speeds. Many of the activities in this book have been designed to identify, correct, or improve the ability to apply more force at the foot during ground contract. A sprinter has about 1/10 second to make this adjustment. The time needed for generating more force at the foot is close to the time required for cracking a whip. The better the sequencing of the limbs of the body, the more effective or louder the pop of the whip or the faster we sprint and play. Table 8.1 shows that the athlete was credited with only 10 percent of the power and work possible. Only the work and power recorded in the allotted time counted.

Similarly, a sprinter's foot is in contact with the ground about .09 to .11 second at a time. Any force that is not applied at the foot during this time is of no use in sprinting faster. Think of the many complicated tasks in your sport to see the importance of this principle. Imagine the complexities of covering an opponent during the game. What if you need to move or cut left, which requires a planting of the right foot, but the right foot is still in the air? Add this delay time to the playing equation to see how far an opponent will be from you in the time it takes to put the foot on the ground to apply appropriate countering force.

Table 8.1 **Power Output**

Total lb. Available	**Total lb. in 10 Seconds**	**Total work in 10 Seconds**	**Total Power**
1,000 lb.	10 X 10 lob. 100 lb.	100 lb. X 1 ft. 100 ft./lb.	100 ft. lb. 10 seconds = 10 ft./lb./second
100%	10%	10%	10%

GROUND CONTACT FORCES

What is the one most important factor to work on to improve the start, acceleration, and maximum speed phases of a short sprint?

The answer is "ground contact forces," which are determined by the speed-strength of the muscles involved in the pushing action away from the ground with each step in all phases of sprinting. This concept has been known and applied for decades by track and field coaches. It was initially viewed as the best way to improve the start and acceleration phase of short sprints such as a 40-yard dash since maximum mph speeds are not reached. It is now evident that ground contact forces also determine the maximum speed an athlete can reach.

As renowned researcher, Ralph Mann, points out, the act of sprinting in football, track and other sports requires the athlete to produce a powerful vertical effort to overcome the effects of gravity and stop downward velocity. Even without gravity in the equation, the ground contact force must equal the athlete's weight just to stand and support the body. The total vertical force needed in sprinting to stop downward velocity, to counter breaking forces, to produce upward velocity, and to overcome the force of gravity is approximately 2.15 X body weight. A 200 pound running back needs to exert a ground contact force with each step of about 430 pounds during the sprinting action. For each pound of weight a football player at any position adds, 2.15 or so additional pounds of ground contact force (pushing action against the ground) are needed to merely maintain starting, acceleration, and maximum speed. A 275 pound lineman who adds 25 pounds of muscle and fat to reach 300 pounds now needs an additional push-off force of approximately 50-52 pounds just to maintain his same speed prior to the weight gain. This increase in ground contact force does not automatically accompany the weight gain, and occurs only with power output training.

Sprinting is a demanding, intense activity requiring a force close to the limit of every athlete's capability on each step. Vertical force requirements are the main factor limiting sprinting performance for athletes in all sports. Ground contact force affects stride rate, the length of the stride, the start (first 2-3 steps), acceleration, and maximum speed. If athletes are to maintain pre-weight gain speed or improve their current speed in short sprints, training must focus on increasing the force of the pushing against against the ground. Speed-strength training, such as sport loading (resistance provided by sleds, harnesses, weights, inclines), free weights (dead lift, clean) and plyometrics are all designed to increase contact forces to the ground.

The ratio between body weight and ground contact force is also an important factor. Adding too much weight and not improving the strength of the pushing action off the ground with each step negatively changes this ratio. Losing body weight and merely maintaining your present ground contact force with each step has a positive effect on this ratio and will improve speed in short sprints. A 10, 15, 20 or 25 pound weight loss (body fat) with no reduction in ground contact force is a desirable goal for over fat football players in any position.

Athletes must be aware that horizontal velocity during the sprinting action and mph speed is determined by the amount of vertical force that can be applied during ground contract. Increasing this force against the ground each step by strength-power gains and increased mechanical efficiency will improve speed. An accurate, practical test is also needed to measure the ground contact force exerted on each step for every athlete to determine the effectiveness of various power output programs.

What do coaches mean when they refer to "triple extension"?

Triple extension exercises increase the amount of force an athlete can apply to the ground, such as the pushing action away from the ground in executing a short sprint. These exercises activate the joints and muscles of the hip, knee, and ankle. Sprinting is a classic example of triple extension that occurs with a forward (sprinting) or lateral (faking and cutting) movement on one leg. The three joints move from a flexed to an extended position to create the thrust to begin and carry out the sprinting action.

Triple extension exercises include the Olympic Lifts and their variations: *Cleans* (Power, Hang), *Snatches* (Power, Hang), *Clean & Jerk,* and *Squats*. Other training programs discussed in this chapter such as *plyometrics* and *sport loading* involve triple extension during the specific act of sprinting.

Didn't one study conclude that the time spent in the air when sprinting was insignificant and that all training should be directed toward improving ground contact force?

In the Weyman study (Weyman, et. al. 2000), the mechanics of 33 subjects of different sprinting abilities running at top speed on a level treadmill were compared. Then, the mechanics of declined (6°) and inclined (+9°) top-speed treadmill running in five subjects were also compared. For both tests, a treadmill-mounted force plate was used to measure the time between stance periods of the same foot (swing time, tsw) and the force applied to the running surface at top speed. To obtain the force relevant for speed, the force applied to the ground was divided by the weight of the body (Wb) and averaged over the period of foot-ground contact (Favge/Wb).

The top speeds of the 33 subjects who completed the level treadmill protocol spanned a 1.8-fold range from 6.2 to 11.1 meters per second. In contrast, the time taken to swing the limb into position for the next step (tsw) did not vary (P = 0.18). Declined and inclined top speeds differed by 1.4-fold (9.96 ± 0.3 vs. 7.10 ± 0.3 m/s, respectively), with the faster declined top speeds being achieved with mass-specific support forces that were 1.3 times greater (2.30 ± 0.06 vs. 1.76 ± 0.04 Favge/ Wb) and minimum tsw that were similar (+8%). The study concluded that human runners reach faster top speeds not by repositioning their limbs more rapidly in the air, but by applying greater support forces to the ground.

Note: Subjects sprinting at only 6.2 m/s (meters per second) or even less than 8-9 m/s are moving at a rather slow speed. The fastest athlete in the study covered 11.1 m/s.

Do the results of the Weyman study mean that "air time" to reposition the legs is not important for team sport athletes?

The finding that faster top speeds are reached by applying greater support forces to the ground, not by repositioning the limbs more rapidly in the air, does not suggest that we should eliminate training to decrease air time. Differences of 2/100th and 3/100th of a second in air time between elite and other athletes are quite significant. Since this difference occurs each step, it may amount to as much as 2/10 - 3/10 of a second for team sport athletes depending on the racing distance. At a pace of 10-11 yards per second, this difference places an athlete 2-3 yards behind an opponent. Covering a wide receiver in football or an opponent on the basketball court from several yards behind means you will arrive to the ball 2-3 yards late in soccer, rugby, lacrosse, and field hockey, or reach first base after an infield ground ball 1/10 second late. In a 40-yard dash, the small time difference in an NFL combine may cost an athlete millions of dollars.

Research at Virginia Commonwealth University from 1970 to 1998 (Dintiman) supported the use of sprint-assisted and sprint-resisted training as a technique that significantly improved 40-yard dash times. The object was to improve ground contact force through speed-strength training and sprint-resisted training and alter neuromuscular patterns through sprint-assisted training. *Contrast training,* the alternate use of sprint-assisted and sprint-resisted training, was also shown to be an important component.

How is ground contact force increased?

The main objective is to increase the speed-strength of the muscles involved in the pushing action against the ground without adding body weight in the form of fat. Although a slight weight gain may occur due to hypertrophy of the muscles involved in this pushing action, the speed-strength increases more than counteract the weight gain by providing a "bigger engine" and additional pushing force.

Table 8-2 points out the differences between strength training programs designed to add muscle weight and those attempting to increase ground contact force by adding speed-strength without gains in body weight.

The key training programs to accomplish this objective are *speed-strength-training* in the weight room, *plyometrics* (weight room and outdoors), and *sprint-resisted training* using the Austin Leg Drive Machine®, heavy sleds, heavy resistance cords, weighted vests and body suits, and staircase and uphill sprinting.

The dead lift and other weight room exercises that require a pushing action are most important. Some coaches follow each set of the dead lift with sprint-specific plyometrics in the weight room. According to Ross (2005), this approach "tricks" the body into creating increased energy stores, and the additional compensation improves the conditioning effect of the workout.

The minimum hypertrophy (growth) program described in table 8.2 increases ground contact force without adding body weight. The maximum hypertrophy program is not only less effective in increasing ground contract force, it also adds body weight, thus increasing the amount of force needed to merely maintain an athlete's current speed.

It is also important to make certain that both feet are exerting maximum and similar force against the ground during the pushing action of each exercise. Speed-strength imbalances between the right and left leg and foot reduce overall driving force and negatively affect sprinting form and technique. Muscle Imbalances identified from the test battery described in Chapter 2 must receive top priority and be corrected immediately.

Does additional force increase ground contact time?

When speed-strength is increased, slightly more time is required to deliver the force, however, maximum speed is determined by both the amount and speed of the force. The increased push-off power lengthens each stride and also moves the athlete faster to the next phase of sprinting.

Hasn't the USA been slow to change their approach to speed improvement training for team sport athletes.

This may have been true for track coaches prior to the early 1970s when the Olympic 100, 200, and 400-meter dash was dominated by American sprinters. In 1972, Russian, Valeri Borzov dethroned American sprint supremacy by winning the Olympic 100-meter dash and may have helped coaches move beyond their over emphasis on genetics, anaerobic conditioning (speed endurance) and form and technique training. Borzov's rapid improvement from the previous year was attributed to a then new technique of training referred to as plyometrics, a program specifically designed to increase ground contact force.

Speed-strength training, sprint-resisted training, plyometrics, and sprint-assisted training are now part of a holistic approach in the USA in track and field and team sports.

Table 8.2 Comparison of Minimum and Maximum Hypertrophy Speed-Strength Training Programs

Training Variables	**Minimum Hypertrophy** (Minimum mass & weight gain)	**Maximum Hypertrophy** (Maximum mass and weight gain)
Intensity (Load/Weight)	90-100% of 1 RM	70-80% of 1 RM
Volume (Reps/Sets)	1-5 repetitions, 1-5 sets	8-12 repetitions, 3-4 sets
Rest Interval (between Sets)	5 minutes	1 minute or less
Speed of Completion	Explosive through the range of motion; slower on negative return.	Less emphasis on explosive movement through the range of motion.
Exercises	*Weight Training* (Push-force stressed): dead lift, kick-back, Olympic lifts, ankle press *Sprint-resisted training* (heavy resistance): Austin Leg Drive Machine, Sleds, Incline sprinting Modified Sprint Resisted Training: Light-to-medium to moderately heavy weights *Plyometrics* (in weight room following lower body exercises) *Core strengthening*	Numerous upper and lower body exercises stressing full body development. Use of periodization, changing the selection and order of exercises, Super setting, compound setting, use of a 4- or 6-day split routine for body sculpting, and a number of variations of the above.

Isn't the current approach to the development of college and pro football linemen making players slower?

For players in certain positions, such as interior linemen, some slowing in the "first three steps" and the 5, 10, 20, and 40-yard sprint may occur from the large amounts of weight gain commonly seen in football. This trend toward larger linemen is continuing at the college and professional levels as teams either recruit or develop 300-375 lb. athletes to enhance blocking and rushing performance. Unfortunately, not all added weight is muscle and athletes often accumulate considerable adipose tissue and exceed the recommended percent of body fat for optimum speed and health.

As indicated previously, this added weight requires much more ground contact force to maintain the pre-weight gain speed in the first three steps and acceleration phase of interior linemen (5-20+ yards during the pass rush). Adding 25 pounds, for example, will not automatically increase ground contact forces by the needed 50+ additional pounds of thrust each step to maintain speed. Without this increase to handle the additional weight (muscle and fat), slowing occurs.

A recent study of retired NFL 300-375 pound linemen has also revealed considerable health consequences such as reduced life span and an increase in the incidence of diabetes, cardiovascular disease, and other illnesses.

What is sprint-strength training and how is it used?

Sprint-strength training (sport loading) adds specificity to speed-strength training through the use of parachutes, sleds, harnesses, slopes, staircases, surgical tubing, and other methods that allow all phases of the sprinting action to be performed against resistance. Sprint-strength training is an effective method of increasing the muscular force applied to the ground without adding muscle-mass weight.

After coaches correct strength imbalances and develop a solid strength foundation in their athletes, training concentrates on various ways to turn strength into speed. The transition from base strength to sprint strength is made through the use of weight training, plyometrics and sprint resisted training.

To be effective, sprint-strength training should simulate the sprinting action as closely as possible. Sprint-strength training requires explosive efforts against moderate and high resistance while performing movements used in the start and acceleration phases of sprinting. Repetitions should remain fairly low in the 2-4 range. Higher repetitions of 8, 10 and over are not compatible with the training goal of speed-strength and move into the category of speed endurance loads.

As the competitive season approaches, the volume of sprint-strength training is reduced, longer rest intervals between repetitions and sets are used, and emphasis is placed on high quality repetitions.

HOW STRENGTH COACHES TRAIN ATHLETES

What type of speed-strength training programs are used by University strength coaches?

We recently surveyed the speed-strength training practices of five strength and conditioning coaches at major universities to help answer this question. The responses to the questions asked are listed below and were interpreted and summarized by Andrea Hudy, strength and conditioning coach, University of Kansas Basketball, and George B. Dintiman.

What is your basic philosophy of speed-strength training to improve speed in team sports?

Simply put, you must work at high intensity for speed, work hard and fast. "To be faster one must train with methods that are fast, using exercises that develop the nervous system as well as the muscular system. Speed improvement is a long, dedicated and constant refinement process. This is applicable to all areas of training."

Size-principle chart--Athletes must work at a high intensity to target the fast twitch glycolytic fibers; otherwise, the pathways are never available to be utilized.

Force-velocity curve--Plyometrics may shift the force-velocity curve to the right. Sprint-resisted training is also an important program.

Energy Systems --Coaches must train the proper energy system.

Fatigue--Rest intervals between bouts of exercise must allow adequate recovery unless the objective is to improve speed endurance.

Technique--Quality repetitions, mechanical efficiency and safety should be stressed.

What specific exercises do you use?

The concept of specificity is applied in terms of the types of exercise and rate of contractions. Explosive exercises are used that emphasize *triple extension* of the ankles, knees and hips such as the Olympic lifts and their variations. Speed-strength exercises, such as dead lifts, squats, and Olympic lifts are used to increase ground contract force.

Exercises target the muscles used in the act of sprinting at the same angle of the sprinting action. These exercises are designed to increase contraction force in the proper direction of movement and involve the prime movers. Exercises specific to muscular movements in sprinting keep the muscle contraction along the neural pathway. Specificity of exercise selection and training results in neural adaptation and an increase in the number of active motor units and allows athletes to complete exercises faster and with more power

The Olympic style lifts such as pulls, cleans, snatches, split snatches and split jerks using free weights are important. Sprint-simulated movements are also used with exercise machines such as the kick back, knee block (drive phase), paw down, sprint arm exercise, cycling, and walking lunge. Squatting exercises such as dynamic lunges, squat jumps, explosive step-ups, and fast (repetitive) step-ups and complexes involving some lifts coupled with a plyometric style exercise (e.g., squat/double leg stair bounds, lunge/split or scissors jumps, etc.) are used by some strength coaches. Knee extension, hip extensions, ankle plantar flexion and knee curls with the iron boot; calf raises, leg raises, and traditional upper body exercises involving the muscles that transfer upper torso energy to lower torso energy in sprinting are used.

In what order are exercises completed?

1. Total body synchronous movements that focus on power development (Olympic movements and/or plyometric exercises involving the upper and lower body).

2. Functional strength exercises for the upper and lower body such as the squat and lunge.

3. Single joint strength exercises.

4. Injury prevention exercises

What is the load and how many repetitions are completed?

Minimum hypertrophy--90-100% of 1RM, 1-3 repetitions, 5 min. recovery

Power development--70-90% or higher of 1RM, 1-6 repetitions.

Strength development--A load of 80-90% of 1RM, 1-5 repetitions.

Hormone/hypertrophy--A load of about 70% of 1RM, 10 repetitions.

Muscle endurance--A load of approximately 50-60% of 1RM, 12 repetitions or higher.

What muscle groups should be targeted?

Four muscle groups have a close correlation to sprinting speed: quadriceps, plantar flexors, hamstrings, and dorsiflexors. For explosive power, the flexor muscles of the legs overcome limb weight and need to be trained with high speed contractions and low weight. The extensor muscles need power training with heavy weight and low repetitions. Performance is closely related to how fast a sprinter can move the knee from the highest point to midway through the support phase. This involves the hamstrings, knee extensors, abductor magnus and gluteus maximis muscle groups. To minimize touchdown distance, muscles active in this phase of sprinting, such as the hamstrings and gluteul muscles, must be very strong to pull the body over the touchdown point during the initial part of ground contact. The strength of these muscles is critical to fast sprinting.

The upper body (biceps, triceps, deltoid, rotator cuff muscles, pectoralis major, trapezius, and rhomboids) also play a role in generating force that is transferred from the mid-torso to the lower-torso.

How fast are repetitions performed?

To improve speed-strength, the load is moved as quickly as possible in executing the Olympic lifts and other heavy strength training exercises. Although heavy weight will move slower through the entire range of motion than lighter weight, athletes should attempt to rapidly complete each repetition.

How many sets are completed?

The more sets completed, the greater the gains in strength, power and performance. As the number of sets increase, the number of exercises is reduced. Five to eight sets are commonly used. with some coaches using as many as 10. For athletes in positions where speed is of primary importance, a minimum hypertrophy speed-strength program is used.

What is the length of the rest interval between sets and exercises?

With a rest period of 3-5 minutes, near complete recovery occurs (ATP/CP is almost restored). A minimum hypertrophy speed-strength program requires a full 5-minute rest period between each set if maximum effort is reached. Thirty seconds results in a recovery of about 50% of depleted stores. To train the neuromuscular system for speed improvement, the 5 minute range is used by most coaches, with some allowing 6-7 minutes to guarantee recovery of the central nervous system including the motor nerve which carries impulses to muscle fibers. In sports that force athletes to handle high levels of lactic acid because of the short rest interval (25-30 seconds or less in football, under 15 seconds in soccer, field hockey, rugby, lacrosse), some strength training sessions with the shorter rest intervals are used.

What is the length of the rest interval between workouts?

To be certain that full restoration occurs, workouts are scheduled no closer than 48 hours (two days) or every other day. If strength training is the only type of activity completed in a workout, recovery occurs faster. Six day workouts that alternate muscle groups are used by some coaches.

WEIGHT ROOM SPEED-STRENGTH EXERCISES

Olympic Lifts

Is it necessary to use the Olympic Lifts?

The Olympic lifts are used in all sophisticated power and speed training programs. In a study of the heaviest successful lifts in the snatch and the clean and jerk for five Olympic gold medalists, Garhammer (1991) showed that "athletes trained in the Olympic style of weightlifting have an extremely high capacity to develop power, which is necessary for success in the sport." The clean portion of the clean and jerk, like the dead lift, is one of the single most important exercises for athletes to increase ground contact force (pushing force against the ground) with each stride. The Olympic lifts focus on optimum starting speed and quickness in movements from power positions and in recovery to catch the weight. They train the mind and body to develop peak force, aid in increasing the amount of time peak force is applied, develop force in a short period of time, and emphasize good body position and movements that transfer to other sports.

Can you describe the proper form for each of the Olympic Lifts?

The Olympic lifts are shown in Figures 8.2 to 8.4. The *Clean* is performed by assuming a comfortable stance with the feet spread slightly wider than shoulder-width apart. The bar is grasped with an overhand grip slightly wider than shoulder-width with the butt down and the head and chest up. An overhand hooked strap can also be used. The legs are bent to begin the lift. A straight back is maintained as the bar is brought up close to the body. The shoulders are placed 8 to 12 centimeters over the bar and the legs are bent once again after the bar clears the knees. Arms remain straight throughout. Athletes jump vertically into the lift with the legs, pulling the bar as high as possible and driving the elbows up. The body drops quickly as the athlete catches the bar on the shoulders while bringing the elbows quickly under the bar. Near maximum weight requires a deep knee bend to catch the bar; therefore, leg and back strength are essential to good lifting. The "1.3 times the clean" rule is used for estimating squatting strength (maximum clean in pounds X 1.3 = squat weight).

To complete the *Jerk*, take the bar from the rack to work primarily on the jerking movement. Assume a comfortable stance with the feet hip-to-shoulder-width apart. Grasp the bar with palms facing up and the hands slightly wider than shoulder-width. Rest the bar on the shoulders. Keep the back vertical and tight. Bend the legs with a quick dipping action. Experience will help athletes find the proper depth for a quick explosive return (a depth of 10 to 15 percent of the athlete's height is recommended). Jump explosively into the bar and try to drive the bar as high as possible. The bar should move vertically overhead. The action of the shoulders and arms will blend into the explosive leg jumping action. Drop directly beneath the bar, catching it straight over the shoulders. In the catch phase, the legs can be kept shoulder-width apart or in a stride position. Experiment to determine which foot to place forward. Both feet should be turned in. Straighten both arms vertically, holding them and the entire body rigid. Return to the erect position by moving the front foot back first with a slight jab step to shorten the distance, and then forward with your back foot.

To complete the *Snatch*, assume a comfortable stance with the feet shoulder-width apart. Widen the Clean grip so that at full extension the height of the bar will be lower and require less vertical work. Experience helps determine the optimal grip to use for a traditional lift. The close grip can be used as a variation. Bend both legs before lifting the bar and use them to get the weight off the ground. The back should be held straight with the arms medially rotated as far as possible to place the shoulders over the bar. Keep the bar close to the body and rebend the legs after the bar clears the knees. Keep the arms straight to allow the legs and back to lift the bar as high as possible. The arms fit into the action after the legs and back have done their part. Drive the elbows up, drop the body quickly, and catch the bar directly over the head and shoulders. Keep in mind that leg and back strength is essential in all aspects of lifting, but extremely important in the recovery phase when lifting maximum weight.

Weight Throwing Exercises

Are weight throwing exercises helpful?

Weight throwing is a practical, effective conditioning program for team sports that has been used by track and field coaches for decades. Plagenhoef's research (1971) showed that hammer throwing produces the greatest forces in sports. Before specialization entered the athletic world and redirected conditioning programs, many football programs used track and field as a part of their off-season and preseason conditioning programs.

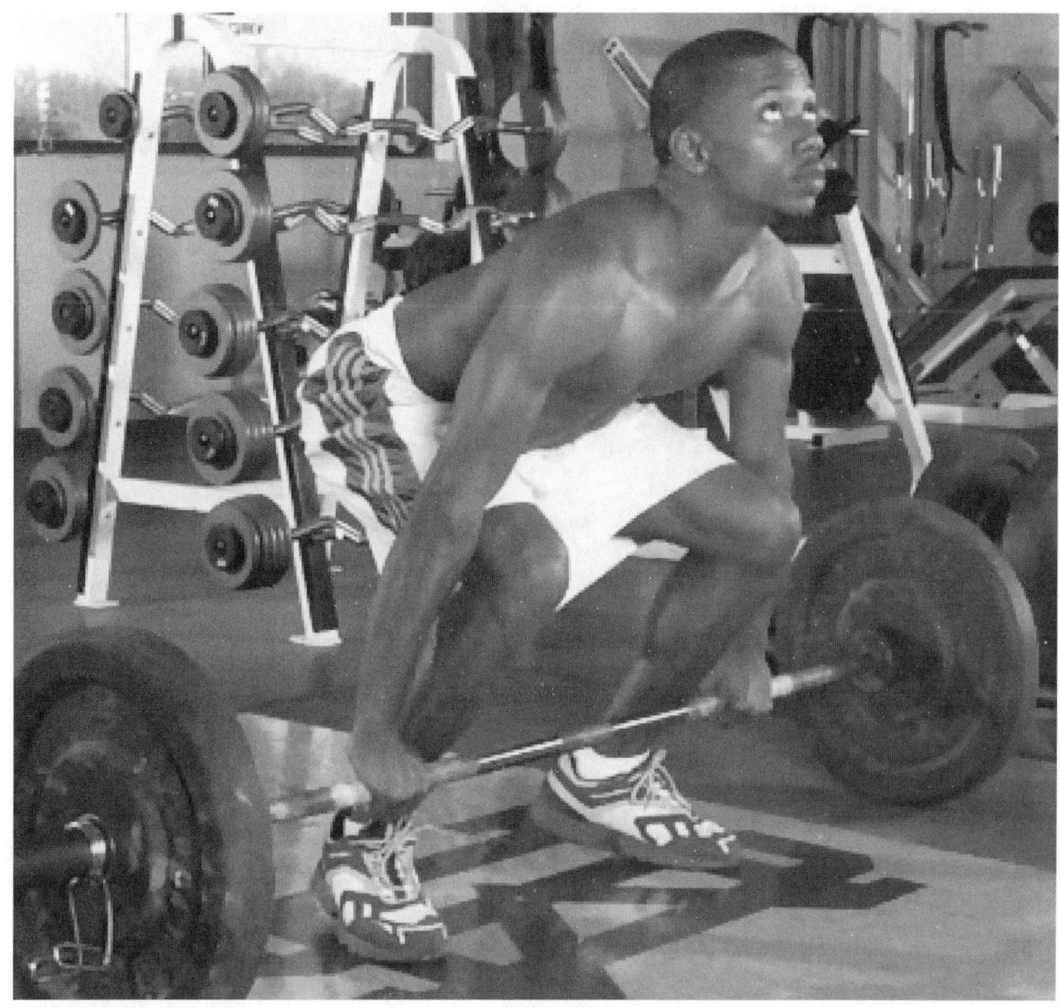

a

Figures 8.2 a, b, c Clean

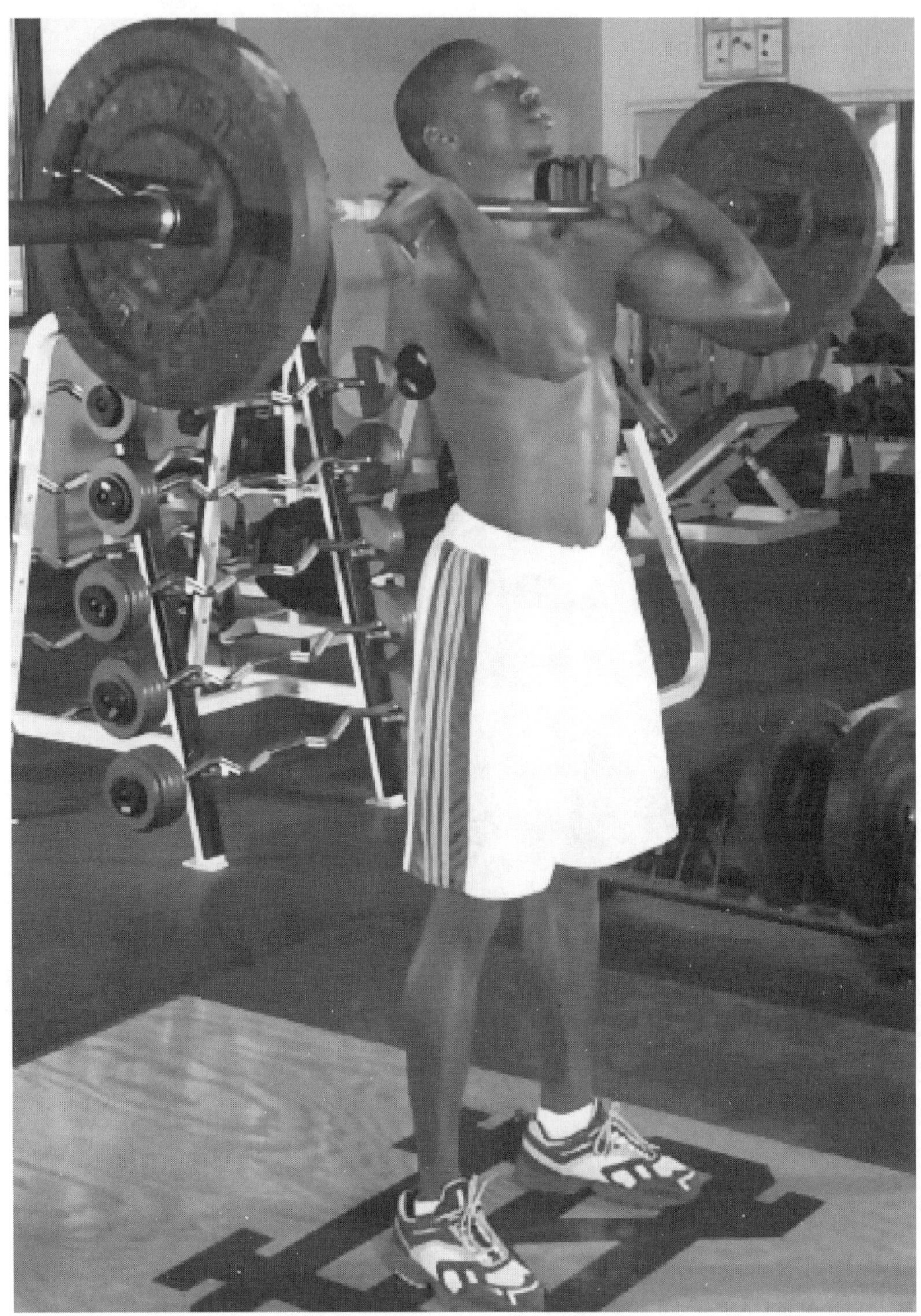

b

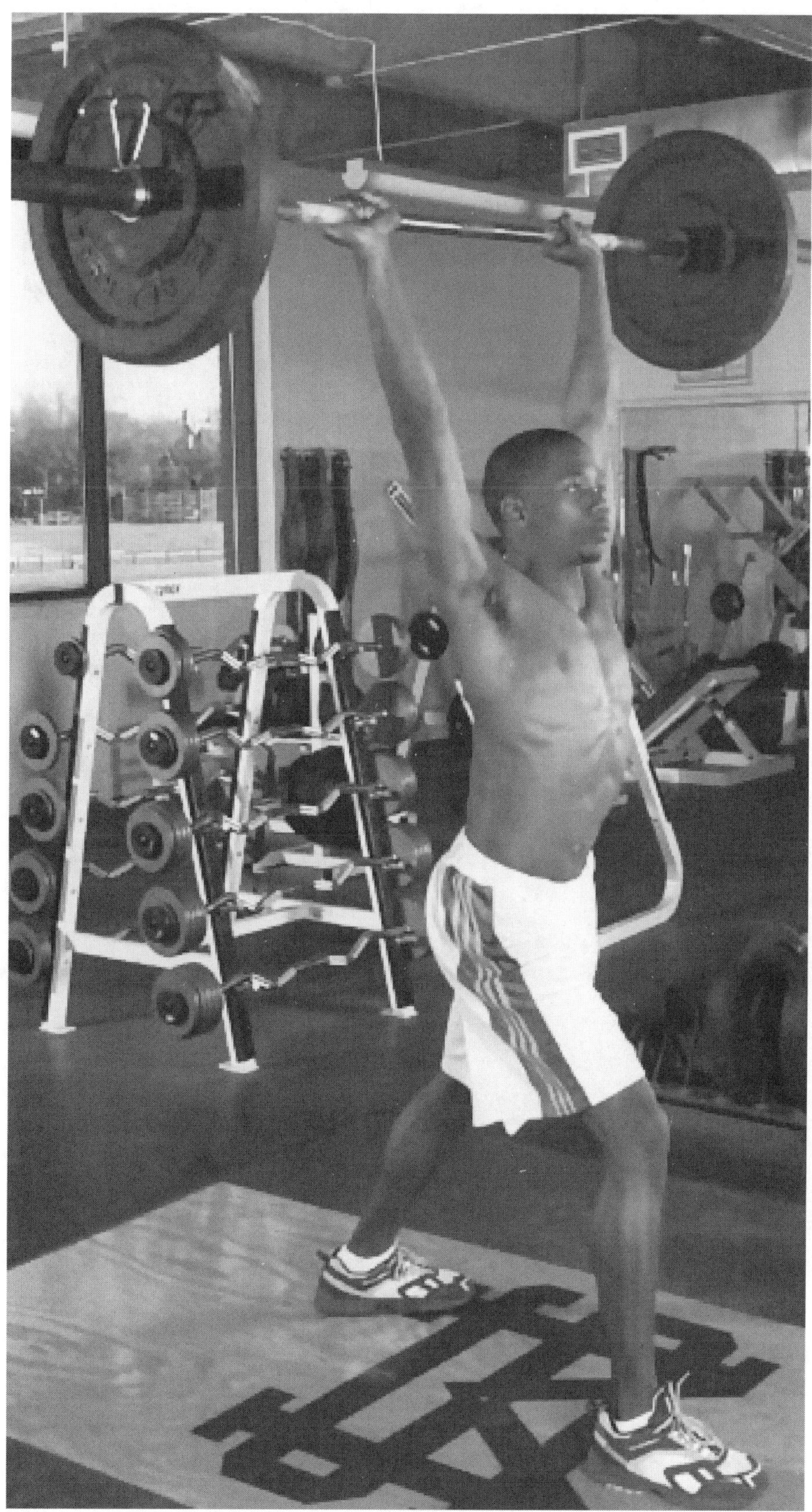

c

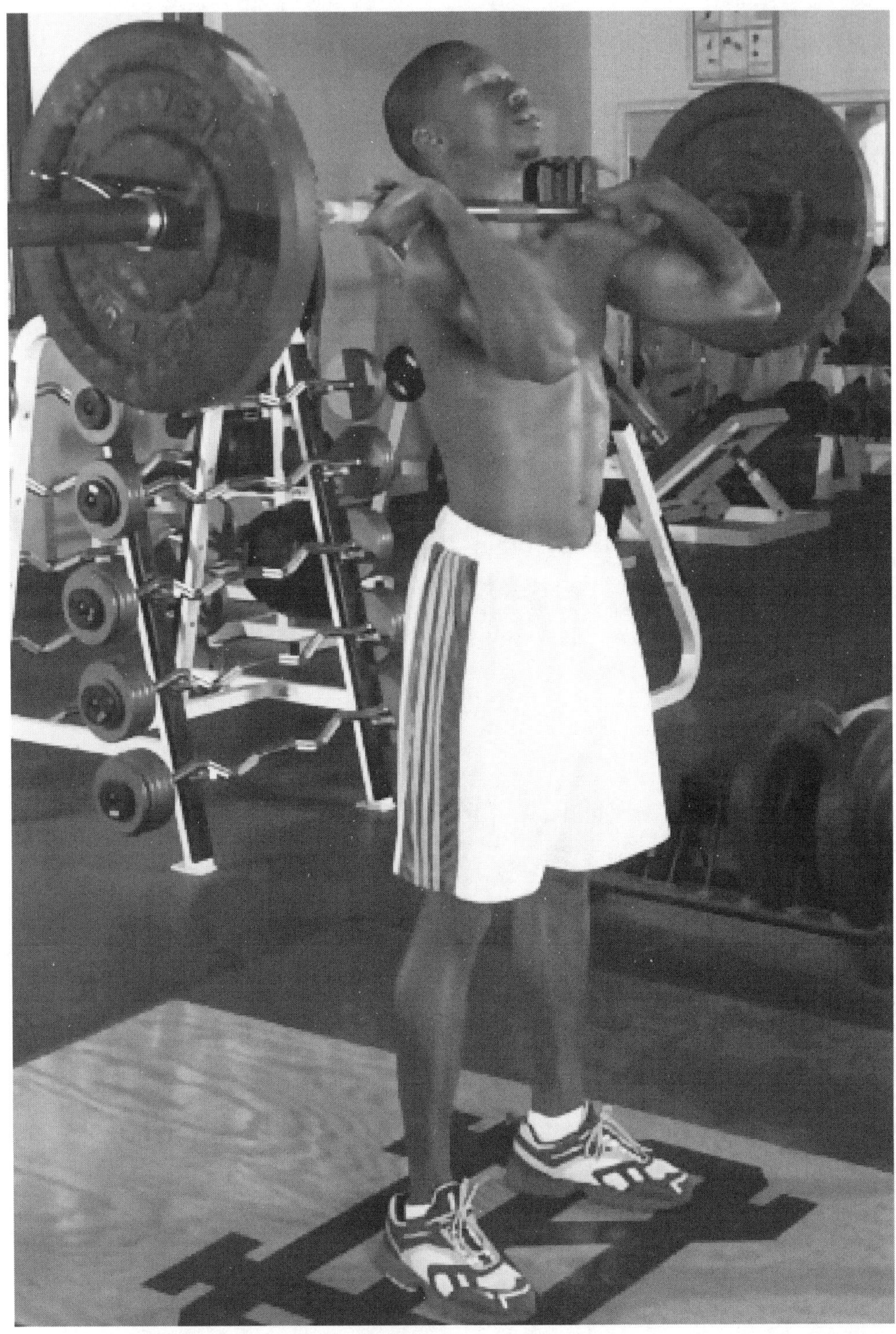

a

Figure 8.3 a, b Jerk

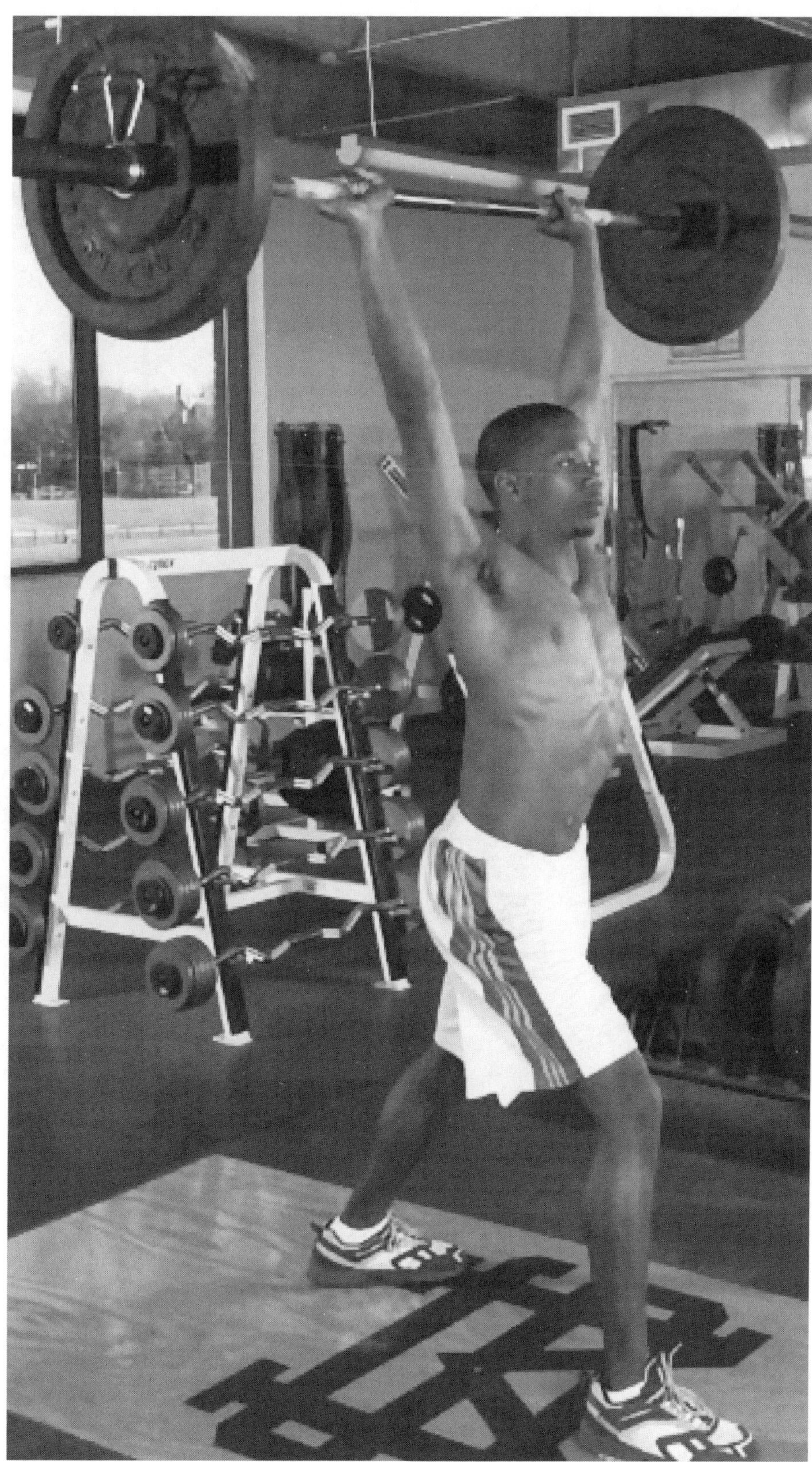

b

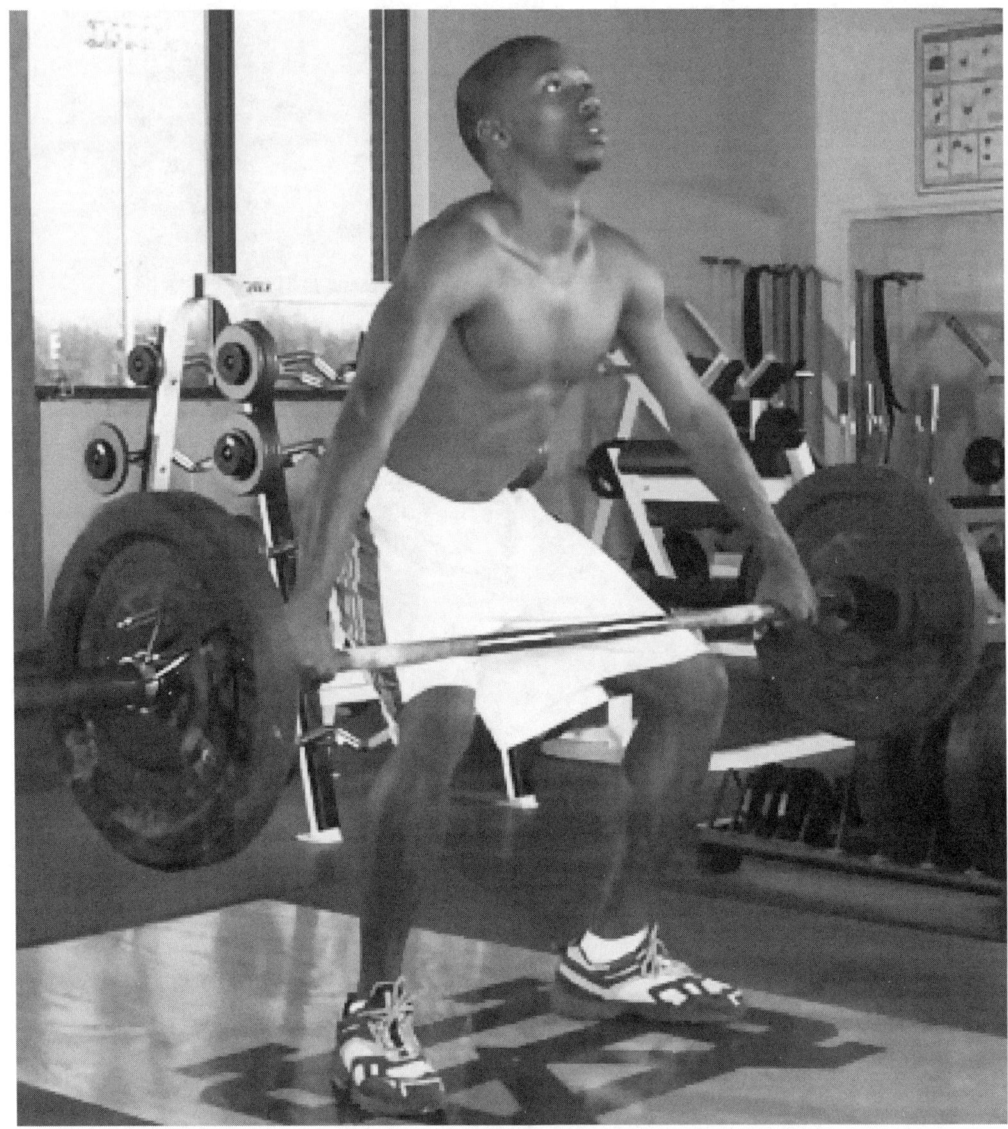

a

Figure 8.4 a, b Snatch

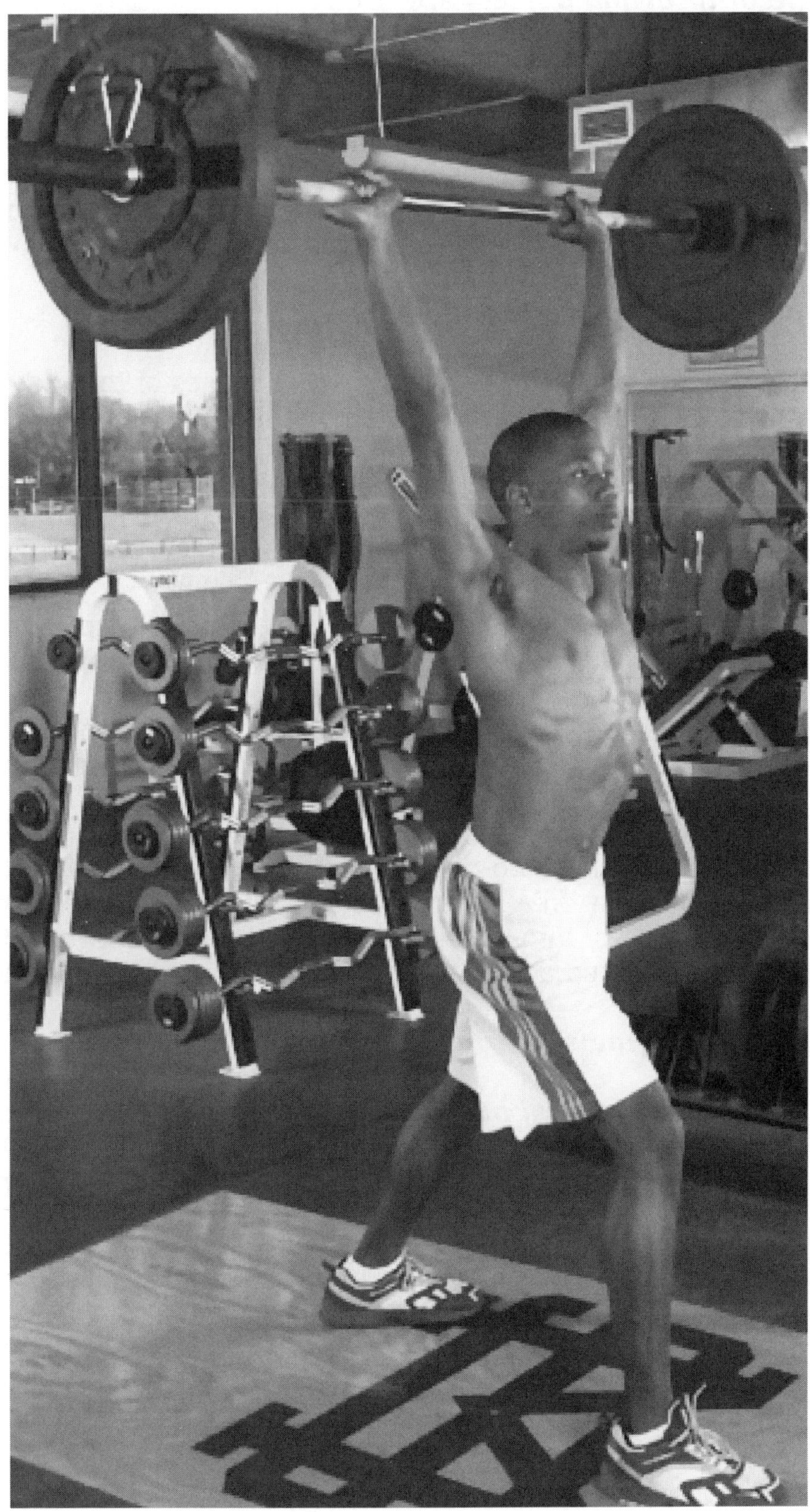

b

What type of throwing objects are used?

The Pud is a device of varying weights that is thrown from an area about the size of a shot put circle. Any level surface, ground, cement, or shot ring can be used. The standard Pud has a fixed handle attached to a weight that can be gripped with one or two hands. The Pud was designed by Lance Deal, American record holder in the hammer. *On Tracks* (www.ontrack.com) carries the Puds in 14-, 21-, 29.- and 35-pound sizes.

What types of throws are recommended?

A comprehensive program includes throwing in all planes of the body through all angles, using an equal number of left and right throws to keep the body balanced. Include Pud throwing after skill work and prior to weight training. Warm-up properly before throwing hard. Start with the lightest weight and move up to the heaviest. Complete one set of four throws from the left and right side or per each throwing action if all four throwing weights (1 rep per weight) are available. On speed days, use lighter weights.

Three stances are used: square with feet shoulder-width apart facing the throwing area, feet shoulder-width apart with the front foot closer to the throwing area, and rear facing as in the square dance.

Swing the weight back, turning the shoulders around and bending the legs on the back swing (figure 8.5). Take a number of swings with the weight before throwing it to develop good rhythm and timing. Try performing left and right one-handed throws to the side, left and right two-handed throws to the side, two-handed throws over the head while facing away from the throwing area (extend your body up and back during the throw), and two-handed throws after swinging the Pud between the legs and extending the body up and back as the throw is completed (figure 8.6).

Power Output Programs

Can you describe a general power output program for athletes?

A power exercise program using Olympic Lifts should be performed on Monday and Wednesday each week after completing the sprint-assisted training and Sport Loading program. The one-repetition maximum (1RM) is used for each exercise as the basis for loading. To determine 1RM, find the maximum weight that can be lifted for only one repetition for each exercise. Table 8-3 shows six levels of workout intensity based on the percent of 1RM. Strength training with heavy weights, near maximum muscle contractions, low repetitions, and full recovery between sets have been shown to produce greater increases in the cross sectional area of fast-twitch fibers than slow-twitch fibers.

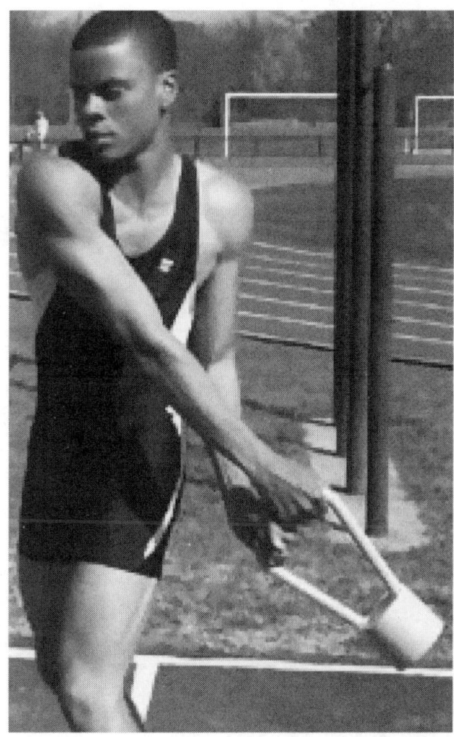

Figure 8.5 Two-handed side throw with the Pud.

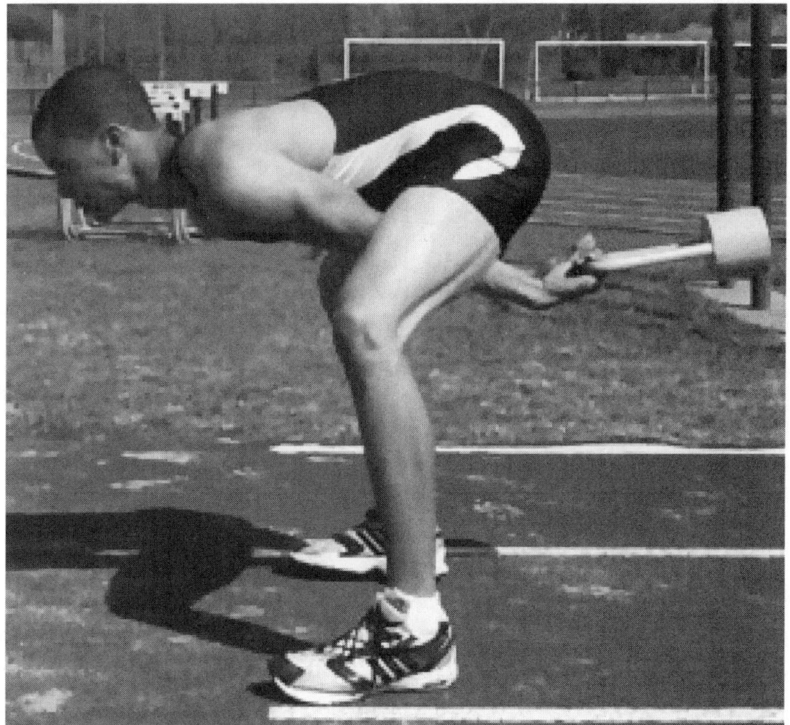

Figure 8.6 Two-handed Pud throw, swing between leg.

Table 8.3 Rating Intensities of the 1RM for Exercise Prescription

1 RM	Rating	Quality Developed
90+	Very heavy	Strength
80 to 90	Heavy	Strength and strength-endurance
70 to 80	Medium	Power and strength-endurance
60 to 70	Medium light	Power and muscle endurance
50 to 60	Light	Power and muscle endurance
40 to 50	Easy	Threshold of training effect

The sample program in table 8-4 shows how Olympic lifts are incorporated into a program to increase strength. It is apparent that a wide range of intensities, with loads increasing to or close to the 1RM exists. Maximize rest between sets to minimize the effects of fatigue as a limiting factor. It is recommended that the lift emphasis varies on Monday and Wednesday. For example, the clean can be at higher intensities and volume on Monday and the jerk can be at higher intensity and volume on Wednesday.

Table 8.4 Sample Program Using Olympic Lifts

Monday	Wednesday
CLEANS 3 to 6 sets 1 to 3 repetitions per set 66 to 100% of 1 RM 1.5 to 5 min. rest between sets	SNATCHES 3 to 6 sets 1 to 5 repetitions per set 66 to 100% of 1 RM 1.5 to 5 min. rest between sets
JERKS 3 to 6 sets 1 to 3 repetitions 66 to 100% of 1 RM 1.5 to 5 min. rest between sets	CLEANS 3 to 6 sets 1 to 5 repetitions 66 to 100% of 1 RM 1.5 to 5 min. rest between sets

Can you describe a typical speed-strength training program?

The components of the complete workout schedule remain the same during the preseason, however intensity and duration increase during the second half. In Phase A of the preseason, most exercises should begin at about 50 percent of each athlete's maximum level as a general guide. The rate of increase should vary, such as from 8 to 10 percent per week above previous maximum levels.

Phase B is composed of many sets and repetitions at a high percentage of the 1RM for each lift. An increased intensity in muscle endurance is also an objective during this period. The increase in workout intensity will require a comparable increase in the number of sets (at least 5 sets in most areas) and the length of the workout will increase from two to three hours. Table 8.5 outlines a standard program.

Table 8.5 **Sample Speed-Strength Program**

Warm-up, flexibility, body control, running or jumping techniques a. Jogging one-half mile or jumping rope (5 min.) b. Speed bags (boxing bags of various sizes (15 min.) c. Running and jumping for flexibility (10 min.)
Power position exercises (40 min.) a. Snatch: power b. Snatch: split squat c. Clean and push jerk d. Pull
Legs and back (23 min.)--3 to 5 sets, 3 to 5 repetitions a. Dead lifts b. Squats: front c. Squats: back
Shoulders and arms (18 min.)--3 to 5 sets, 3 to 5 repetitions a. Incline b. Bench c. Curls
Abdominal muscles and neck (9 min.) a. Four-way neck: 1 set of 8 to 12 repetitions b. Rotary neck: 1 set of 6 repetitions each way c. Abdominal muscles: 3 sets of 25 repetitions per set

A minimum of two sessions weekly, preferably every other day, is needed to improve speed-strength. One workout per week during the season will nearly maintain off-season gains. During the first two weeks of a newly started program, more recuperation time is needed. Using maximum and near maximum weight also lengthens recovery time. Short (45 minutes or less) highly intense workouts allow athletes to train more often.

Can you provide sample speed-strength programs for athletes at various stages of conditioning?

Table 8.6 shows a sample program for beginners. Three sets of the leg press exercise is performed, the first set with 60 percent of maximum for 10 repetitions, the second at 65 percent of maximum for 8 repetitions, and the third at 70 percent of maximum for 6 repetitions. The same sequence is followed for each exercise.

Table 8.6 Sample Functional Strength Program for Beginners

Exercise	RM	Monday	Wednesday	Friday
LEGS/BACK				
Leg press		L	M	M
Knee extension		L	M	H
Knee flexion		L	M	H
Toe raises		L	M	H
SHOULDERS/ARMS				
Lat pull-down		M	H	L
Bench press		M	H	L
Press (seated)		H	M	L
Press (standing)		H	M	L
Curls (dumbbells)		M	H	L
TRUNK/ABDOMEN Sit-ups (bent knee)		3 X 5	3 X 5	3 X 5
NECK Partner four-way neck		3 X 8 to 12	3 X 8 to 12	3 X 8 to 12

Percent RM, sets, and repetitions
Light (L): 60% RM, 1 X 10; 65% RM, 1 X 8; 70% RM, 1 X 6
Medium (M): 60% RM, 1 X 10; 70% RM, 1 X 8; 80% RM, 1 X 6
Heavy (H): 60% RM, 1 X 10; 70% RM, 1 X 8; 85% RM, 1 X

A sample program for the athlete at the intermediate stage of strength development is shown in table 8.7. A workout involves three sets of five to eight repetitions of each exercise with the first set at 60 percent of maximum, the second at 65 percent of maximum, and the third at 70 percent of maximum.

The advanced program shown in Table 8.8 is programmed for high intensity. Four sets are performed. The first set is completed at 60 percent of maximum for five repetitions, the second set at 75 percent of maximum for three repetitions, the third set at 85 percent of maximum for three repetitions, and the fourth set at 90 percent of maximum for two repetitions.

Table 8.7 **Sample Functional Strength Program for Intermediate Athletes**

Exercise	RM	Monday	Wednesday	Friday
POWER CLEAN		H	M	L
LEGS AND BACK				
Squat		L	M	H
Dead lift		M	H	L
Knee extension		M	H	L
SHOULDERS				
Bench press		H	M	L
Press (seated behind neck)		M	H	L
Rowing (bent-over)		L	M	H
TRUNK/ABDOMEN				
Sit-ups (medicine ball)		2 X 12	2 X 12	2 X 12
Sit-ups (crunches)		3 X 25	3 X 25	3 X 25
Trunk (hypertension)		2 X 12	2 X 12	2 X 12
NECK				
Partner four-way neck		3 X 8 to 12	3 X 8 to 12	3 X 8 to 12

Percent RM, sets, and repetitions
Light (L): 60% RM, 1 X 8; 65% RM, 1 X 8; 70% RM, 1 X 8
Medium (M): 50% RM, 1 X 5 to 8; 70% RM, 1 X 5 to 8; 80% RM, 1 X 5
Heavy (H): 60% RM, 1 X 5 to 8; 75% RM, 1 X 5; 85% RM, 1 X

Athletes in most sports must develop multi-directional speed-strength. Counsilman (1994), one of the most successful and analytical coaches in history, stated that the Russian and East German coaches felt so strongly about explosive power that they monitored training sessions and stopped their athletes if speeds decreased below the desired speed of movement in any direction.

Advanced athletes can train this quality by performing the clean, jerk, or snatch one time at 70 percent in one session (Monday or Wednesday), by working with weights at fast speeds with 70 percent 1RM for 12 repetitions, and by working with weights at fast speeds with 50 to 60 percent 1RM for 16 to 20 repetitions.

Table 8.9 lists performance standards for men as a percent of body weight for various speed-strength exercises.

Table 8.8 **Sample Functional Strength Program for Advanced Athletes**

Exercise	RM	Mon.	Tue.	Wed.	Thur.	Fri.
POWER						
Clean (power)		M		H		
Snatch (power)			M		H	
Jerk (rack)		H		M		
LEGS AND BACK						
Pull, clean		M		L		H
Dead lift		H		M		
Squat		L		M		H
Squat (front)						M
SHOULDERS, CHEST AND BACK						
Bench press		H				
Incline press			M		H	
Rowing		H				L
Flys, supine				L		M
TRUNK/ABDOMEN						
Trunk hyperextrension				3 X 25-60%		3 X 10-70%
Sit-ups (bent knee)		3 X 25		3 X 25-60%		3 X 5-70%
NECK						
Partner four-way neck		3 X 8 to 12		3 X 8 to 12		3 X 8 to 12

Percent RM, sets, and repetitions

Light (L): 60% RM, 1 X 5; 65% RM, 1 X 5; 70% RM, 1 X 5

Medium (M): 60% RM, 1 X 5; 70% RM, 1 X 5; 80% RM, 1 X 5

Heavy (H): 60% RM, 1 X 5; 75% RM, 1 X 3; 85% RM, 1 X 3; 90% RM 1 X 2

Table 8.9 **Sample Speed-Strength Performance Standards by Percent of Body Weight**

Level	Snatch	Clean	Clean and jerk	Power curl	Pull
Very poor	.50	.90	.90	.70	1.10
Poor	.70	1.10	1.10	.90	1.30
Average	.90	1.30	1.30	1.10	1.50
Good	1.10	1.50	1.50	1.30	1.70
Excellent	1.30	1.70	1.70	1.50	1.90

Legs and Back

Level	135o 1/4 back squat	90o 1/2 back squat	Full 3/4 back squat	Front squat	Dead-lift	Good morning
Very poor	1.70	1.50	1.30	1.20	1.30	.30
Poor	2.00	1.80	1.80	1.40	1.60	.40
Average	2.30	2.10	1.90	1.60	1.90	.60
Good	2.60	2.70	2.50	2.00	2.50	.70
Excellent	2.90	2.70	2.50	2.00	2.50	.70

Arms and Shoulders

Level	Military	Incline	Bench	Dips (20 sec.)	Push-ups (20 sec.)
Very poor	.40	.50	.80	4 reps	11 reps
Poor	.60	.80	1.10	12 reps	19 reps
Average	.80	1.10	1.40	20 reps	27 reps
Good	1.00	1.40	1.70	28 reps	35 reps
Excellent	1.20	1.70	2.00	36 reps	43 reps

Notes: Numbers indicate percent of body weight; weight times percent equals the weight lifted.

Female athletes should also use this table. For a more accurate interpretation of performance, use the category one level above your score. For example, a snatch using .90 (90 percent of body weight) would be a rating of GOOD for the female athlete rather than AVERAGE.

WEIGHT ROOM EXERCISES

Leg and Back

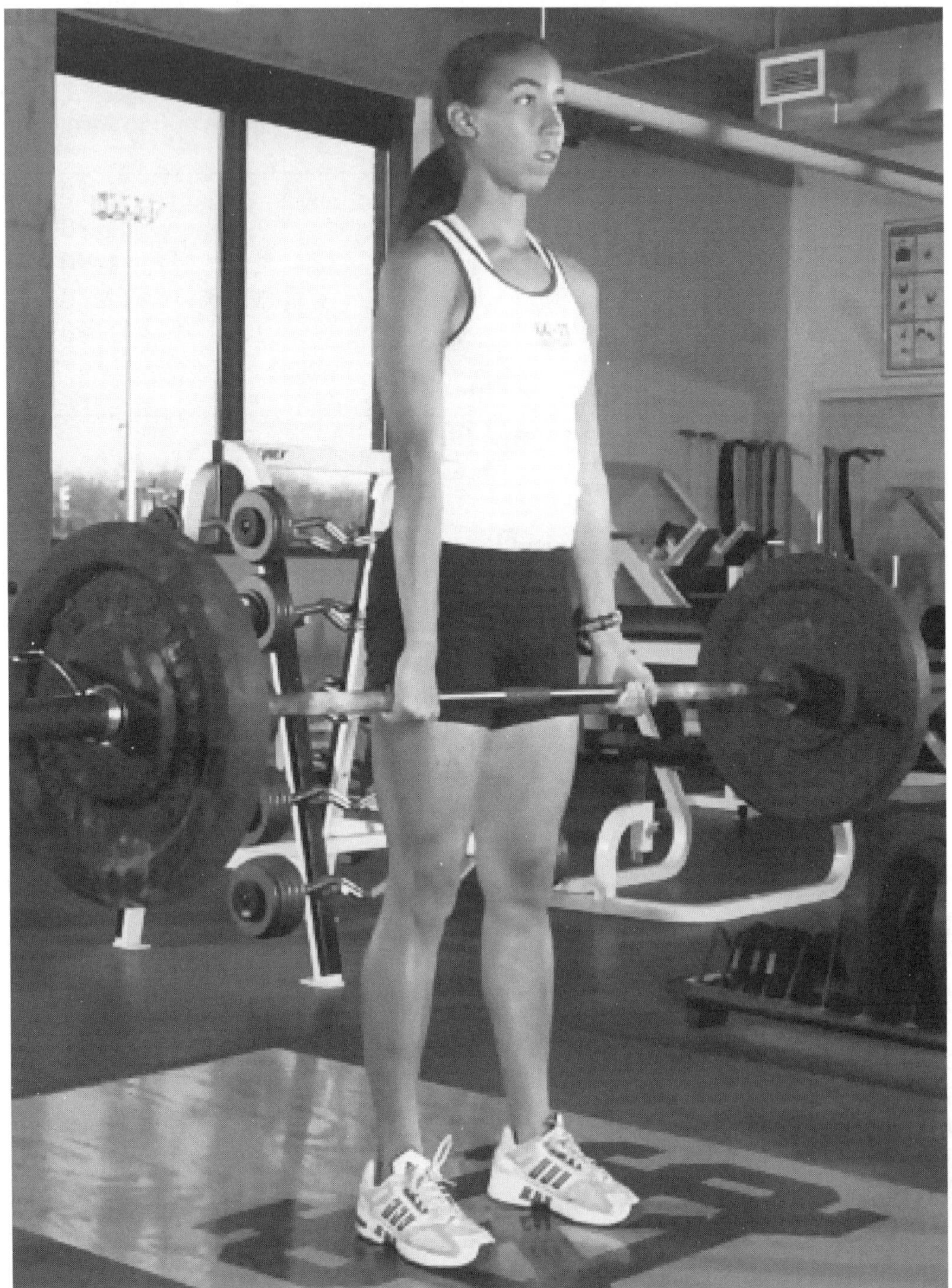

Figure 8.7 Dead lift with alternate grip

See Figure 8.2a for the proper starting position. Assume a comfortable stance with feet slightly more than shoulder-width apart. Bend the knees, grasp and lift the bar from the floor keeping the back straight. Hold the bar at the thighs before bending the knees to place the bar back on the floor.

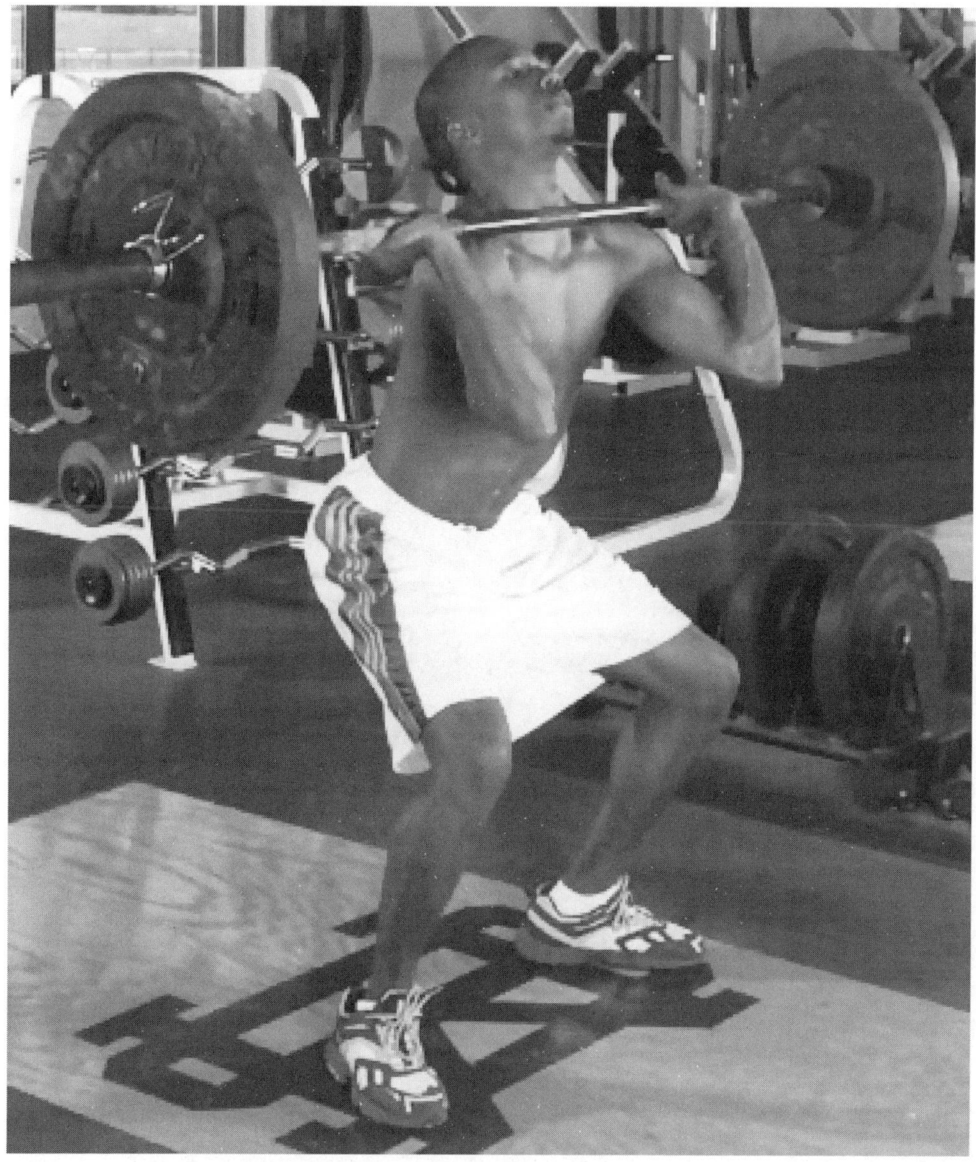

a

Figure 8.8 a, b Front squat

Take the bar from a weight rack, using a weight belt to support the back. For the *front squat*, position the bar on the shoulders so it rests evenly on the deltoids. Spread the feet comfortably with toes slightly out. Placing the toes in various positions will work different parts of the thighs. Keep the neck and back straight and elbows lifted high throughout the lift. Inhale to support the trunk at the start and bend the knees as far as possible until the upper thighs are parallel to the ground. Exhale and return to a standing position until the upper thighs are slightly below a position parallel to the ground. A thick board or weight can also be placed under the heels. The added height will work the front part of the thighs more.

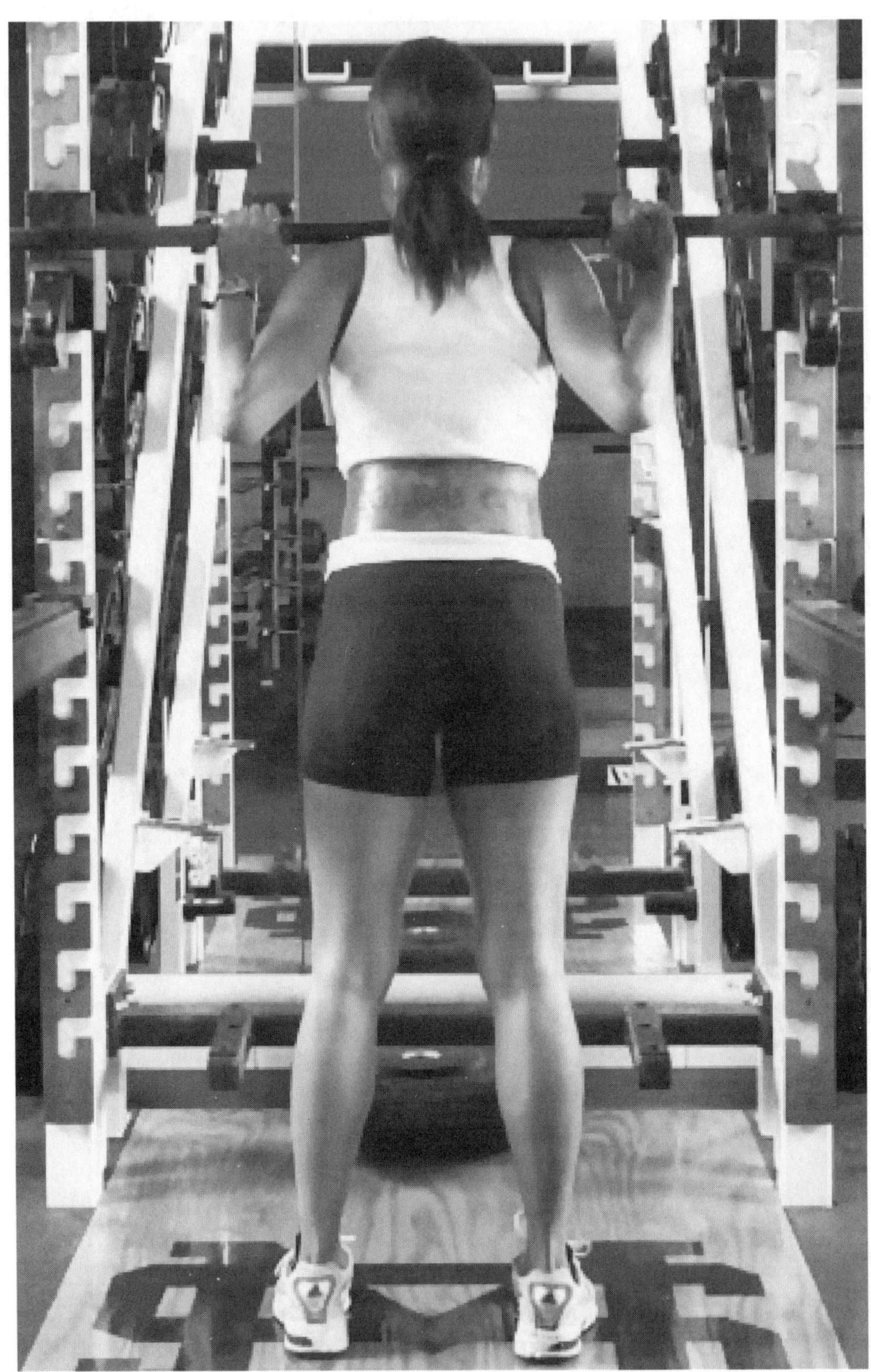

b. Back Squat

For the *back squat*, position the bar on the shoulders behind the head and execute the same movements as the front squat.

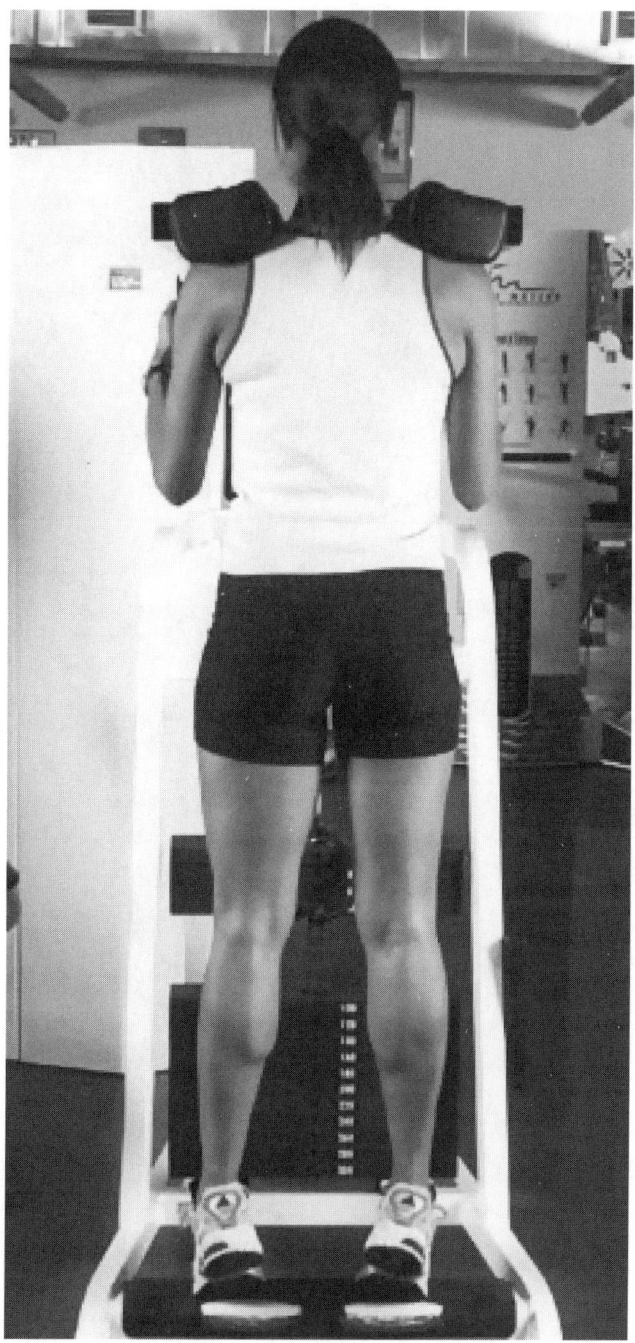

Figure 8.9 Toe raises

Toe raises can be done on a machine, using a padded barbell, or with a partner sitting on your back. Repeat the exercise with the feet in the following three positions to develop all aspects of the calf: heels out, heels straight, and heels in. The clean, snatch, hi-pull, sprinting drills, and plyometrics also all work the calves and reduce the need for toe raises.

Shoulder and Arm

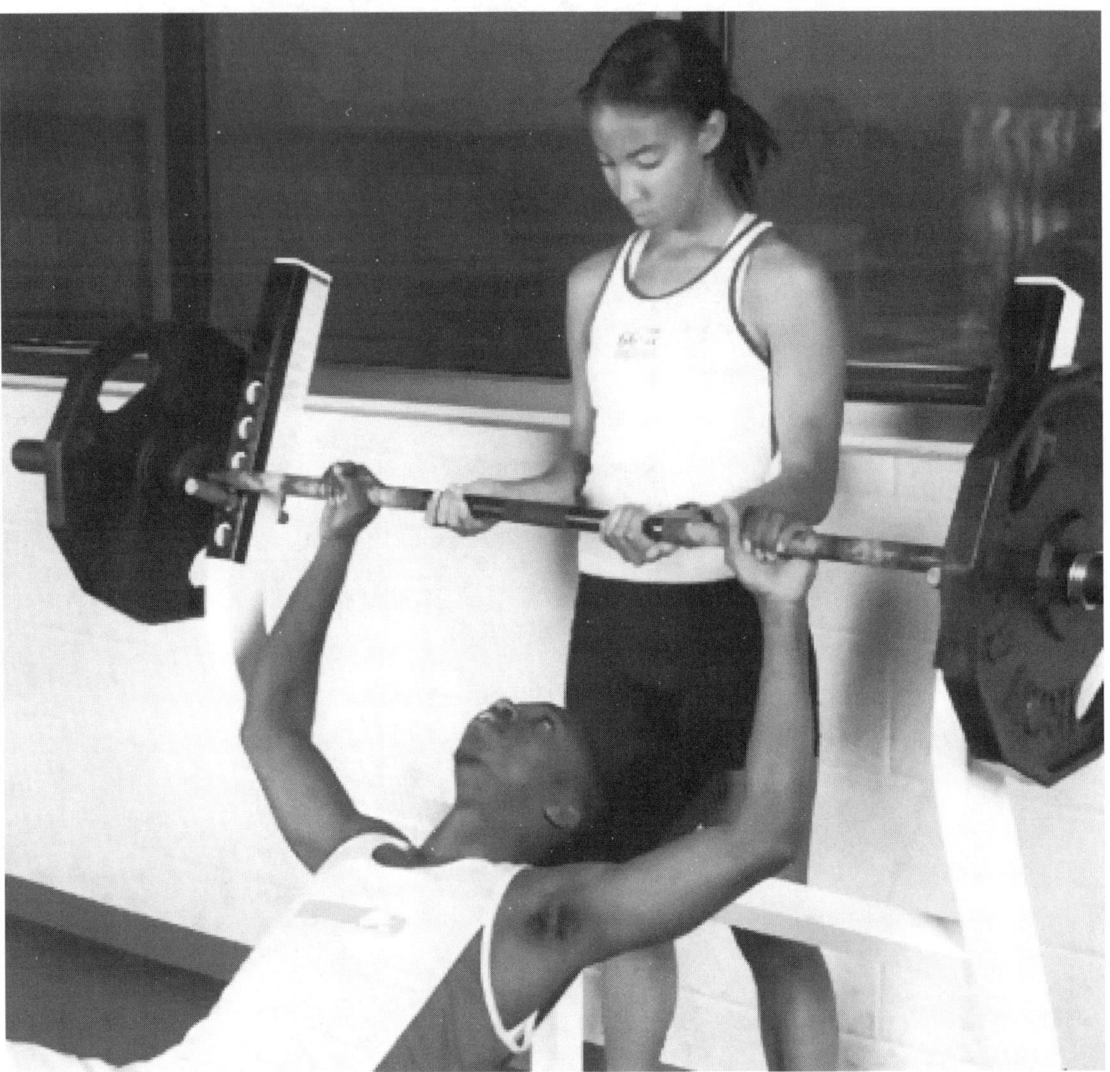

8.10 Incline press (dumbbell and barbell)

The incline press develops the chest, shoulders and arms. It also closely simulates the working angles of the muscles in many sports. With the bench in an incline position, place both hands on the bar at or slightly wider than shoulder-width. Hands that are spread wide work the shoulders and chest; whereas hands positioned closer together on the bar work the triceps more. Inhale as the elbows bend and bring the bar to the chest. Exhale as the arms are straighten and returned to the starting position.

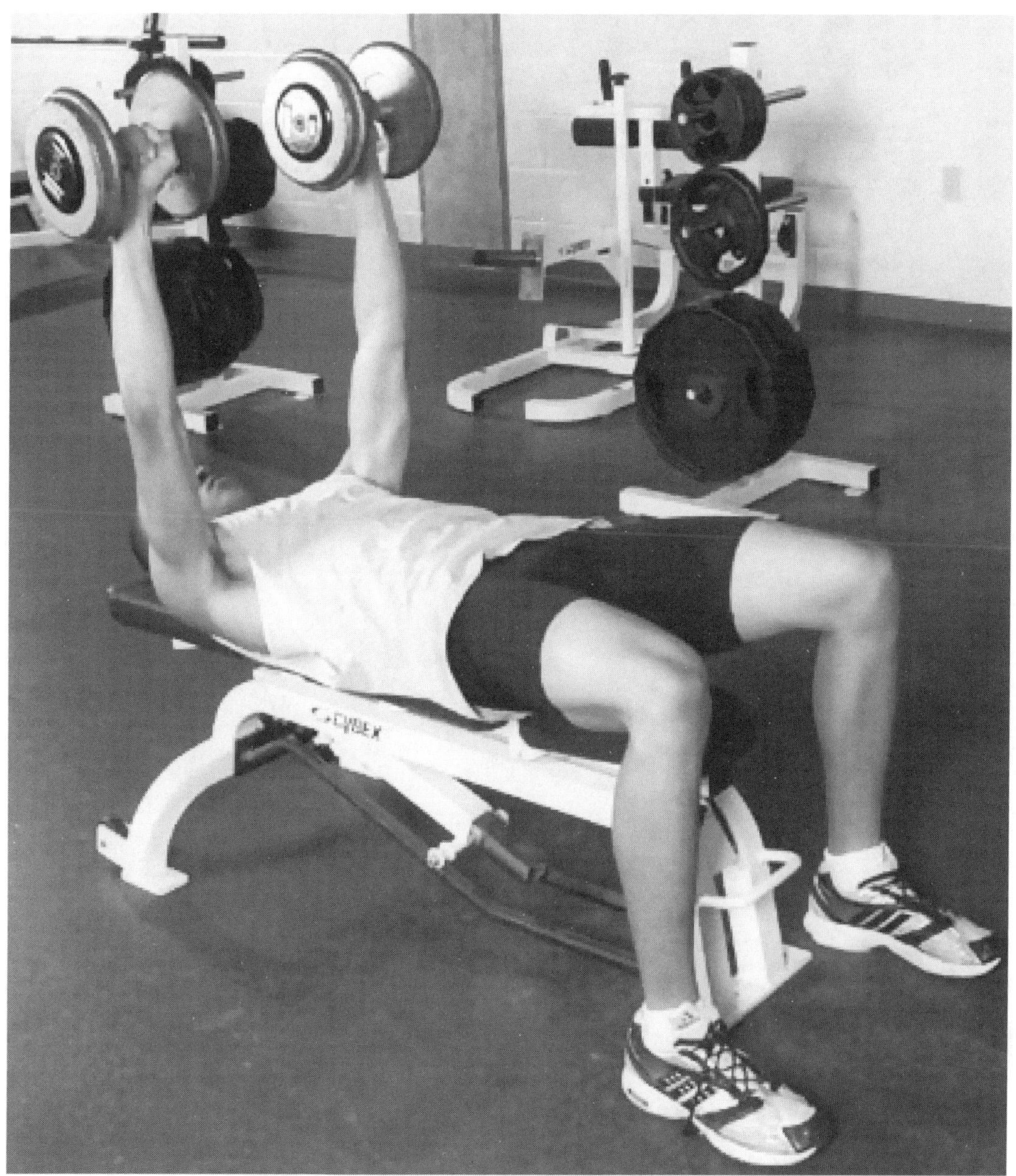

Figure 8.11 Bench press

The bench press strengthens the shoulders and arms for optimal shoulder girdle protection. With the bench flat, position the hands at or slightly wider than shoulder-width. Inhale and lower the weight to the chest. Exhale as the arms are straightened and returned to the starting position.

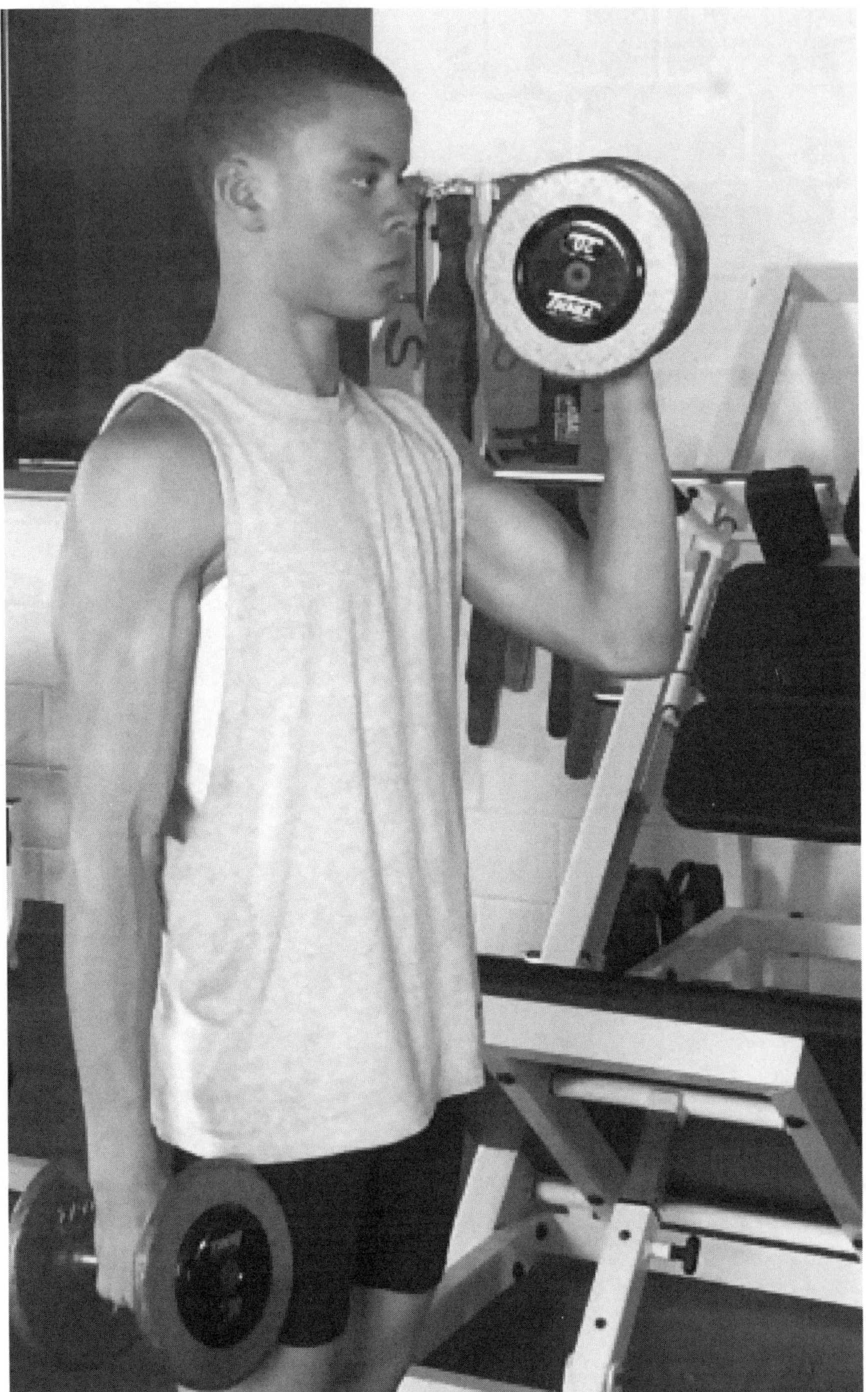

Figure 8.12 Dumbbell arm curls

Dumbbell curls develop arm strength and help maintain proper left-to-right muscle balance. For the alternate curl, hold each dumbbell at the side with palms facing the body. As each arm curls forward one at a time, rotate the palm upward. The curling arm moves down as the opposite arm moves up. Take one breath for each cycle of left and right arm curls. Also, complete several sets of this exercise by starting with the palms facing backward (reverse curl) to work the biceps more as the palm is rotated.

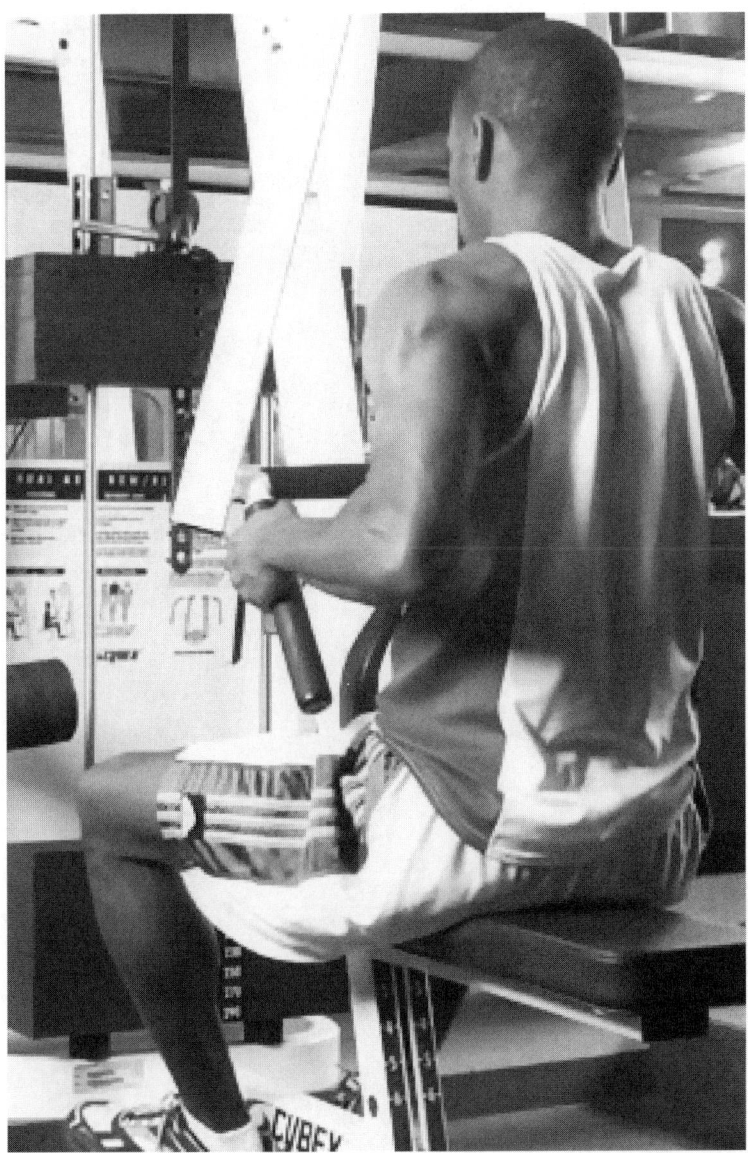

Figure 8.13 Lat row (machine, dumbbell or barbell) or bent over rows

The lat row strengthens the chest, back, shoulders, and arms. Execute the lat row using different hand positions to isolate different muscles. Exhale as the cable is pulled toward the chest, making sure the trunk is vertical. Inhale as the arms return to the starting position, following the same path as the pull. Completely extend the arms at the end of each repetition to stretch the lats.

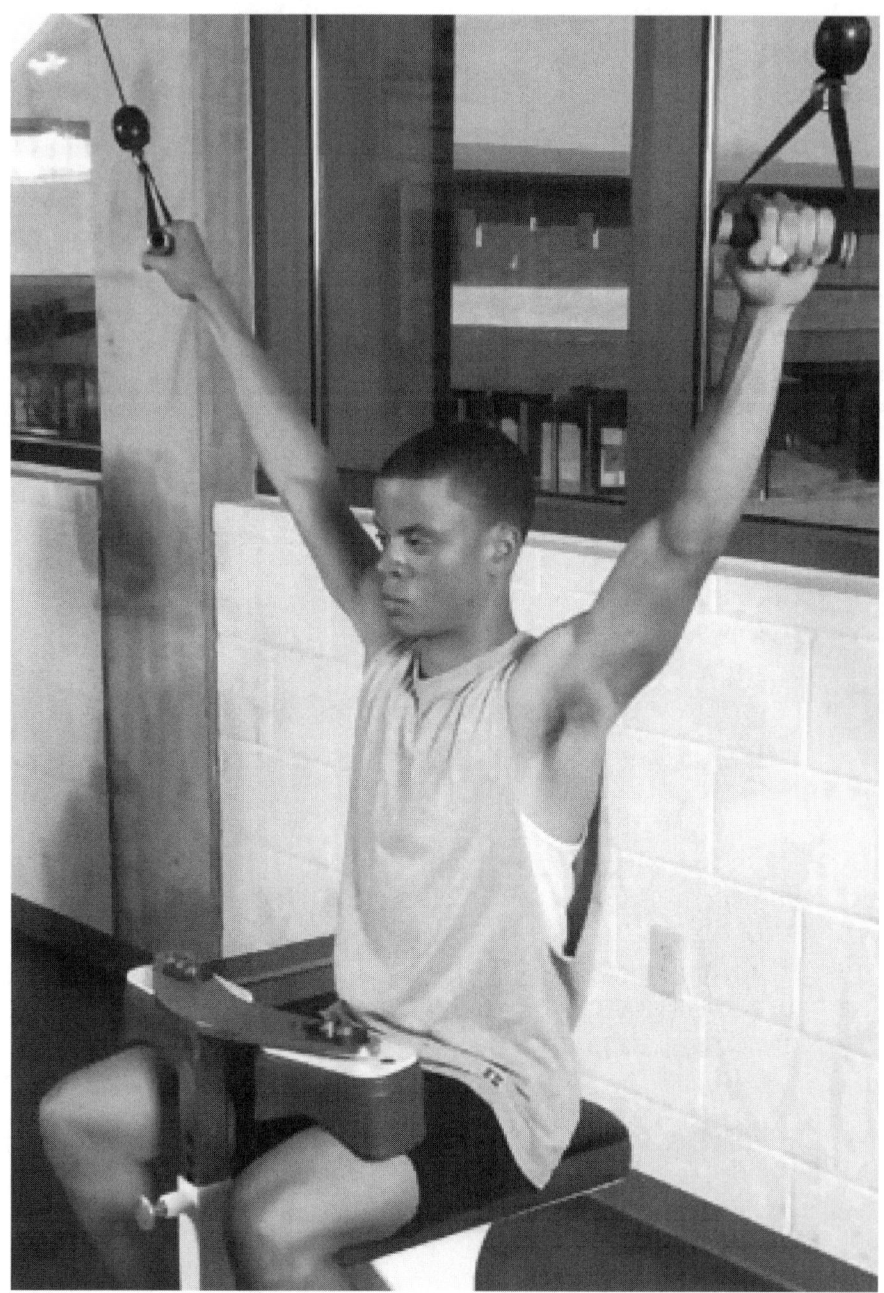

Figure 8.14 Lat pull-down

The lat pull-down strengthens the chest, back, shoulders, and arms. As in the lat row, try a variety of grips (palms away, toward, or alternated) and hand widths. Exhale while pulling the cable down to the chest or to the shoulders (concentric phase) and inhale on the upward movement (eccentric phase). Be sure to completely extend both arms at the top of each repetition to stretch the lats.

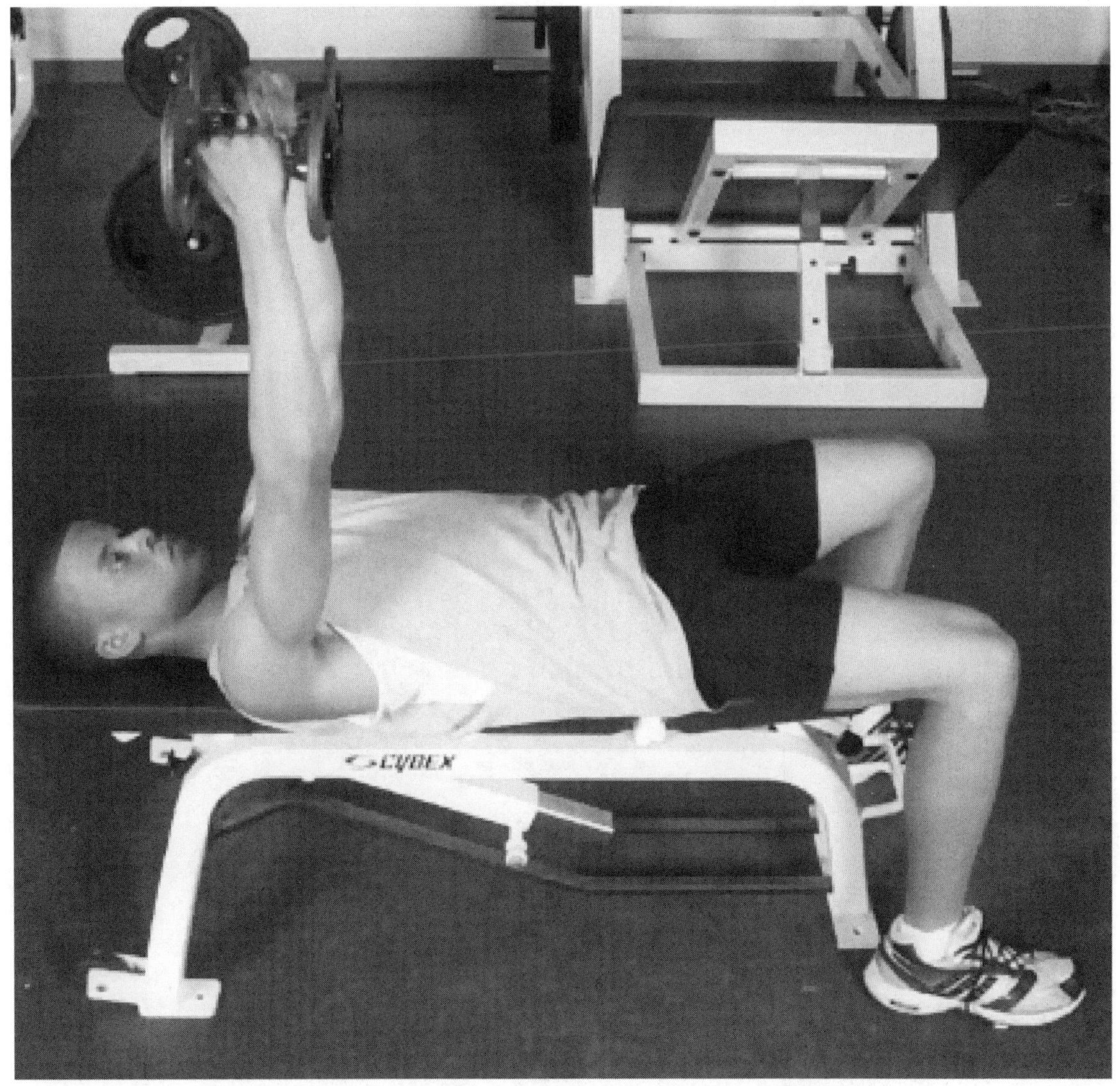

a

Figure 8.15 a,b Flys (supine)

Flys are perfect for maintaining the proper muscle balance of the chest, shoulders, and arms. The actions of this lift should cover a wide variety of shoulder movements. Lie on your back on a flat, incline, or decline bench. Hold the dumbbells over the body, arms extended with a slight bend at the elbow. Inhale as the dumbbells are lowered to the side, keeping the arms slightly bent until reaching a maximum range of motion. Exhale and return to the starting position.

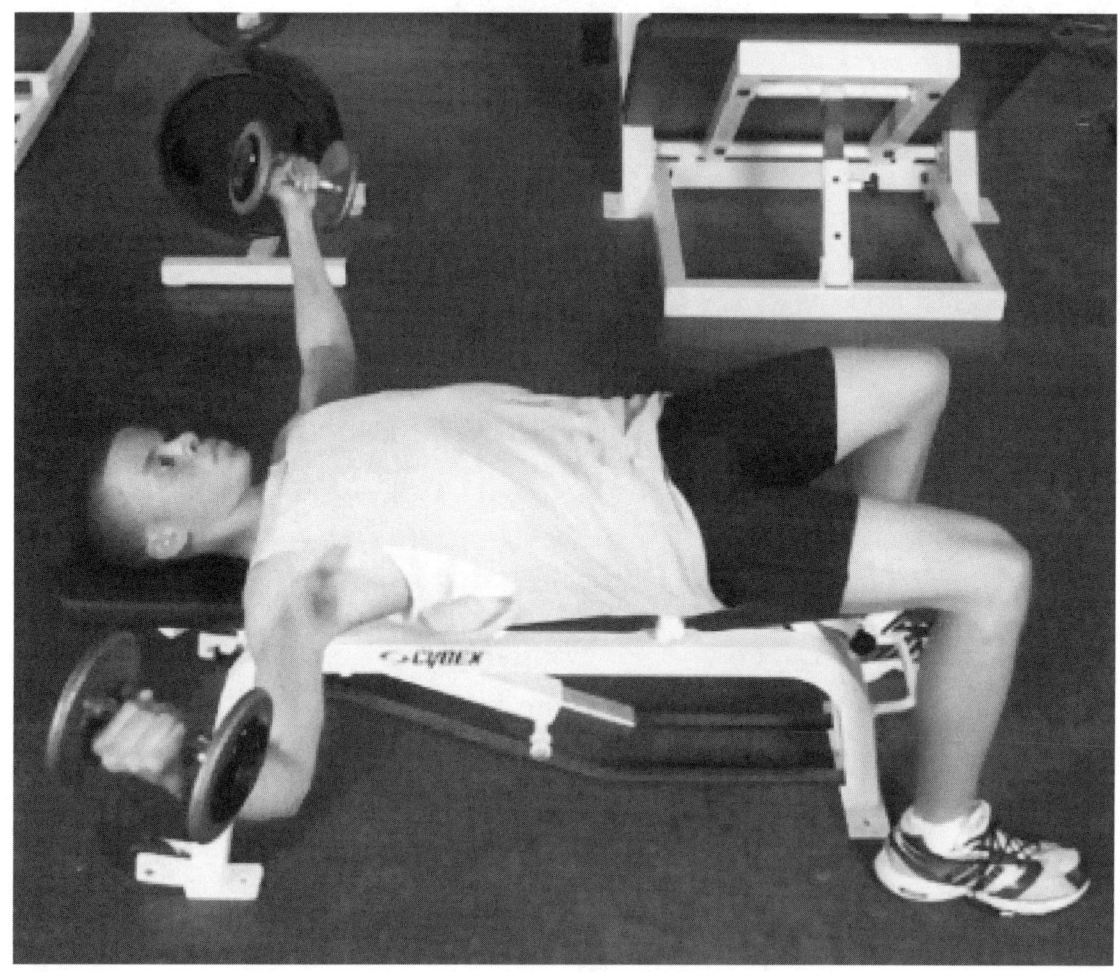

b

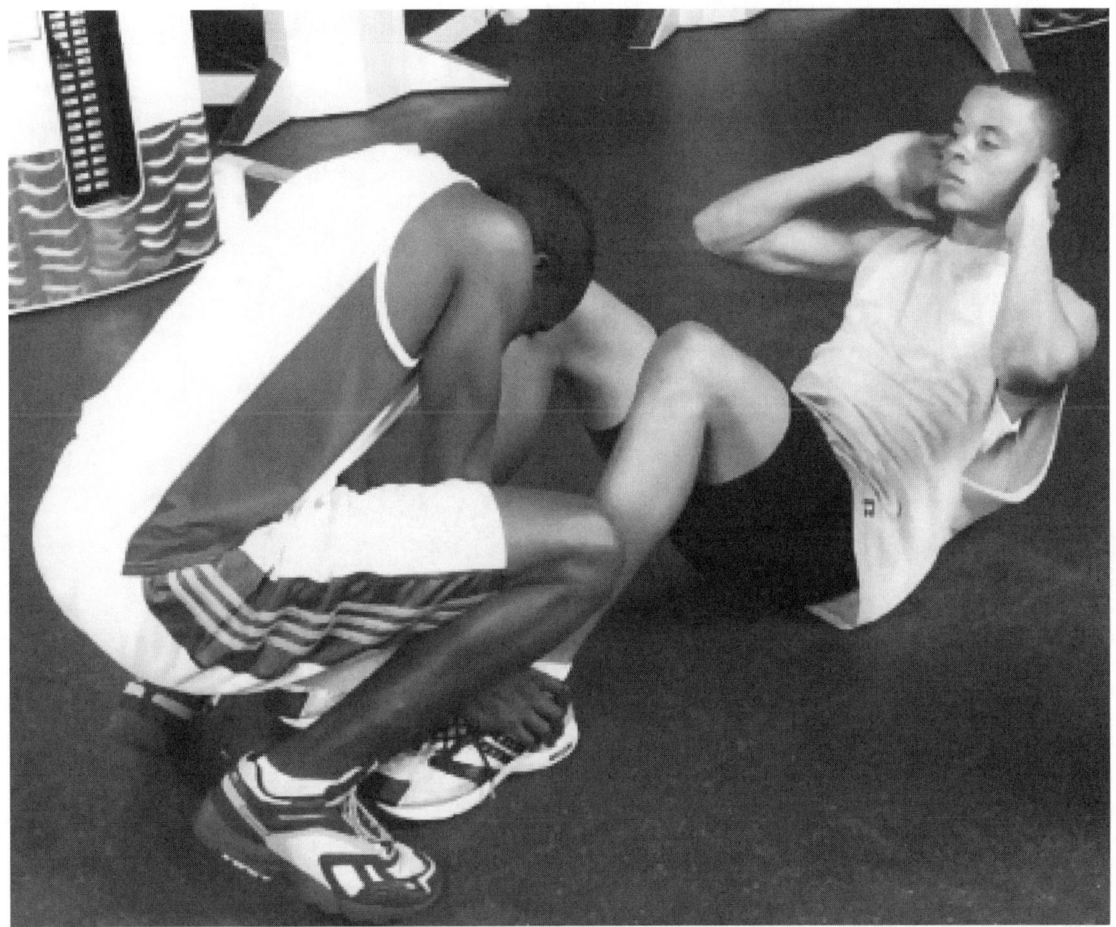

Figure 8.16 Abdominal crunches

Flex the abdominal muscles and force out air as the body is curled. The shoulders should clear the floor slightly. Hold and exhale while returning to the floor. Use twisting actions in the curl to work all aspects of the trunk.

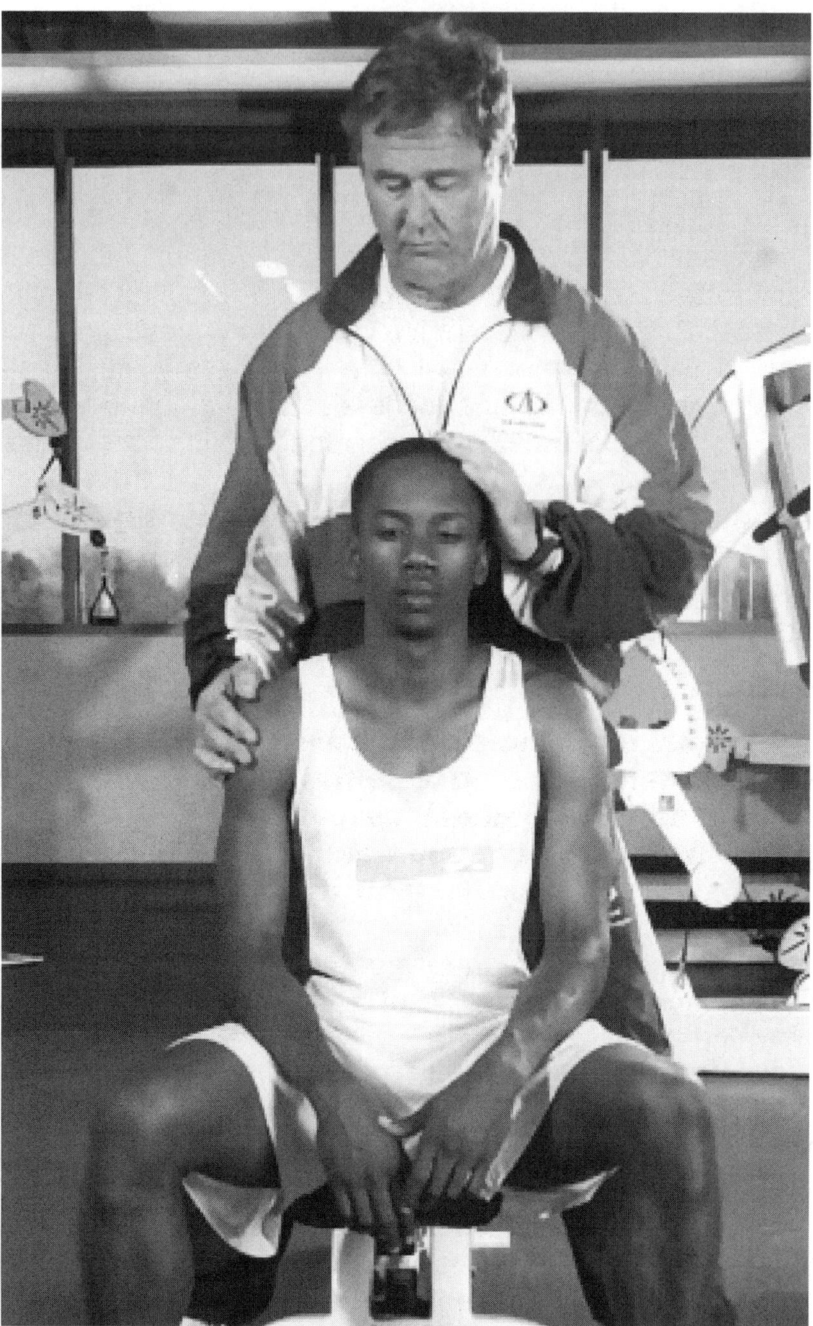

Figure 8.17 Neck strengthening

Many athletes often fail to develop their necks adequately. The two-person exercise shown above prepares the neck for the movements that occur during competition in most sports. Front, back, and side movements are used. A partner places his hands in a position that permits a good pushing surface to provide resistance without discomfort. The partner applies even pressure as you push against the resistance.

How is the strength of the hamstring muscle group improved?

The hamstring-to-quadriceps ratio using the double and single leg extension and the double and single leg curl presented in Chapter 2 do uncover gross differences in quadriceps and hamstring strength as well as identify left and right leg imbalances. Results also point out the need for further testing at different joint angles. Most athletes, however, need additional training to increase the speed-strength of the hamstring muscle group.

Many experts feel that the hamstrings are the sprinters weakest link. This is also true for team sport athletes. Very few are equally strong in both muscle groups (e.g., some elite sprinters, power lifters such as former world champion Dr. "Squat" Fred Hatfield, and some defensive backs in football). In over 35 years of conducting speed camps, we've seen only *one* athlete who possessed equal strength in both muscle groups. The large majority of athletes failed to meet our minimum standard (hamstring strength should equal 75 percent of quadriceps strength).

The Olympic Lifts and the leg curl are very effective in improving hamstring strength. Isometric exercises are also effective since the angle of exertion can easily be altered. One key exercise is performed by lying on the back with one foot extended to a point several feet up a wall (different angles are used). Athletes exert a downward isometric pull with a straight leg and hold that contraction for 8 to 10 seconds, repeating the exercise three to five times before moving to the opposite leg. This downward pull is similar to the "paw down" movement used during the sprinting action.

Sprint-resisted training (weighted suits, vests, or pants) using backward sprinting can be added to the drills described in Chapter 11 for extra loading of the lower extremities. University of Massachusetts Strength Coach, Bob Otrando recommends that defensive backs in football end each workout with repetitions of backward sprinting to improve back pedaling skills. Training loads should be kept light enough to allow athletes to reach high backward sprinting speed. Backward high speed sprinting repetitions without added weight are also an important aspect of improving the speed-strength of the hamstring muscle group.

Roller skates or inline skates offer a unique method of training the muscle groups at the hip, knee, and ankle (gluteus, hamstrings, quadriceps, calf muscles) responsible for the driving force behind high levels of sprinting. Four areas of conditioning are recommended using skates.

- Moving the hips and legs in all directions while holding onto a chair and completing 8 to 12 repetitions. Athletes progress to three sets over a period of 3 weeks.

- High speed sprint-assisted drills using surgical tubing and both forward and backward movement.

• Overspeed skate leg cycling. Athletes hold on to a support and move the legs as fast as possible in a back and forth motion completing 3 to 5 sets of 3 to 12 repetitions with maximum rest (full recovery) between each set. After an initial adjustment period, athletes are able to complete each set without holding on.

• Speed endurance exercises. Athletes move back and forth at high speed for 10 to 30 seconds, working up to 60 seconds. A gradual build up occurs to 8 to 12 repetitions in sets of four, resting 30 seconds to several minutes depending upon the sport.

Strengthening the Knee

What type of training should athletes do to prevent knee injuries?

According to most orthopedic surgeons, it is important to have strong legs from the ankle to the hips. There are 13 muscles that provide the tension to support the knee. Each must be properly strengthened to give the knee maximum support throughout the total range of motion. A review of the literature in the September/October 2008 issue of *Sports Medicine Reports* suggests that the risk of knee ligament tears and other injuries can be decreased by strengthening the muscle groups surrounding the knee.

The following knee functions should be included in every program: flexion, extension, medial rotation, and stabilization. Quadriceps and hamstrings are the major muscle groups that affect knee stability and motion. Quadriceps are related to straightening of the knees and movement of the kneecap. Hamstrings are related to bending of the knees and the pushing action against a surface. The strengthening of these muscles are the key to injury prevention. The squat, dead lift, power clean, and leg curl exercises are four of the most important exercises to accomplish this objective.

In spite of the best conditioning efforts, the knee remains very vulnerable to injury in team sports from twisting, torque, and contact while a foot is firmly planted.

BALLISTIC TRAINING

Dr. Bob Ward, strength and conditioning coach of the Dallas cowboys during the entire Landry coaching era, is a strong supporter of ballistic training for athletes in football, basketball, rugby, lacrosse and soccer. Bob introduced numerous innovative methods into the Dallas Cowboy off-season and in-season workouts. One of his favorites was ballistics.

What is ballistic training and how is it used?

The ability of body tissues to deliver, transmit, and absorb energy is fundamental to human performance and survival in football and other sports. Not all tissues are capable of managing energy at the same level. In fact, the ability ratings for energy absorption capacity of the most important tissues shown in Figure 8.18 may surprise you.

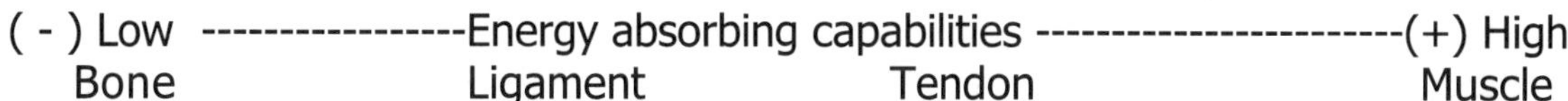

Figure 8.18 Energy absorbing capabilities of bone, ligament, tendon, and tissue

Ballistics are a needed supplement to traditional speed-strength training since the program improves the energy absorbing capabilities of bone, ligament, tendon and muscle tissue in a different way and involves movements and actions not found in other training programs. There are three categories of energy management:

1. *Sending energy away from the body.* This category includes all types of hitting, kicking, and throwing various implements, from footballs to medicine balls, to assorted weights.

2. *Receiving energy from outside sources.* Forces that come into the body in the form of a ball or opposing player are included in this category. Any form of catching develops the necessary sensitivity needed for receiving outside forces.

3. *The zone or flow state.* Whatever this state is finally discovered to be, most athletes who claim they have "been there" report that it feels effortless. Time and motion slow, and performance approaches an almost spiritual level. All of these factors permit athletes to perform at levels closer to their maximum potential. It is important to recognize that there are degrees and levels of flow. Furthermore, each level or amount of time in the zone will bring a different degree of performance enhancement. The higher the level, the higher the level of energy management. Many off-season training programs fail to systematically toughen the body in preparation for the level of sending and receiving energy that occurs in sports such as football and other sports that have some physical contact even if physical contact is not part of the game. Although speed-strength programs do have a toughening effect, other methods such as ballistics are needed to move the body to higher levels of toughness. Boxers have used medicine balls for

decades. The Dallas Cowboys used medicine balls on a regular basis to sensitize the neuromuscular system to respond instantly to contact. Many present-day systems fail to recognize the importance of delivering and redirecting these outside forces to the athlete's advantage. Very few of the many outstanding high school, college, and professional players we have coached demonstrated skill in the sophisticated unity of resisting and yielding.

What special equipment is needed?

Medicine balls or sandbags weighing 2 to 25 pounds and a mini trampoline is commonly used. Sandbags can be made from the inner tube of an automobile by tying the tube off at one end, filling with sand, then tying it off again after the desired weight has been achieved.

What exercises are recommended?

Many different movements involving the arms, legs, and torso are used in team sports. Some key exercises and drills are listed below.

- *Medicine ball toughening catches.* The medicine ball is thrown in the air or at the mini-trampoline and caught with the body. The object is to catch the ball and absorb the shock with body movements and various body parts. Catches can be done alone, with a partner, or group.

- *Medicine ball throws and toughening catches.* Complete 8-10 seated throws, forward throws (underhand and overhand), backward throws (overhead), and side throws (left side and front, right side and front; left side and back, right side and back).

- *"Overweight" implement programs for all throwing actions.* Designed for pitchers, quarterbacks, javelin throwers, and any athlete who needs to improve the throwing action. Begin with the heavy ball for foundation and progress to lighter balls. The heavy ball strengthens the muscles and joints used in throwing, establishing a sound foundation; lighter weights allow the high-speed throwing action needed to improve throwing skills. Throwing into a net is a high intensity workout that allows more throws and less wasted time.

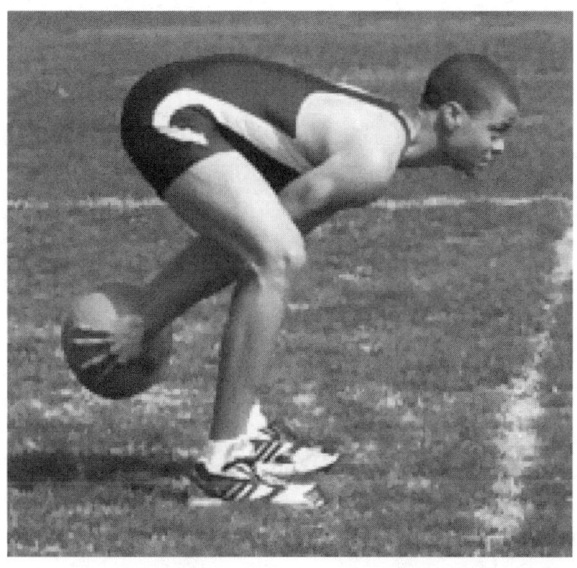

Figure 8.19 Underhand throw

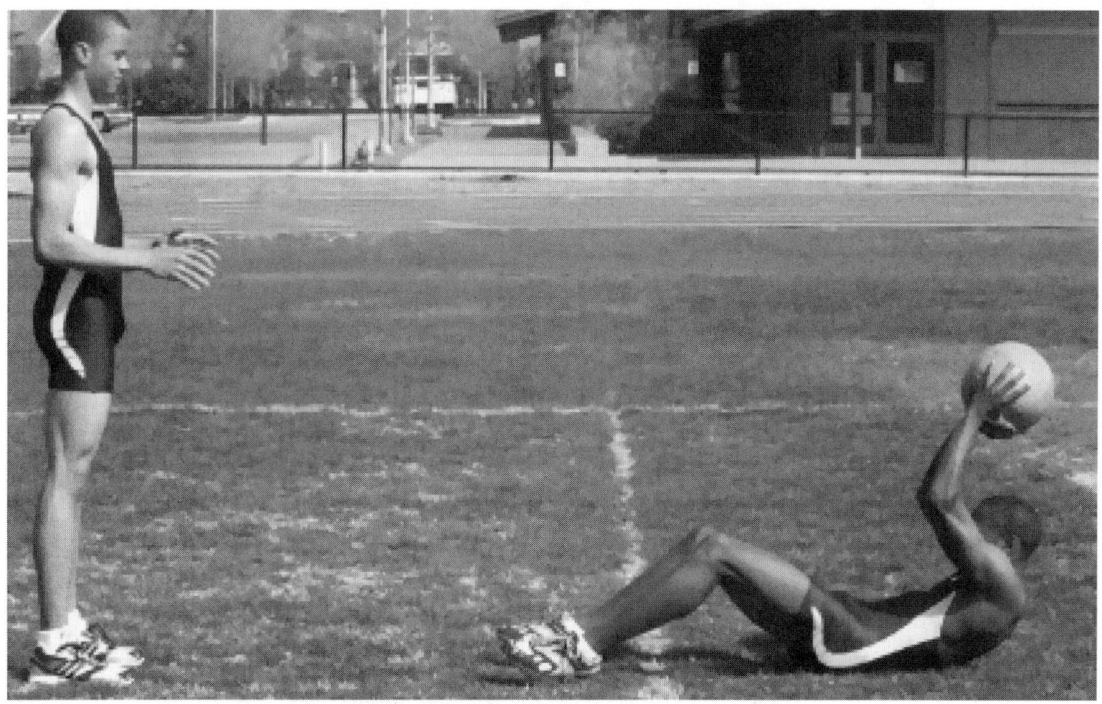

Figure 8.20 Seated throws

PLYOMETRICS

The word plyometric is derived from the Greek word pleythyein, meaning "to increase" or from the Greek roots *plio* and *metric* meaning "more" and "measure." Plyometrics refers to exercises that enable a muscle to reach maximal strength in as short a time as possible. Plyometric exercises are important in sports requiring high levels of speed-strength (ability to exert maximum force during high-speed activity) to complete movements such as starting, stopping, cutting, accelerating, sprinting, jumping, and throwing.

The term was first used in the United States in 1975, by Fred Wilt, former Olympic runner and women's track coach at Purdue University. Coach Wilt got the term from European track and field coaches who had already used plyometrics for more than a decade in the training of sprinters and athletes in jump events. Yuri Verhoshansky, coach in the Soviet Union, is credited as being one of the early pioneers and leading researchers of plyometric training. Although plyometric training was slow to be accepted in the United States, numerous articles, books, and videos produced in the 1980s and early 1990s have led to its widespread use in baseball, basketball, football, lacrosse, rugby, soccer, and other team and individual sports.

How does Plyometric Training Work?

Although plyometrics take several different forms, activities usually revolve around jumping, hopping, and bounding movements for the lower body and swinging, quick action push-off, catching and throwing weighted objects (medicine balls, shot put, sandbags), arm swings, and pulley throws for the upper body. The medicine ball throws presented in this chapter are similar to some of the ballistic exercises described in the previous section; however, the emphasis is placed on loading the abdominal and arm muscles prior to the movement or toss rather than on catching the ball. Exercises that simulate specific movements in a particular sport or activity are chosen.

Plyometrics develop both strength and power (speed-strength) in the muscles involved in sprinting. An athlete may have superior strength, yet be unable to produce the needed power to sprint a fast 20-60-yard dash. The completion of some movements in sports, such as sprinting, involve less time than it takes for the muscle to develop a maximal contraction. Evidence suggests that for such actions, an athlete will use only 60 to 80 percent of his or her absolute strength (maximum force a muscle group can produce). The key to plyometric training is to display strength as quickly and as forcefully as possible.

The unusual progress and success of Russian sprinter Valeri Borzov, 100-meter gold medal winner (10.14) in the 1972 Olympic Games, is partially attributed to the use of plyometric exercises during the six-year period prior to the games. Borzov progressed from a 100-meter time of 13.0 seconds at age 14 to 10.0 at age 20. Although all athletes will not show such dramatic improvement, the hops, jumps, bounds, leaps, skips, ricochets, swings, and twists that make up plyometrics should be an important part of a speed improvement program.

Plyometrics focus on two key aspects of speed strength: *starting strength*, which is the ability to instantaneously recruit as many muscle fibers as possible, and *explosive strength*, which is the ability to keep the initial explosion of a muscle contraction going over a distance against some resistance. Starting strength is the key to sprinting a fast 20 to 100 yards, throwing or kicking a ball, and similar movements requiring little more than body resistance to be overcome. Examples of explosive strength are football blocking, throwing the shot put or hammer, Olympic weight lifting, power lifting, and other movements requiring considerable resistance. As Yessis and Hatfield point out in their book on plyometrics (1986), "the lighter the implement you have to move and the shorter the distance, the more your starting strength becomes important; the heavier the resistance and the longer the distance, the more important your explosive strength becomes.

The main objective of plyometric training is to improve an athlete's ability to generate maximum force in the shortest time. This is accomplished by first loading or coiling muscles to accumulate energy before unloading this energy in the opposite direction. The force of gravity (such as the action of stepping off a box) is used to store energy in the muscles that are immediately released in an opposite reaction (bounding or jumping up or forward upon landing). In other words, plyometric exercises involve powerful muscular contraction in response to the rapid, dynamic loading (stretching) of the involved muscles.

Most athletes already apply the basic concept of plyometrics (loading and unloading) when they cock their wrist or ankle before throwing a baseball or football, hitting a baseball, shooting a basketball, kicking a soccer ball or football, swinging a golf club, or executing the forehand or backhand stroke in tennis. The rapid stretching (loading) of these muscles activates the stretch reflex, which sends a powerful stimulus to the muscles causing them to contract faster and with more power. In the actions listed above, athletes are rapidly stretching a muscle group and then transferring the energy by immediately contracting that same group. A rapid deceleration of a mass is followed by a rapid acceleration of the mass in another direction. The loading or stretching action is sometimes called the *yielding* phase, and the reflex contraction of the muscles is called the *overcoming* phase. The object is to obtain a maximum eccentric contraction (muscle develops tension while lengthening) to load the muscle, and switch this contraction to concentric (muscle develops tension while shortening), which produces the desired explosive movement.

Rapid loading of the muscles (yielding phase) must occur just prior to the contraction phase of these same muscles. When jumping from an elevated platform to the ground, for example, the legs bend under the g-force (kinetic energy), and an immediate reactive jump occurs. How much the legs bend depends upon the g-force and the stored energy that will be used to release the powerful contraction to jump.

What plyometric training guidelines should be followed?

The following guidelines and concepts will improve the effectiveness of your program:

- Plyometrics is merely a type of resistance training to develop strength and power. The force of gravity is used to store energy in the muscles that are then immediately used in an opposite reaction causing the elastic properties of the muscle to produce kinetic energy.

- Athletes should be strong enough to squat 1.5 X body weight before starting any program.

- Exercises should correspond to the form, muscle work, and range of motion in a sport or activity. The main goal is to rapidly apply overload force to the muscles to improve speed-strength.

- Exercises should correspond to the correct direction of movement. Because the leg moves toward the rear in one phase of sprinting, some plyometric movements should also be directed toward the rear.

- The rate of the stretch is strongly tied to the effectiveness of plyometric training; the higher the stretch rate, the greater the muscle tension and the more powerful the concentric contraction in the opposite direction.

- Workouts begin with low impact plyometrics followed by higher impact.

- Exercises to improve sprinting speed should explode at the beginning of the movement and allow inertia to move the limb through the remaining range of motion. In one phase of sprinting, for example, maximum effort is exerted at the point athletes begin to pull the thigh through and diminishes as the leg passes underneath the body.

- Too much weight (vest, ankle spats) may increase strength without much effect on power and make it impossible to jump or sprint explosively, which defeats the purpose of the plyometric workout. The body already provides considerable resistance. Adding excessive weight is unnecessary. Light weight or body weight is recommended to develop quick force. Alternating light (1 to 2 percent of body weight, no more than 2 to 3 pounds) and heavier weight (5 to 6 percent of body weight, no more than 10 to 12 pounds) in the same plyometric exercise is also an excellent technique.

• Whenever possible, a plyometric exercise should be performed at a speed faster than one is capable of producing without some assistance. The object is to use a "down time" (the time the feet are on the ground, the amortization or "paying off" phase of plyometrics) that is less than the down time in sprinting. The faster a muscle is forced to lengthen, the greater the tension it exerts. Also, the closer the stretch of the muscle is to the contraction, the more violent the contraction. When jumping from boxes or bleachers, there is no hesitation after ground contact. The object is to be on the ground as little time as possible by shortening the span between contact and takeoff. The use of box jumps to increase the loading phase and surgical tubing to decrease the resistance to be overcome in speed hops are examples of techniques that allow a more forceful load or a faster contraction speed. This method conditions the nervous system to experience the higher speed so it can duplicate it later in competition without any assistance.

• Athletes must make a strong effort to handle the forces of landing with as little flexion of the joints as possible. When jumping on a flat surface or off boxes, too much flexion of the legs upon landing increases the time spent on the ground, absorbs most of the force, and allows very little pre-loading or tensing. As soon as the balls of the feet touch the floor, the knees are rapidly flexed to a comfortable jumping position (never beyond right angles). This proper knee flexion position also prevents excessive ankle flexion.

• Correct form is emphasized for each exercise. A key aspect of proper technique is assuming a knee/thumbs-up position (knees bent just above a right angle, elbows to the sides with hands in front of the body and thumbs facing upward) to help maintain balance and center the workload around the hips and legs. For upper body exercise, proper follow-through is also stressed. For each specific exercise, the quality (proper form and speed) of each jump rather than the quantity is most important.

• Coaches differ in the order of their placement of plyometric training in a workout. Some are careful to use the program near the end of the workout since a plyometric session is so demanding and interferes with high speed drills and scrimmage that may need to be completed in the absence of fatigue. In the off-season, the use of selected sprint-specific plyometric exercises can be used in the weight room program during the recovery period after each speed-strength set involving an exercise to improve ground contact force.

• A highly explosive movement in sports does not occur automatically. Athletes do not sprint at maximum speed, serve at 120+ miles per hour in tennis, kick a ball 60+ yards, or jump 25+ feet without being "psyched" prior to the movement. It takes a concentrated mental effort to perform these actions and this should be emphasized during plyometric workouts.

- Adequate recovery is necessary between each high-intensity plyometric workout. A minimum of 48 hours is recommended. Alternating light-intensity and high-intensity workouts permit the use of additional workouts weekly if necessary.

Safety Precautions

What safety precaution should be followed o prevent injury?

Although surveys reveal that plyometric training is not likely to result in injury, unsound and/or unsupervised programs could potentially cause shin splints and knee, ankle, and lower back problems. These injuries are often a direct result of too many workouts per week (one session weekly may be sufficient), too many jumps per workout, poor form, jumping on hard surfaces, and using plyometrics at too early an age or without the necessary strength and conditioning base. To reduce the chances of injury, follow these guidelines:

- Preadolescent boys and girls should avoid plyometrics, unless other factors indicate more advanced maturity, because of greater susceptibility to injury prior to puberty.

- Plyometrics should also be postponed for athletes who do not have a sufficient strength and conditioning base. Lower body plyometrics should be avoided until an athlete can leg press 2.0 to 2.5 times their body weight, and upper body exercise until five consecutive clap push-ups can be performed. Athletes weighing more than 260 pounds should also be capable of bench pressing their body weight; athletes weighing less than 160 pounds should be capable of bench pressing 1.5 times their body weight. Athletes falling between 160 and 260 should be able to meet the gradations of these guidelines (160-184: 1.4, 185-209: 1.3, 210-234: 1.2, 235-259: 1.1).

- Experts recommend that large athletes over 250 lb. avoid high volume, high intensity exercises since they may be more susceptible to injury. Very large football players such as interior linemen must also take extra precautions.

- Athletes who do not respond well to the instructions of coaches are also at greater risk of injury and over training.

• A general warm-up period consisting of walk-jog-stride-sprint cycles for one-half to three-quarters of a mile, followed by dynamic stretching exercises should precede each plyometric workout.

• Footwear should provide good ankle and arch support, lateral stability, and a wide, non-slip sole, such as a basketball or aerobic shoe. Running shoes with narrow soles and poor upper support can lead to ankle problems and are not recommended. Heel cups may be needed for those who are prone to heel bruises.

• Plyometrics should be performed only on surfaces with good shock-absorbing properties, such as soft grassy areas, well-padded artificial turf, and wrestling mats. Asphalt or gymnasium floors should be avoided.

• Boxes should be sturdy and have a non-slip top.

• Depth jumping from objects that are too high increases the risk of injury, particularly to larger athletes, and prevents the rapid switch from eccentric to concentric activity. The average recommended heights for depth jumps are 0.75 to 0.8 meters. Athletes over 250 pounds should use heights of 0.5 to 0.75 meters.

• Plyometric training should be supervised at all times. The number of sessions weekly should not exceed 2 for a maximum of 15-20 minutes each session, and the total number of quality jumps per session should be carefully controlled.

How often should athletes engage in plyometric training?

Plyometric workouts should be scheduled no more than two times weekly during the off-season period in most sports and once weekly during the in-season period as part of a maintenance program.

How much volume or number of jumps should be completed each workout?

To date, there is no magic number of jumps (foot or feet contacts with the surface) that are known to produce the best results. Coaches at various levels use different number of repetitions, sets, and total jumps in a single workout and realize that taking too few jumps is better than taking too many. Ideally, the number of jumps should not exceed 80 to 100 per workout session for beginners and athletes in early workouts, 100 to 120 per session for intermediate-level athletes, and 120 to 140 per session for advanced athletes who have completed four to six weeks of plyometric training.

How is the intensity of a plyometric workout controlled?

The amount of stress placed upon the muscles, the connective tissue, and the joints is referred to as *intensity*. Skipping movements provide minimum stress and are considered low-intensity exercises; box jumping, two-foot takeoff and landing exercises, high-speed movements, and using additional weight, all increase the intensity of the workout. A program should progress from low-to high-intensity exercises, and low-to-high volume.

It is important to remember that the objective is to improve speed-strength, not speed endurance. Thus, adequate rest (recovery) between repetitions and sets during a workout is required. For example, recovery for box jumping may take 5 to 10 seconds between repetitions, and two to three minutes between sets. In repeated jumps where limited ground contact is stressed, there is no recovery period between repetitions since the athlete immediately "unloads" into the next repetition. Adequate recovery is needed, however, between sets.

How much recovery time is needed between workouts?

Plyometric training is extremely strenuous and a minimum of 48 hours of rest is needed to fully recover. Recovery between workouts is generally two to four days, depending on the sport and time of year. Two days is generally sufficient during the preseason; a period of three to four days is appropriate during the competitive season. The key to a successful program is to do each explosive movement with perfect form.

How is the progressive resistance exercise principle (PRE) applied to make certain improvement in speed-strength occurs?

Exercises progress from low-intensity, in-place exercises for beginners to medium-intensity, and then to high-intensity levels for advanced athletes. Table 8.10 outlines a 10-week off-season program that moves from low- to medium- to high-intensity exercises over a period of six weeks. Numerous variations can be developed using this table and selecting exercise choices from the low-, medium-, and high-intensity exercises. In six to eight weeks, when high-intensity plyometric drills become the foundation of the program, the volume of exercises should decrease. A plyometric program begins eight weeks from the start of the competitive season in a sport, using a program such as the one shown in table 8.11.

WHAT THE EXPERTS SAY ABOUT PLYOMETRICS

The interview responses to the questions below from Russ Ebbets, track coach, were made by a leading expert on plyometrics, Dr. James Radcliffe, Strength and Conditioning Coach, University of Oregon 1985-Present; author of *Plyometrics: Explosive Power Training* and *High-Powered Plyometrics.* These responses are helpful in understanding the importance and role of plyometric training in sports.

What does the term plyometrics mean to you?

Plyometrics means a style of training utilizing exercises that are explosive and take advantage of the elastic-reactive components of the neuromuscular system. This includes any form of jumping, bounding, hopping, throwing, and tossing movements that combine the effects of eccentric loading and the rate of concentric execution.

At what point do you feel an athlete is ready for plyometric work? Is there safe plyometric work for a novice or Junior Olympian?

Researchers support utilizing plyometrics in 12-14 year olds as preparation for future strength training, suggesting moderate training progressions. The "1.5 times body weight" criterion was initially suggested for depth jumps and shock training, yet doesn't need to be applied to the successful performance and training of other plyometric progressions. In our research (Radcliffe, 1996), such low correlations were shown to exist between squat performance and depth jump capabilities, that any predictions are extremely insignificant. Use posture, balance, stability, and flexibility assessments as a guide for progression to the next level of training. If any of the criteria are doubtful, maintain until the criteria are met, then progress.

Where do you use plyometrics in your weekly plan? Do the plyometrics come after weight work or before? On the day of weight work or the day after?

Depending upon the emphasis for the day/session, the plyometric work can be placed immediately after the warm-up and before the sprint or strength work, "complexed" with the lifts and or sprint work within the body of the total training session, or placed at the end of the training session, before the cool-down. Work the day of explosive, dynamic, intense work, not the day after or the recovery day.

To improve the force of the pushing action against the ground, plyometrics (box jumps, depth jumps, standing broad jump, standing triple jump, and hops and bounds that closely mimic the sprinting action) should be used twice weekly during the recovery phase following the completion of each set of lower body weight training exercises.

Core strength, from a dynamic stabilization standpoint, is critical to power generation in the extremities. From either a general or specific standpoint, what are some of the moves or muscles you concentrate on in your core strength program?

Our core conditioning focuses on the torso of the body; the torso being the trunk, including the initial portion of the limbs (shoulders, hips, thighs). The concentration is on the proper execution of flexion, extension, and rotation of the torso, especially about the hips, utilizing proper posture, balance, stability, and mobility.

As a general statement--aside from the obvious rotary motions of the shot, disc and hammer, all track and field events have a heavy linear emphasis in their execution. I fully realize there are joints or body torque in any movement but I think the average coach ignores the training for dynamic stability in the medial and lateral plane (coronal plane). How do you address this?

Within the general portions of the workout sessions, care is given to emphasize work in all planes and styles of movement. The warm-up includes dynamic form movements, forward, laterally and backward. The core routines will always include flexion, extension, and rotation in all directions. With strength training, different lunge progression will employ steps out at 45- and 90-degree angles. Medicine ball multi-throw and toss progressions at similar angles are included.

It has been found that dynamic stability is more a product of endurance (red fibers) than of strength. How do you train these two important qualities that are physiologically at odds with each other?

We use assisted exercises that have higher volumes (repetitions or distances) and lighter loads or body weight exercises that involve balancing on one limb or walking/bouncing/skipping certain distances twisting or with an implement locked out over the head. Dumbbell complexes have been used by numerous coaches as another way of attending to this. The alternation of pulls, squats, and pushes in a complex of certain repetition schemes is also used.

Progressive overload is one of the cornerstones of training. How do you quantify plyometric work? Is it by number of repetitions, time of repetitions or some other method? How do you know when the workout is over?

The "quality" of execution should always be favored over quantity. Utilizing repetitions (contacts) is preferred over the amount of time and/or distances. We like to give a range of repetitions for each set. The athlete learns that, with 8-12 repetitions, eight quality repetitions are more useful in elastic-reactivity than 12 sloppy ones. Observing contact time for "dead" landings or releases will be a good indicator for stopping.

The "more is better" mantra when applied to plyometrics work will rapidly negate any training effect, only to produce acute bone, joint, or soft tissues injuries. How do you know when enough is enough?

In keeping with the quality over quantity concept, per session is again a look at the quality of the takeoffs and the response time. Some jump coaches will take weekly jump measurements (standing vertical or horizontal) and if an athlete or group falls 5-8 cm below the baseline or norm, they know progress and recovery needs to be altered. Over the course of a macro cycle, volume increases slightly, then must decrease as impacts (landing intensities) increase.

Most females have a larger quadriceps angle (Q angle) than men that posturally presents with an increased valgus (shin out) stress at the knee. How do you deal with this fact with your female athletes?

There has been considerable research out of Cincinnati, Ohio (Silvers, et. al. 2007) on this particular subject. The findings point directly to teaching female athletes how to land. Use simple teaching and training progressions, as in fuller foot landings, jumping straight, preparing to land as if to takeoff again, and progressing along a continuum of bounces, jumps, bounds and hops, and also look at how well the posture, balance, stability, and joint mobility of the landings are handled. We like to do a good deal of our beginning progressions barefooted to stress these points.

Plyometric drills can be used for various forms of fitness testing. What are some common plyometric tests you like and what information or correlations do you feel the test gives you?

Most coaches use standing countermovement jumps such as the vertical jump, standing long jump, standing triple jump and they are good evaluations of power if athletes are lacking in strength work versus speed. The original "Jumps Decathlon" created by Wilf Paish of Great Britain can still be utilized for many quality evaluations and the norms still fit well. Jumping sheds light on lifting, bounding on acceleration, and hopping evaluations (done correctly) can tell us a lot about sprint needs.

When using medicine balls, how do you determine the appropriate weighted ball for the athlete doing the drill?

It is the drill and the objective that dictates the size of the ball; other times it is a small percentage of the athlete's body weight (5-15%).

Leg drills can be done with double or single support. I once watched Tom Tellez's Houston athletes do a plyometric hurdle workout--all double support (two-footed landings). When I asked Coach Tellez why they only did double support, he stated simply, "It's safer." How do you break things up?

Our teaching and training progressions always begin with both feet landing and taking off, then progress to alternate (true bounding) and single (true hopping) leg drills. As shown by the following continuum:

Low ------------- Moderate ------------- High --------------- Shock ---------------

JUMPS: 1- Pogo, 2- Squat jump, 3- Box jump, 4- Rocket jump, 5- Star jump, 6- Butt kick, 7- Knee tuck, 8- Split Jump, 9- Scissors jump, 10- Scissors double, 11- Stride jump, 12- Stride crossover, 13- Quick leap, 14-Depth jump, 15- Box jumps (MR), 16- Depth leap, 17- Depth jump leap

BOUNDS/SKIPS: 1- Prance, 2- Gallop, 3- Skip progression, 4- Ankle flip, 5- Lateral (SR), 6- Single leg stair, 7- Double leg incline, 8- Lateral stair, 9- Alternate leg stair, 10- Alternate leg bound, 11- Lateral bound (MR), 12- Alternate diagonal bound, 13-Box skip, 14- Box bound

HOPS: 1- Double leg press, 2- Double leg speed (MR), 3- Incremental vertical, 4- Side hops, 5- Hops-sprint, 6- Angle hop, 7- Single-leg butt kick, 8- Single-leg progression, 9- Single-leg speed hop (MR), 10- Diagonal hop, 11- Lateral hop, 12- Decline hop.

Do you do much box work? At what point in the season? How high are the boxes? What would be a sample workout? Do athletes land with double or single support? Do they rebound or "stick the landing?"

Box jumps are different than depth jumps off a box or platform. Along our stress continuum, box jumps can be done early. Ground takeoffs onto a box at mid-thigh level can enhance landing mechanics and decrease impacts.

Depth jumps were designed as "shock" training and landings are stressful. As with the continuum, we won't progress to this area until late in a macro- or mesocycle. The teaching progression begins with landing only, then moves to elastic-reactive takeoffs. Our research suggests that, to work the reactivity needed for short response landings, all you need is a drop from approximately knee level.

You cannot run fast, jump or throw far unless you have a strong foot. How do you prepare the foot for the stresses of plyometrics?

We like to use barefoot training. It may be in the form of recovery strides, backward running, light changes of direction, and/or the simplified bounce, jump, bound, and hop progressions. These are also useful maneuvers for shoulder, elbow, and wrist--rudimentary work using either a wall, stairs, or ground as in push-up positioning.

One of the limiting factors in improved performance is eccentric strength. Are there any special exercisers or drills (medicine balls, boxes, weights, etc.) that focuses on this critical factor?

As on the continuum, by progressing from jumps to bounds, bounding to hopping, towing to throwing, then to catching and throwing, we drill on the concept of eccentric loading. In addition, teaching single response movements first, then multiple response (like a "superball"), we focus on the handling of eccentric loading and the utilization of the reflexes, responses, muscle mechanics, and the proprioception that go into this training.

SAMPLE PLYOMETRIC PROGRAMS

Can you provide a sample off-season plyometric workout schedule that progresses from low to high intensity?

The 10-week general plyometric program recommended by Allerheiligen (1994) in Table 8.10 shows how to progress from low to medium to high intensity in a six week program.

Table 8.10 **Sample Off-Season Plyometric Program**

Week	Drills	Sets/Repetitions	Rest between sets	Sessions per week
1 to 2	4 low intensity drills	2 X 10	2 min.	2
3 to 4	2 low intensity drills 2 medium intensity drills	2 X 10	2-3 min.	2
5 to 6	4 medium intensity drills	2-3 X 10	2 to 3 min.	2
7 to 8	2 medium intensity drills 2 high intensity drills	2-3 X 10 2 X 10	2-3 in. Box jumps - 10-15 sec.	2
9 to 10	4 high intensity drills	Non-box jumps: 2-3 X 10 Box jumps: 2 X 10	3 min.	2

Table 8.11 presents a plyometric cycle designed to improve speed in short sprints that begins eight weeks from competition and assumes that each athlete enters the program with a solid conditioning foundation in speed-strength training. After week six, high-intensity plyometrics become the foundation of the program and total volume (number of jumps) for the lower body is reduced to avoid overtraining injuries, sprint-specific jumps are emphasized, and a series of upper body form plyometric exercises are included.

Table 8.11 Eight-week Plyometric Program for Speed Improvement

Type	Exercises	Sets and repetitions	Rest	Progression
Low intensity Week 1	Squat jump	3 X 6-10	2 min.	Add 1 repetition each workout
	Double-leg ankle bounce	3 X 6-10		
	Lateral cone jump	2 X 6-10		
	Drop and catch push-up	4 X 6-10		
Low to medium intensity Week 2	Lateral cone jump	3 X 8-10	2 min.	Add 1 repetition to each workout until reaching 10
	Split squat jump	2 X 8-10		
	Double-leg tuck	2 X 8-10		
	Standing triple jump	2 X 8-10		
	Medicine ball (overhead backward and underhand forward throw)	2 X 8-10		
	Clap push-up	2 X 8-10		
Medium to high intensity Weeks 3 & 4	Standing long jump	3 X 8-10	2 min.	Add 1 repetition each workout until reaching 10
	Alternate-leg bound	3 X 8-10		
	Double-leg hop	3 X 8-10		
	Pike jump	2 X 8-10		
	Depth jumps	2 X 8-10		
	Medicine ball throw (with Russian twist)	3 X 8-10		
	Dumbbell arm swings	2 X 8-10		Reduce weight each workout; max of 20 lb
Medium to high intensity Weeks 5 & 6	Double-leg tuck	3 X 10-12	2 min.	Add 1 repetition each workout until reaching 10
	Single-leg zigzag hop	3 X 10-12		
	Double-leg vertical power jump	3 X 10-12		

Table 8.11 **(continued)**

Type	Exercises	Sets and repetitions	Rest	Progression
	Running bound	3 X 10-12		
	Box jumps	2 X 8-10		
	Standing broad jump	2 X 6-8		
	Standing triple jump	2 X 6-8		
	Dumbbell arm swings	3 X 12		
	Medicine ball sit-up	3 X 10-15		
	Single-arm Skipping	3 X 25 yards		
	Backward Skipping	3 X 25 yards		
High intensity* Weeks 7 & 8	Alternate Leg Bound	2 X 12-8	60-90 sec	Stress form and maximum explosion; Decrease repetitions from 12 to 8 in two weeks.
	Running Bound	2 X 12-8		
	Single-leg speed hop	2 X 12-8		
	Double-leg speed hop	2 X 12-8		
	Multiple box jumps	2 X 12-8		
	Standing broad jump	2 X 10-8		
	Standing triple jump	2 X 10-8		
	Double-arm Skipping	2 X 12-8		
	Standing Arm Swings	2 X 12-8		Start with 2 lb, reduce to 1 lb. Contrast - complete 12 with 2 lb., 12 with 1 lb. and 12 with no weight.
	Dumbbell arm swings	2 X 12-8		
	Contrast Arm Swings	2 X 12-8		
	Side jump and sprint	5 X 3		
	Decline hops	2 X 12-8		
	Medicine ball sit-up	3 X 15-20		
Maintenance Program	Alternate Leg Bound	2 X 12	90 sec.	Stress form and quality on each repetition.
	Running Bound	2 X 12		
	Double-leg speed hop	2 X 12		
	Side jump and sprint	5 X 5		
	Standing broad jump	5 X 8		
	Standing triple jump	5 X 8		
	Dumbbell arm swings	2 X 15		
	Contrast Arm Swings	2 X 15		
	Medicine Ball sit-ups	3 X 20		

*High-intensity plyometrics now become the foundation of this program. Total volume (number of jumps) for the lower body is reduced, sprint-specific jumps are emphasized, and a series of upper body form plyometric exercises have been added.

PLYOMETRIC EXERCISES AND DRILLS

What plyometric exercises are used to improve speed and strength?

Jumps that involve limited ground contact time and improve ground contact force are used.

(low intensity exercises)

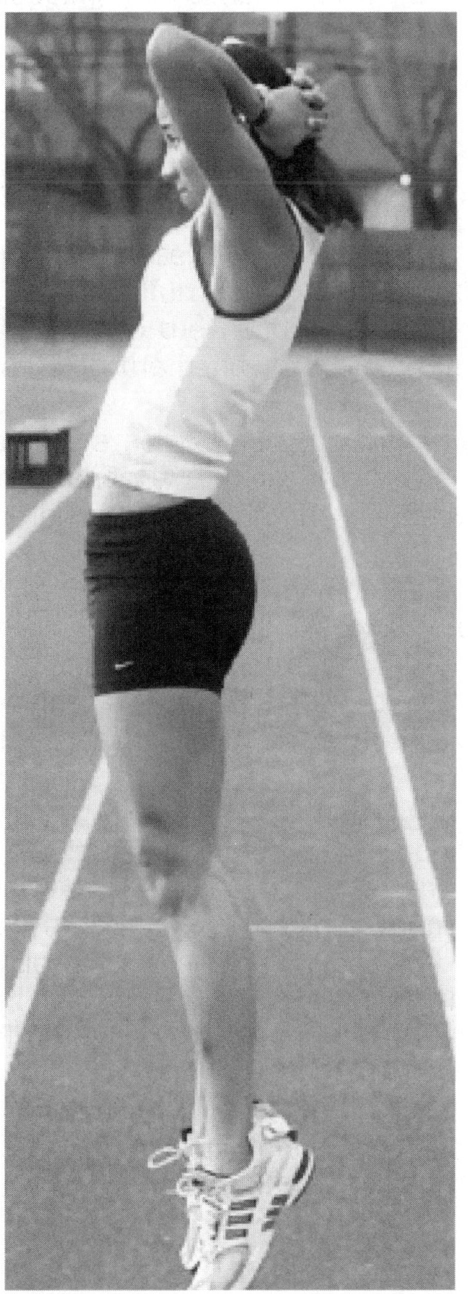

Figure 8.21 Squat jump. Stand upright with hands behind the head. Drop to a half squat and explode upward as high as possible.

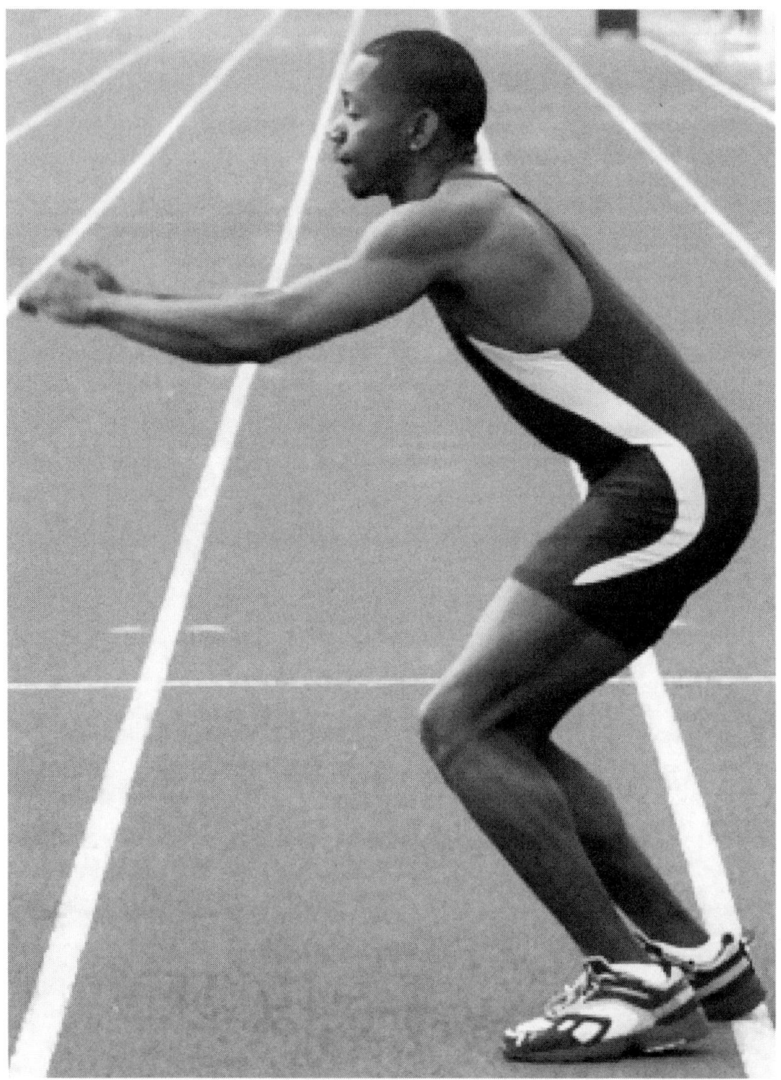

a

Figure 8.22 a, b Double-leg ankle bounce. With the arms extended to the side, jump upward and forward using the ankles. Immediately upon landing, execute the next jump, continuing until completing the desired number of repetitions.

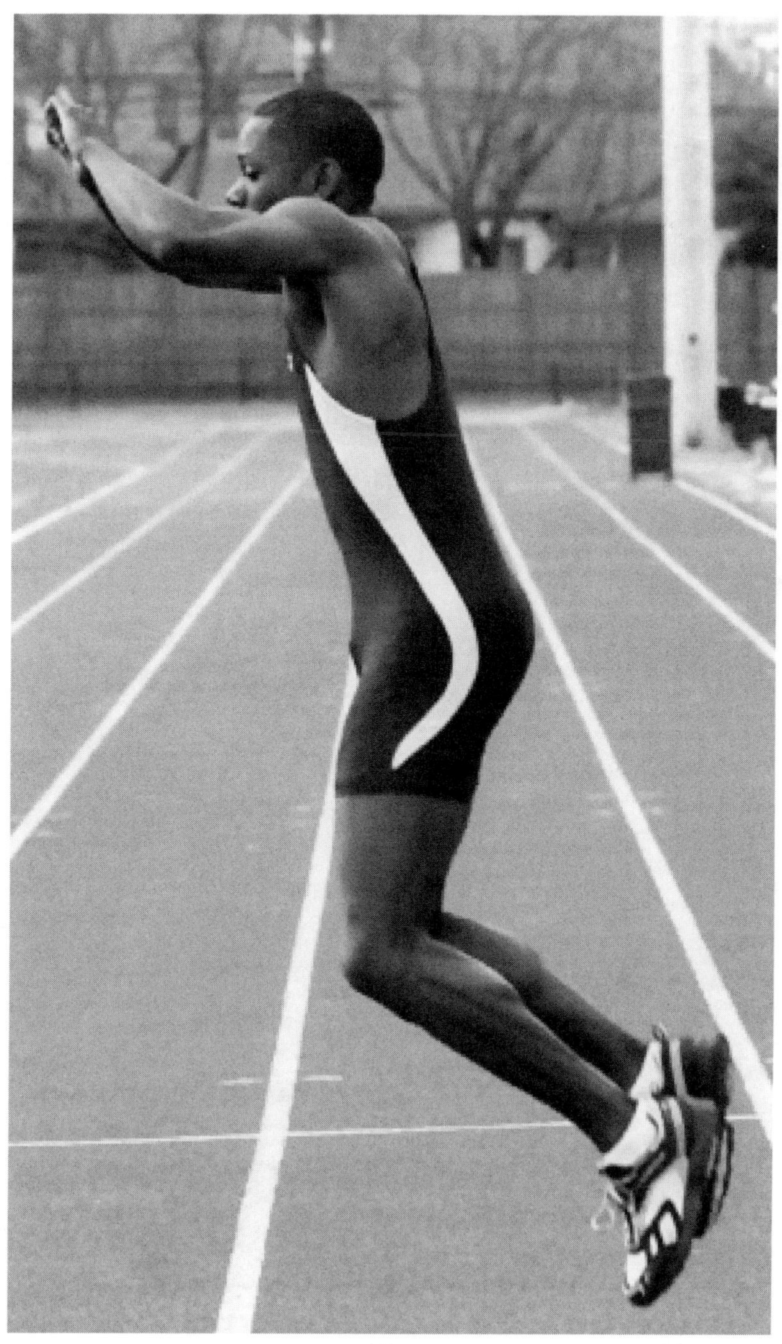

b

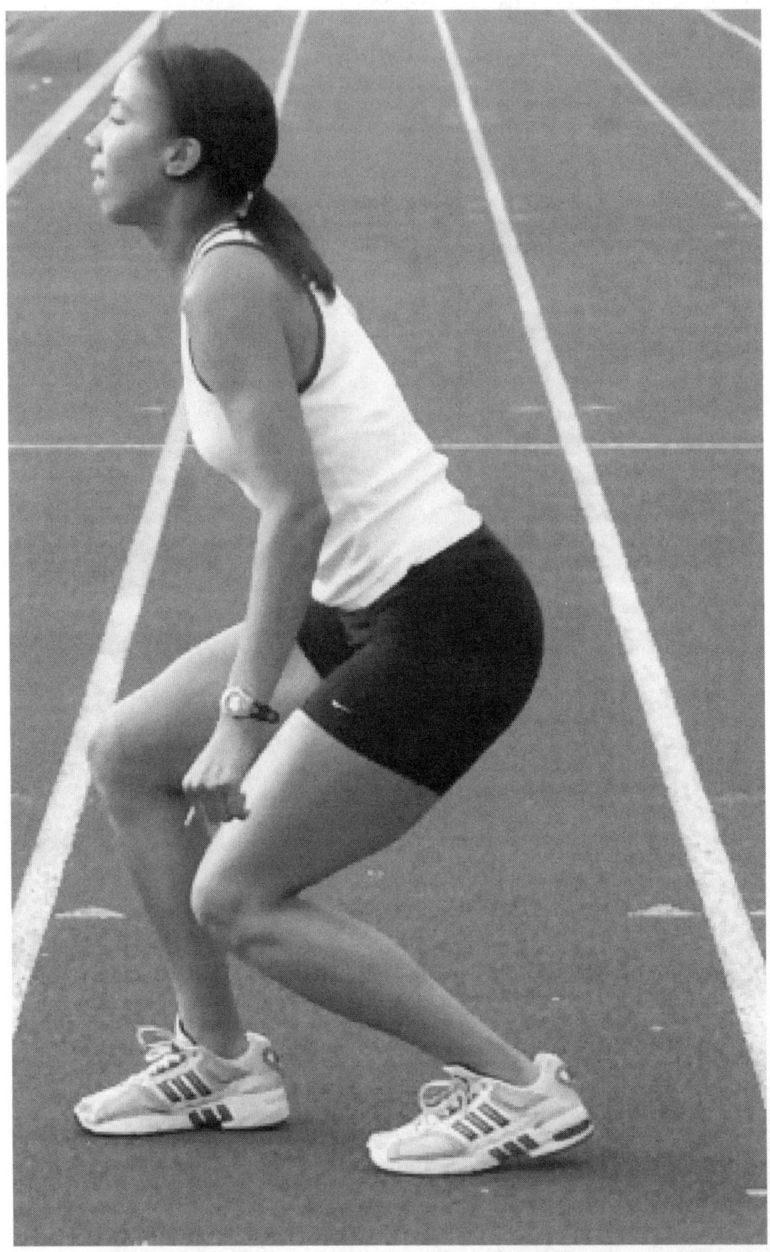

Figure 8.23 a, b. Split squat jump. With one leg extended forward and the other behind the center of the body (lunge position), perform a vertical jump off the front leg landing with the same leg forward. Repeat with the other leg.

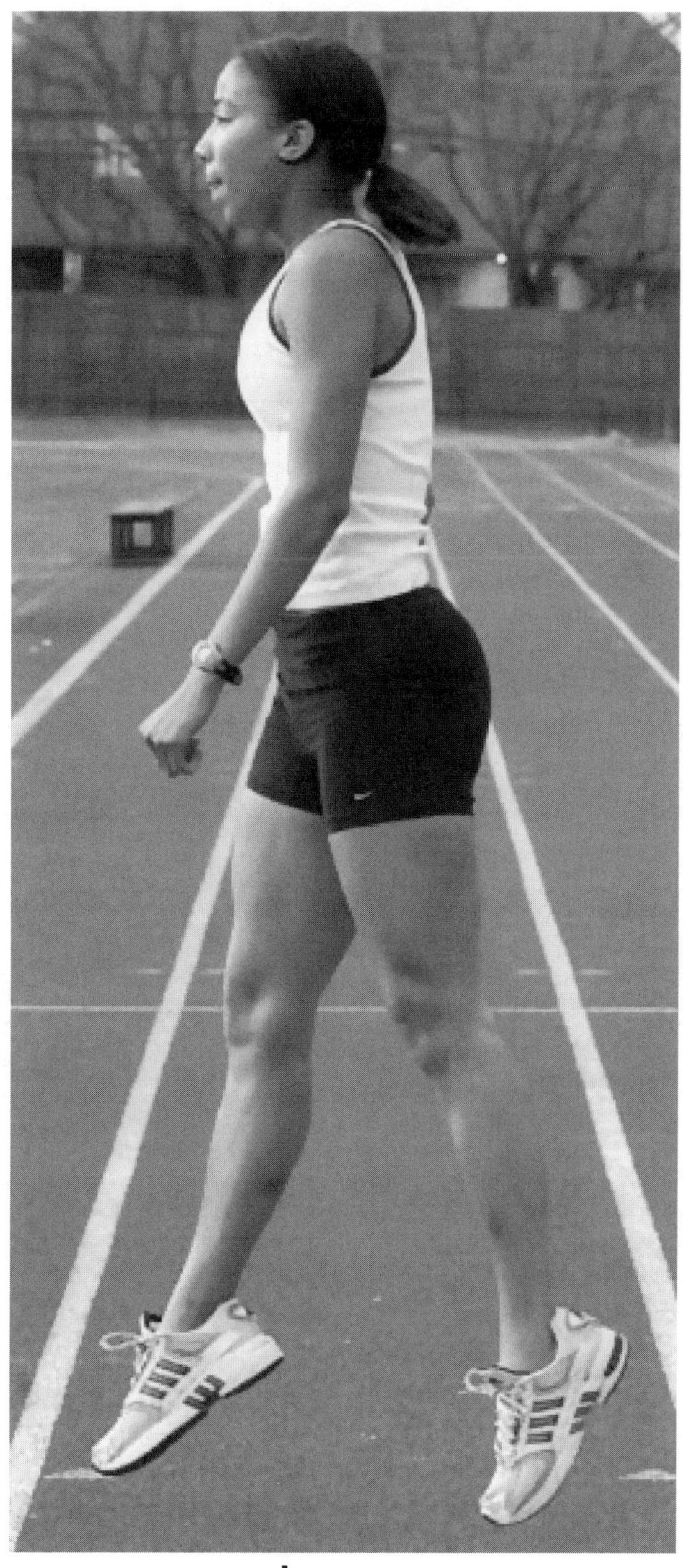

b

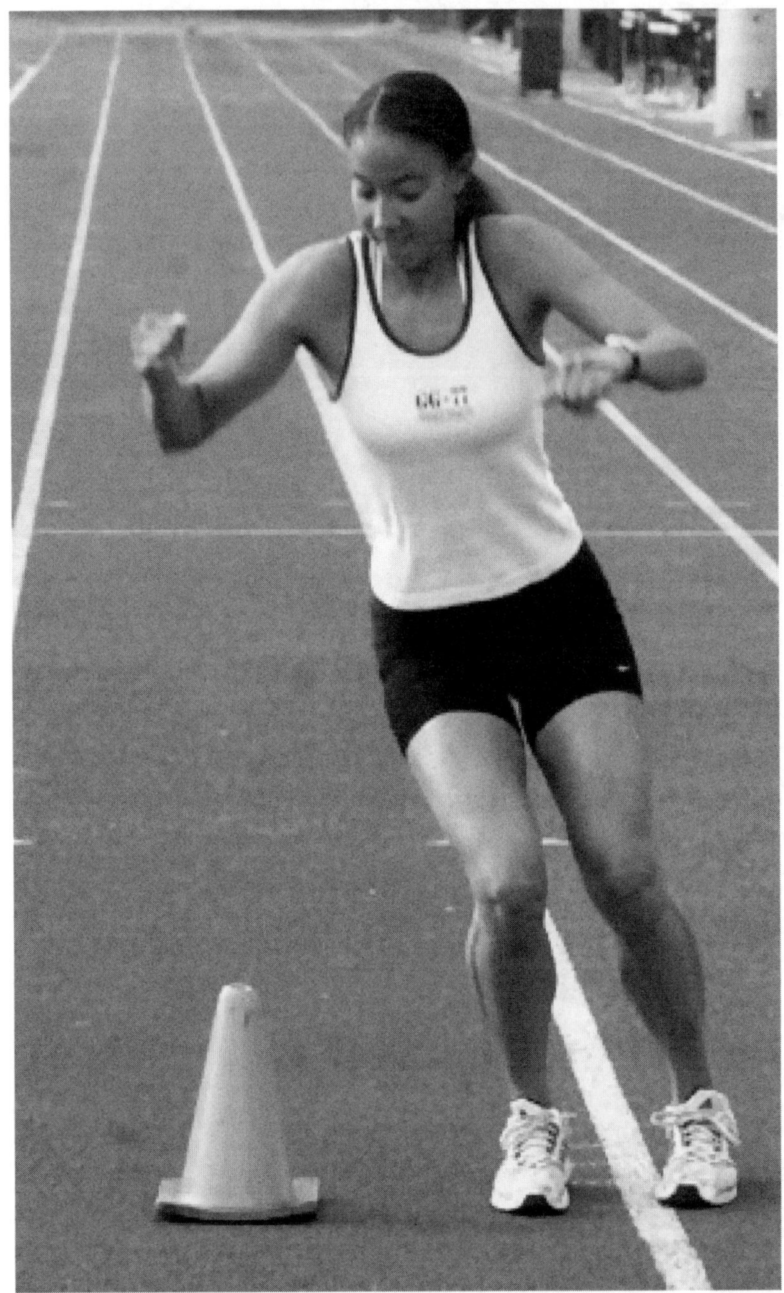

Figure 8.24 Lateral cone jump. Standing to one side of a cone, jump laterally to the other side. Immediately upon landing, jump back to the starting position to complete one repetition.

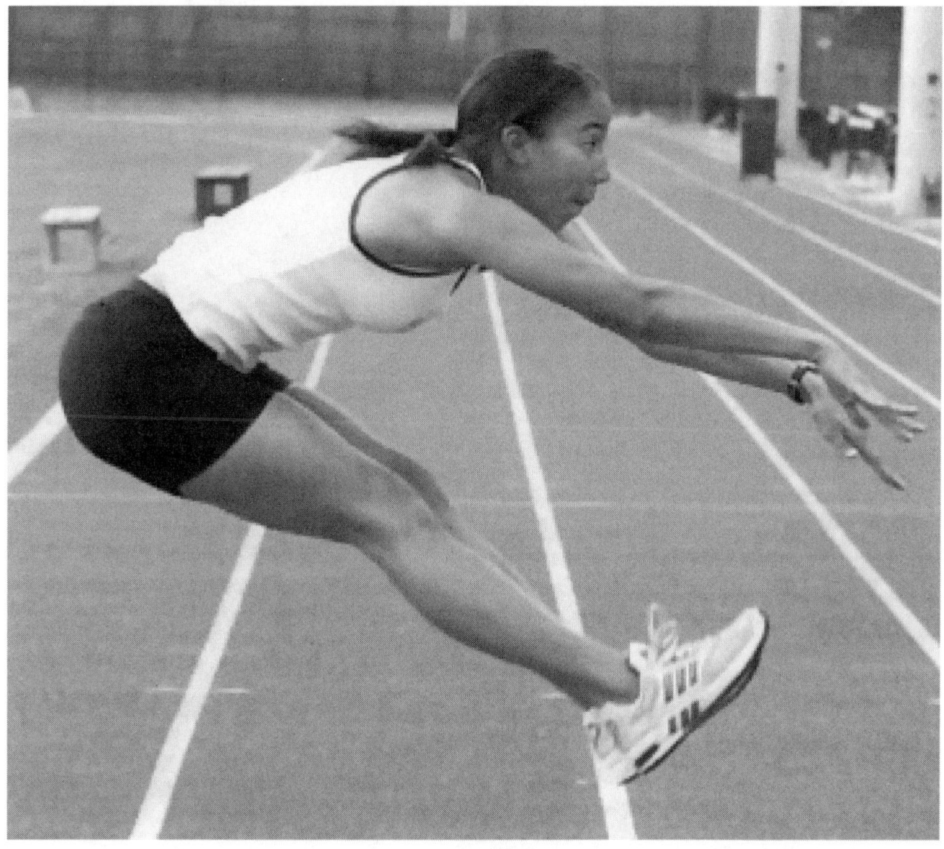

Medium Jumps

Figure 8.25 Pike jump. Assume an upright stance with both arms to the sides, feet shoulder-width apart. Execute a vertical jump, bring both extended legs in front of the body, and reach out with both hands and touch the toes in a pike position. Upon landing, immediately repeat the sequence.

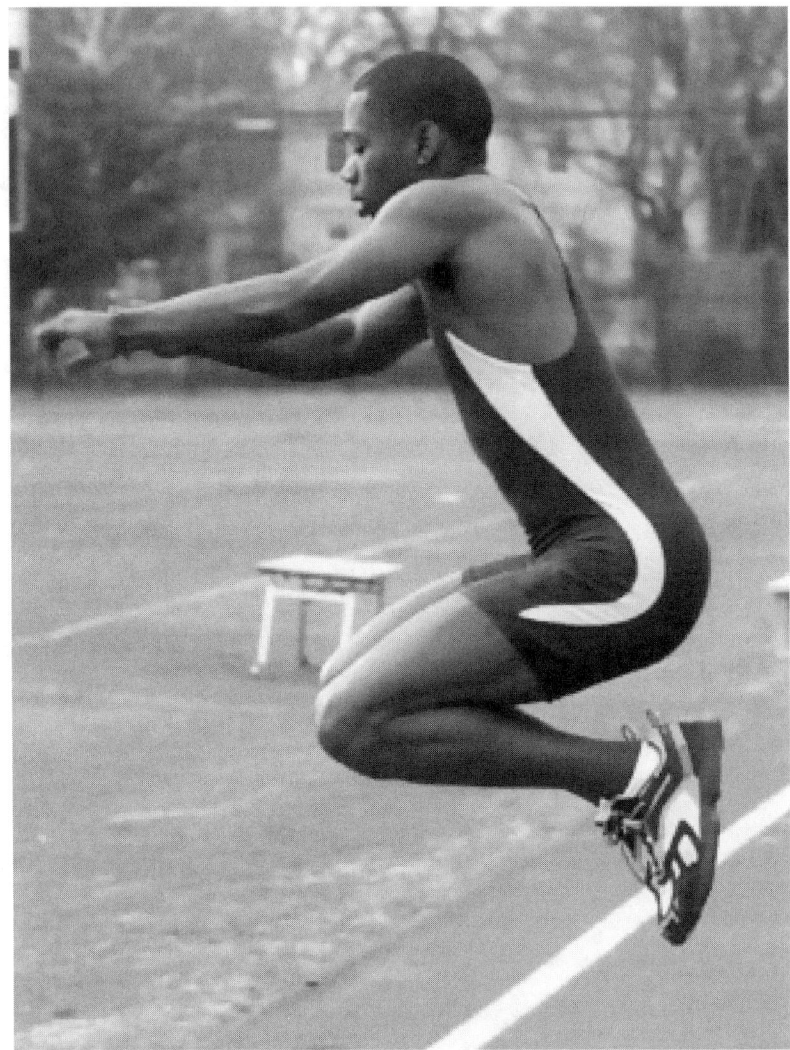

Figure 8.26 Double-Leg Tuck Jump. Assume an upright stance with both arms to the side, feet shoulder-width apart. Execute a vertical jump, grasping both knees while in the air. Release the knees before landing and immediately execute the next jump.

Double-leg vertical power jump. Assume a standing position with the feet shoulder-width apart and the arms to the side in preparation for a vertical jump. With a powerful upward thrust of both arms, jump as high as possible. Upon landing, immediately jump again with as little ground contact time as possible.

Single-leg vertical power jump. Complete the preceding action with a one-foot takeoff. Repeat the action using the opposite foot.

Single-leg tuck jump. Assume an upright stance with both arms to the side and feet shoulder-width apart. Execute a vertical jump with a one-foot takeoff, grasping both knees while in the air. Release the knees before landing on the same foot and immediately execute the next jump. Repeat the jump using the opposite leg.

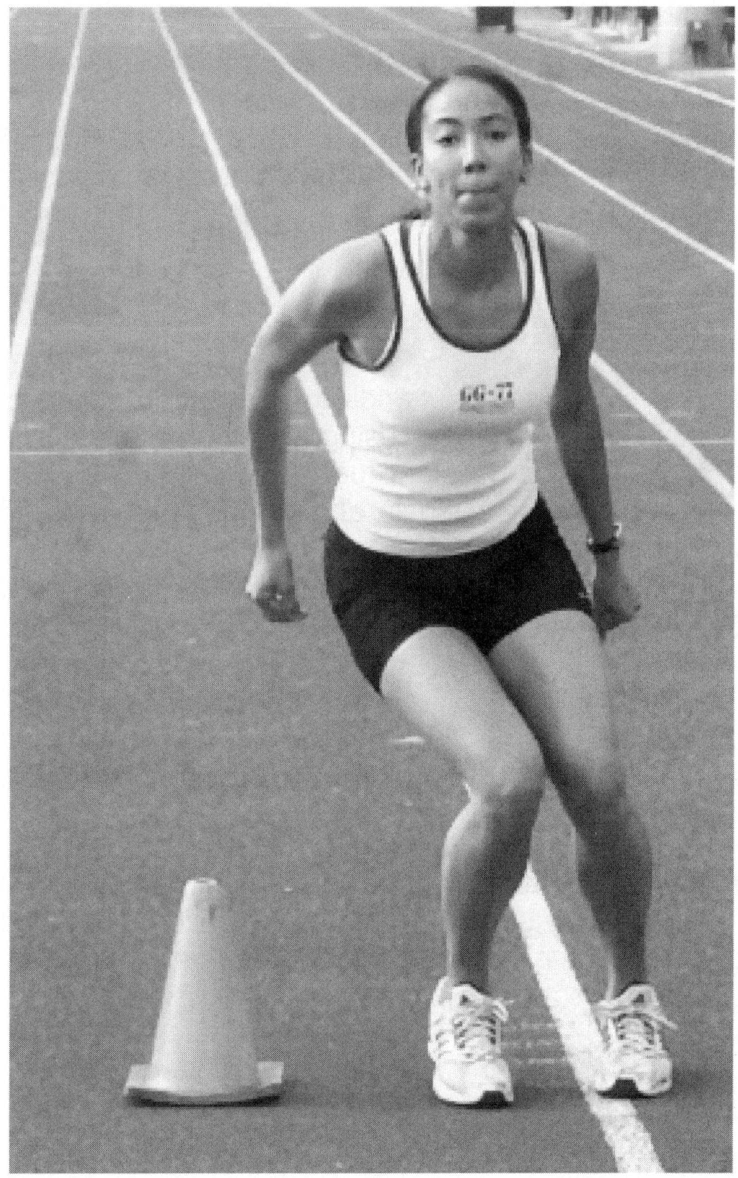

Figure 8.27 Side jump and sprint. Stand to one side of a bench or cone with the feet together pointing straight ahead. Jump back and forth over the bench for 4 to 10 repetitions. After landing on the last jump, sprint forward for 25 yards. Two athletes begin this exercise at the same time. The first to complete the specified number of jumps and reach the finish line is the winner. Benches or cones can be set up for 100 yards. Players perform 4 to 10 jumps and sprint to the next cone before repeating the jumps and sprinting again.

Upper-Body Exercises

Single-clap push-up. Assume a normal push-up position and lower the chest to the floor. Push the body upward with an explosive action, clap the hands and catch yourself in the upright position. Repeat the movement immediately for the desired number of repetitions.

Drop and catch push-up. Kneel on both knees with the upper body erect, as though you are standing on the knees. Place both hands in front of the chest, palms down, and drop the upper body to the floor, catching the weight with both elbows bent in the bottom phase of the push-up position. Immediately push off with both hands to extend the arms and return to the upright push-up position.

Standing Jumps (High Intensity)

Standing triple jump. Assume the standing broad jump position: arms to the side, and feet shoulder-width apart. Using a two-foot takeoff, jump forward as far as possible, landing on the right foot, then immediately jump to land on the left foot. Finally, jump once again and land on both feet. The standing triple jump is identical to the triple jump in track (hop, step, and jump), except for the use of a two-foot takeoff. The object is to generate maximum speed and secure as great a distance as possible on each of the three phases.

Standing long jump. Complete only the initial jump described in the standing triple jump using maximum arm swing. Strive for both vertical and horizontal distance.

Single-leg hop. Assume a standing broad jump starting position with one leg slightly ahead of the other. Rock forward to the front foot and jump as far and high as possible driving the lead knee up and out. Land in the starting position on the same foot and continue jumping to complete the desired number of repetitions.

Short-Response Hops and Bounds (favored exercises to improve ground contact forces and sprinting speed)

Single-leg speed hop. Assume the position described in the preceding exercise with one leg in a stationary flexed position. Concentrate on the height of each jump.

Decline hop. Assume a quarter-squat position at the top of a grassy hill with a one to two-degree slope. Continue hopping down the hill for speed as described for the double-leg hop. Repeat the exercise using the single-leg decline hop.

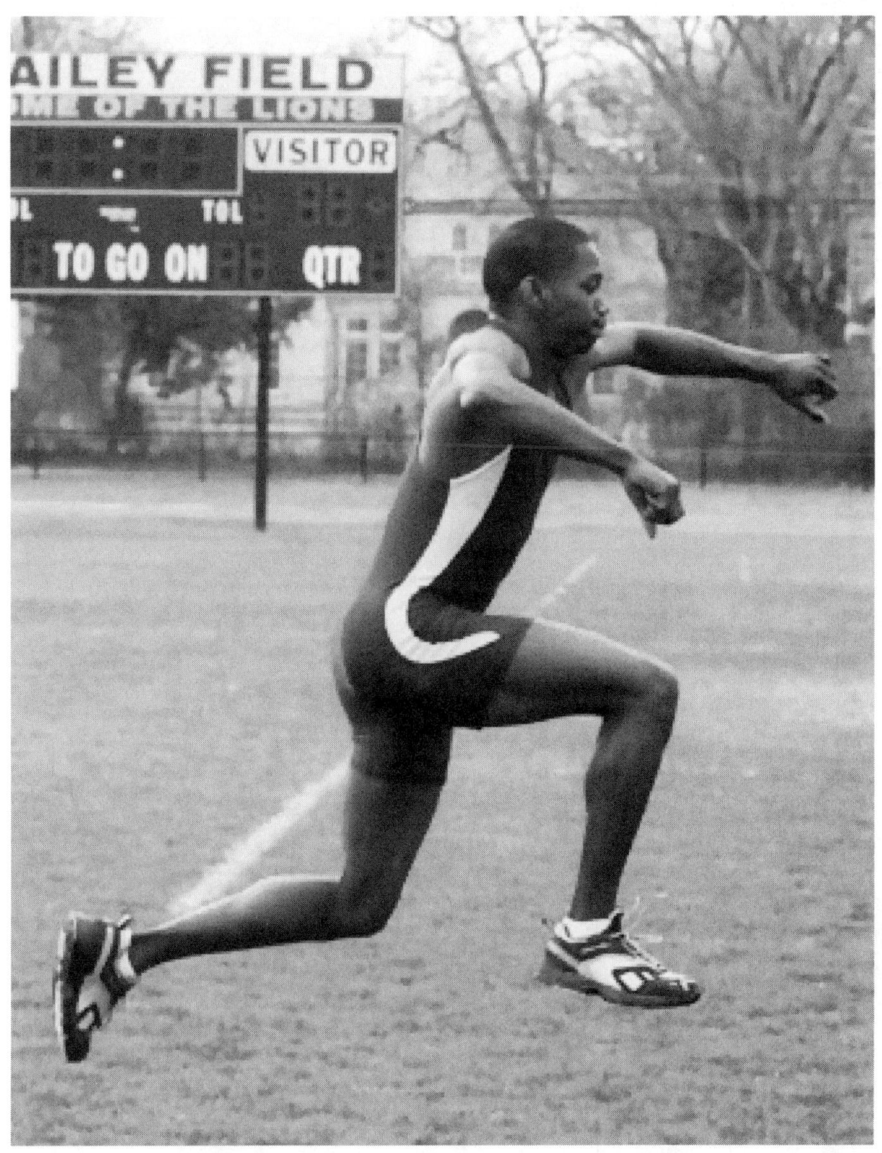

Figure 8.28 Double-leg speed hop. From an upright position with the back straight, shoulders forward, and head up, jump as high as possible, bringing the feet under the buttocks in a cycling motion at the height of the jump. Jump again immediately upon contacting the ground.

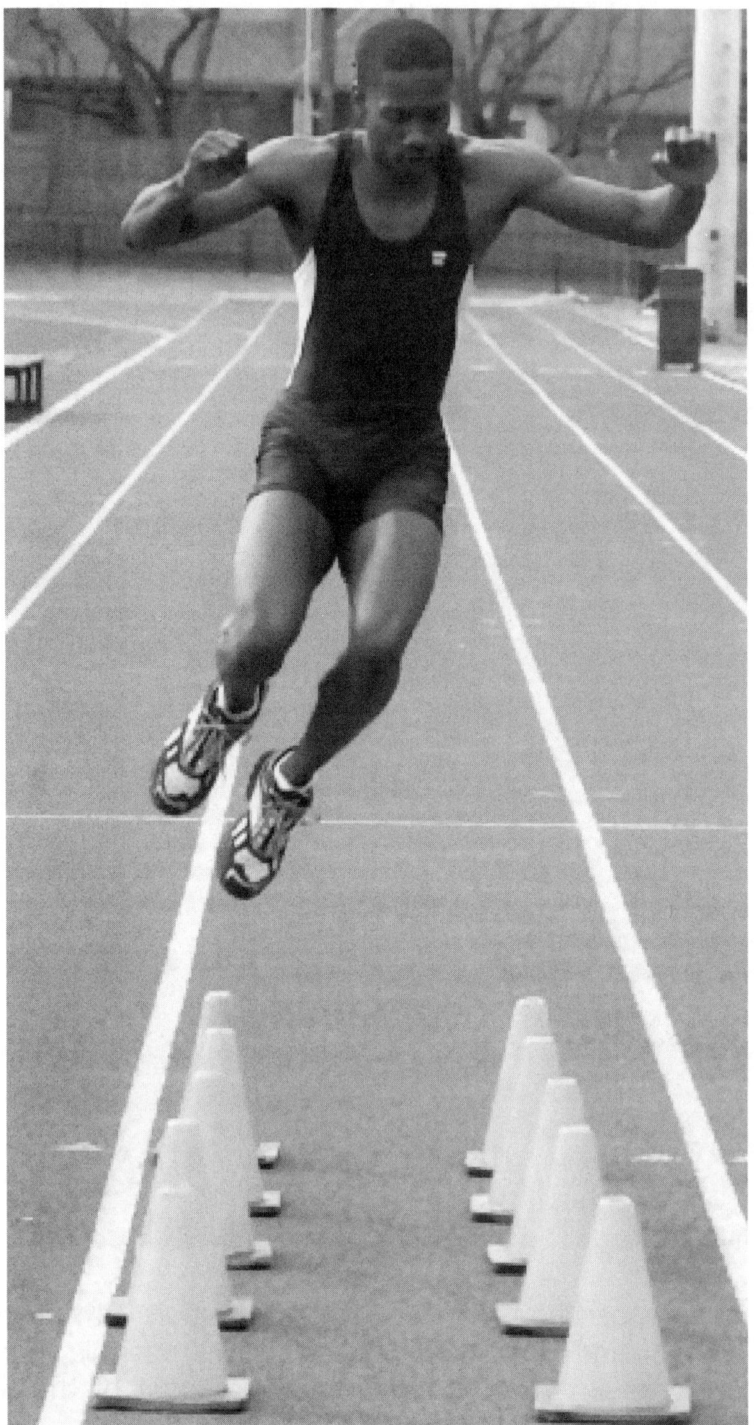

Figure 8.29 Double and single-leg zigzag hop. Place 10 cones 20 inches apart in a zigzag pattern. Jump with legs together in a forward diagonal direction over the first cone keeping the shoulders facing straight ahead. Immediately upon landing, change direction with the next jump to move diagonally over the second cone. Continue until jumping over all 10 cones. Execute the single-leg zigzag hop in the same diagonal direction but using one leg at a time.

Depth jump. From an elevated box, drop to the ground, landing with both feet together, knees bent in an attempt to absorb the shock. Return to the box, repeat the exercise for the desired number of repetitions.

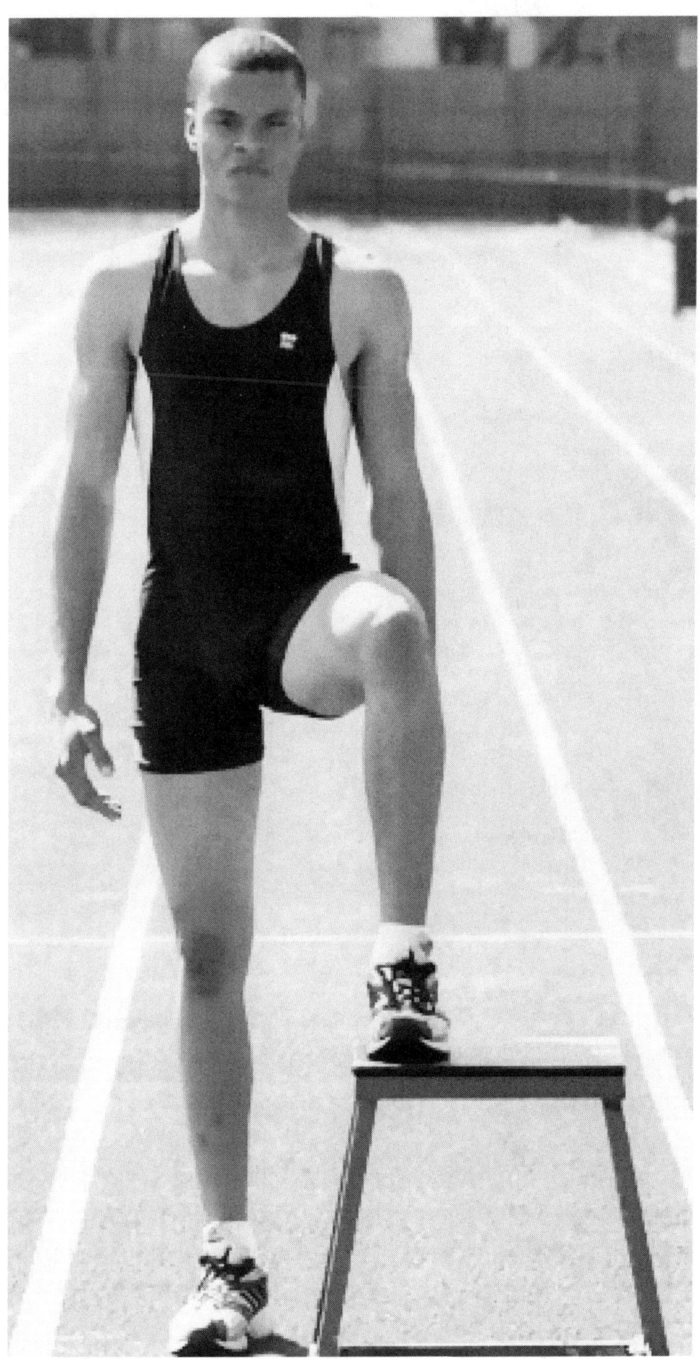

Figure 8.30 Single-leg stride jump. Assume a position to the side and at one end of a bench with the inside foot on top of the bench and the arms at the sides of the body. Drive the arms upward as the inside leg on the bench pushes off to jump as high into the air as possible. Continue jumping until reaching the other end of the bench.

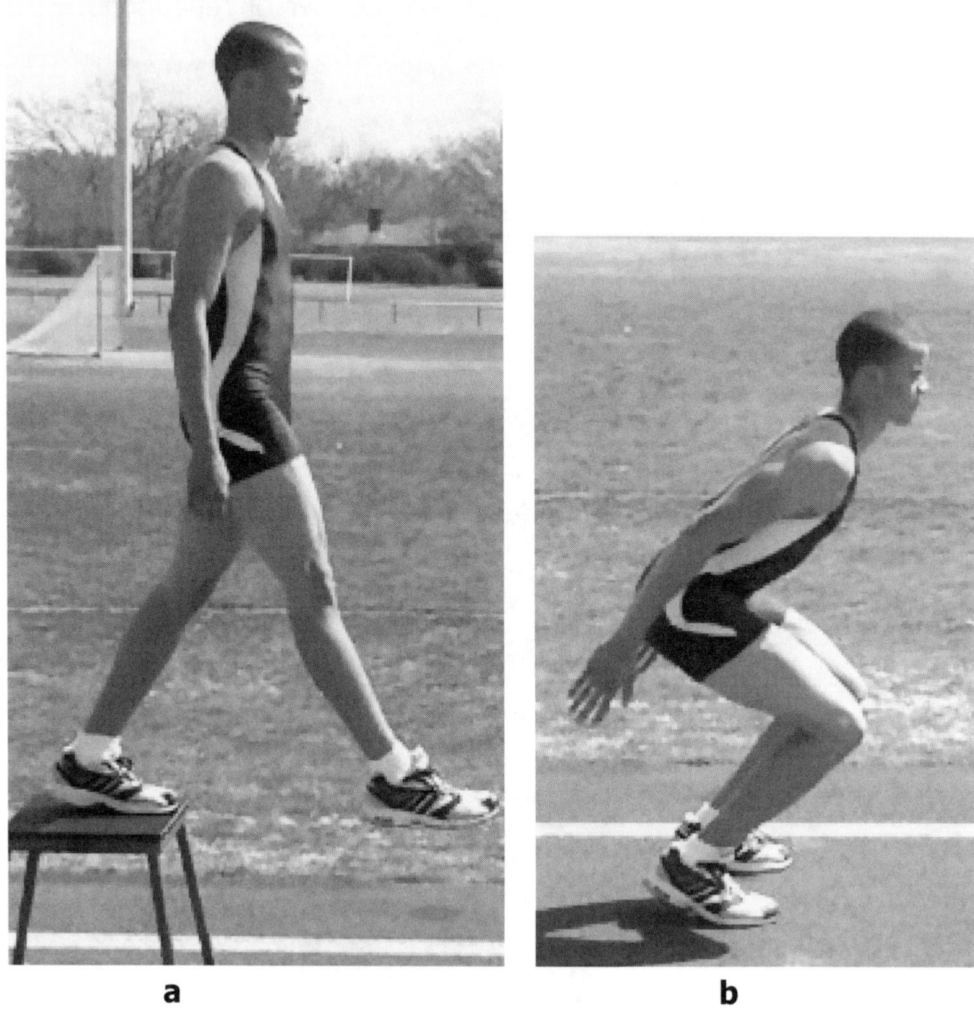

a b

Figure 8.31 a, b Box Jumps. Step off a box that is within the recommended box heights for your weight and age and immediately jump upward and outward upon hitting the ground.

Multiple Box Jumps. Set up five boxes of differing heights 3 to 5 feet apart. Stand on the first box with toes slightly extended over the edge. Step off the first box and, upon landing on the ground, jump upward and outward to land on the second higher box. Repeat the action for the remaining boxes, alternating low and high boxes.

Double-Leg Bound. From a standing broad jump position (half squat stance, arms at sides, shoulders forward, back straight, and head up), thrust the arms forward as the knees and body straighten and the arms reach for the sky.

Alternate-leg bound. Place one foot slightly ahead of the other. Push off with the back leg, drive the lead knee up to the chest and try to gain as much height and distance as possible. Continue by immediately driving with the other leg upon landing.

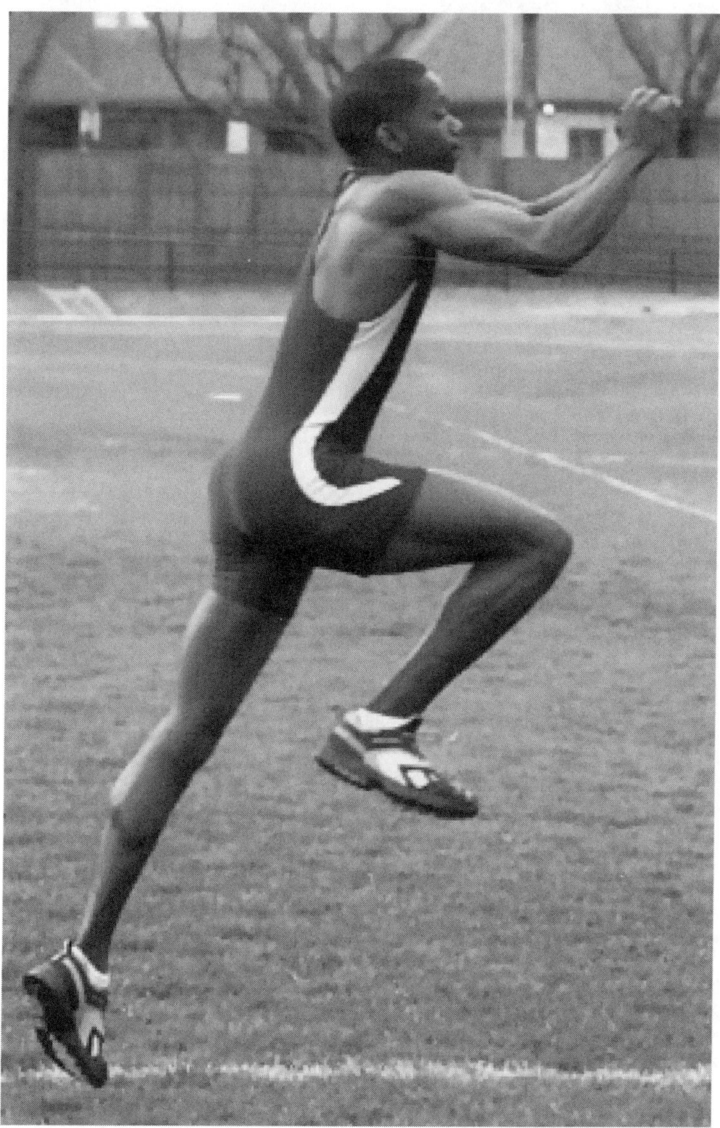

Figure 8.32 Running bound. Run forward jumping as high and far as possible with each step. Emphasize height and high knee lift and land with the center of gravity directly under the body.

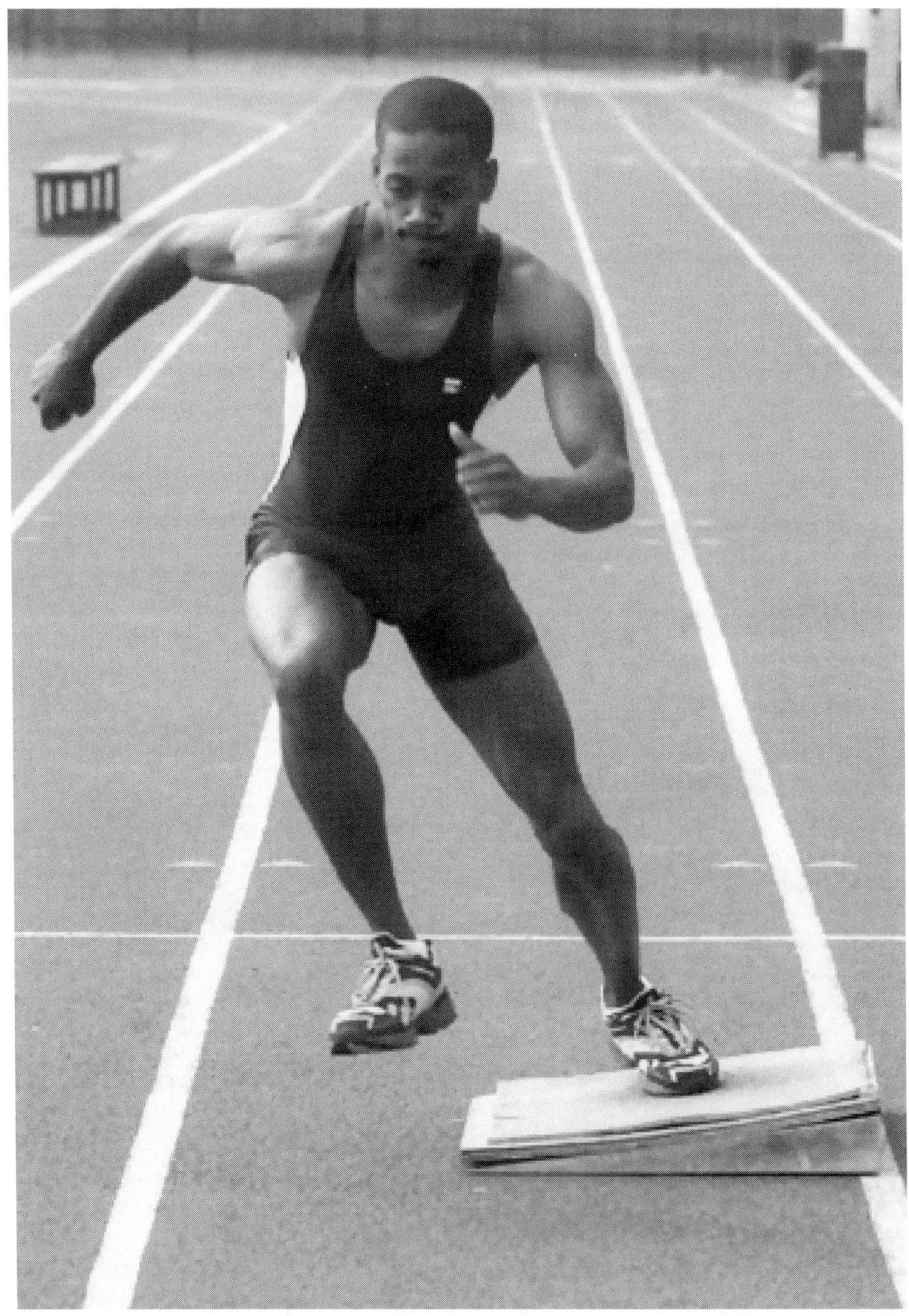

Figure 8.33 Lateral bound. Assume a semi-squat stance about one step from the side of an angled box or grassy hill. Push off with the outside foot to propel the body into the box. Immediately upon landing, drive off again in the opposite direction, stressing lateral distance.

Ricochets

Incline ricochet. Stand facing the bottom of the bleacher steps with the feet together and arms to the sides. Rapidly jump upward to each step as fast as possible by attempting to be "light on your feet."

Decline ricochet. From the top of a one to two-degree grassy hill, take a series of short, rapid hopping movements down the hill. Concentrate on being "light on your feet."

Upper Body

Push-up with weights. Assume a push-up position with the arms fully extended, both hands on top of the weights. Quickly remove both hands, drop to the floor, and catch yourself with the elbows slightly flexed before allowing gravity to flex the arms further until the chest nearly touches the floor. Rapidly extend the arms so the hands leave the floor high enough to again assume the position with the hands on top of the weights.

Double-clap push-up. Perform a normal push-up with enough explosive action to allow you to clap the hands two times while the hands are in the air before again catching the body with slightly flexed elbows.

Dumbbell arm swings. With 5- to 25-pound dumbbells in each hand, assume a stance with the feet apart, hands at the sides, shoulders and upper body tilted only slightly forward, and the head straight. Drive one arm upward to a point just above the shoulder as the other arm drives backward behind the body. Before each arm reaches maximum stretch, check the momentum and initiate motions in the opposite direction.

Sprint-arm action with weights. Place one to 10-pound dumbbells in each hand. Assume a position with the upper body leaning only slightly forward, both arms bent at right angles in the correct sprinting position (left arm raised in front, elbow close to the body with the hand about shoulder height, right arm lowered, elbow close to the body with the hand no further back than the right hip). Swing the arms from the shoulder joint and execute 10 to 15 explosive movements of the arms with the correct form. On the upswing, the hand rises to a point just in front of the chin and just inside the shoulder. As the arm swings down, the elbow straightens slightly and the hand comes close to the thigh.

SPRINT-RESISTED TRAINING (SPORT LOADING)

What is sport loading?

One could take the position that any kind of training is a form of sport loading. As acceleration occurs during a sprint, the amount of force the body has to manage increases, thereby placing an added load on the body. For speed training, sport loading is defined as the systematic adding of weight to the body in any form (uniform, vest, pants, or suit) or to the tools used in a sport such as bats and balls.

Training Objectives. Two basic approaches are used to accomplish two separate objectives. *The first approach* involves the use of relatively light resistance (weighted uniform, vests, and body suits) that allows high speed repetitions. The main objective is to load the involved muscles during the maximum speed phase of sprinting. The majority of information and sample programs presented in this section deal with this objective. *The second approach* involves the use of heavier weight (Austin leg drive machine, weighted sleds, staircase sprinting) and is designed to increase ground contact force during the start and acceleration phase of sprinting when ground contact time is higher. Each program needs to match the range of demands faced by the athlete in these two phases of the sprinting action.

What does sport loading accomplish for the athlete?

Sport loading, along with speed-strength training, plyometrics, speed-endurance training, and overspeed training, produce the greatest changes in the fast-twitch muscle fibers and contribute to the improvement of speed-strength in the muscles involved in the pushing action away from the ground with each step in sprinting.

Sport Loading Programs

What type of sport loading should be used for speed improvement?

Although every athlete may not have access to all the technical equipment found at many colleges or professional facilities, an effective sports loading program can still be devised using alternative methods requiring little or no equipment.

Weighted Body Suits, Vests and Shorts. Stan Plagenhoef developed a weighted strap system to fit around the various segments of the body. Each strap is placed at specific biomechanical segment points. This method distributes the load over each of the segments of the body. Ce'bo, a company from England, manufactures and markets a body suit design (Ce'bo Bodykit) that is available to the general public. In the literature promoting the Ce'bo Bodykit, the company states that the suit is "a weighted exercise garment that increases the gravitational pull on the body of the wearer while exercising." The suit includes four sections: upper body, arms, upper leg, and lower leg and allows the load to be distributed over the entire body to attain more precise loading.

New materials and design changes used in constructing weight vests are improving. More durable, light, tight-fitting vests with the capability to easily change weights are giving athletes a greater range of usability. A weighted vest should become the foundation piece of equipment for a sport loading program. This vest can be safely utilized by male and female athletes of all ages and be adapted to practically any sport.

Research completed by Bosco (1985) indicated that the proper use of sport loading improves power output and aids performance in sprinting. An average improvement of 10 centimeters in vertical jumping ability was also found after three weeks of training. A repeat study of Bosco's designed for female subjects at Brigham Young University (BYU) showed similar positive effects on vertical jumping ability with an average gain of five centimeters for the athletes. Weekly increases in the vest loads were 8 percent of body weight the first week, 10 percent the second week, and 12 percent the third week. Female athletes wore the vests during the day and for practice sessions. BYU researchers also suggested that the vest could influence other aspects of power output.

Some athletes are concerned that wearing a weight vest or shorts will injure the lower back, knee and ankle joints. The other concern is restricting the form, function and range of movement while performing in a sport. Neither is likely to occur in a properly supervised program involving good equipment that fits each athlete well. Correct use will strengthen the key muscles involved in sprinting including the start, the drive and acceleration phase and the maximum speed phase.

Some vests can be incrementally loaded, like The Smart Vest by Training Zone Concepts, Inc. In addition, it is desirable to be able to increase the weight on the vest in increments of a half pound, or one pound (figure 8.34. Table 8.12 summarizes the major purposes and weight ranges of the three vests in the Smart Vest System. Vest I (heavy weights) is used primarily to improve speed-strength and ground contact force. Vest II (moderate weight) provides an opportunity to develop speed endurance, and Vest III (lighter weight) to allow performance at higher rates of speed to improve maximum mph speed.

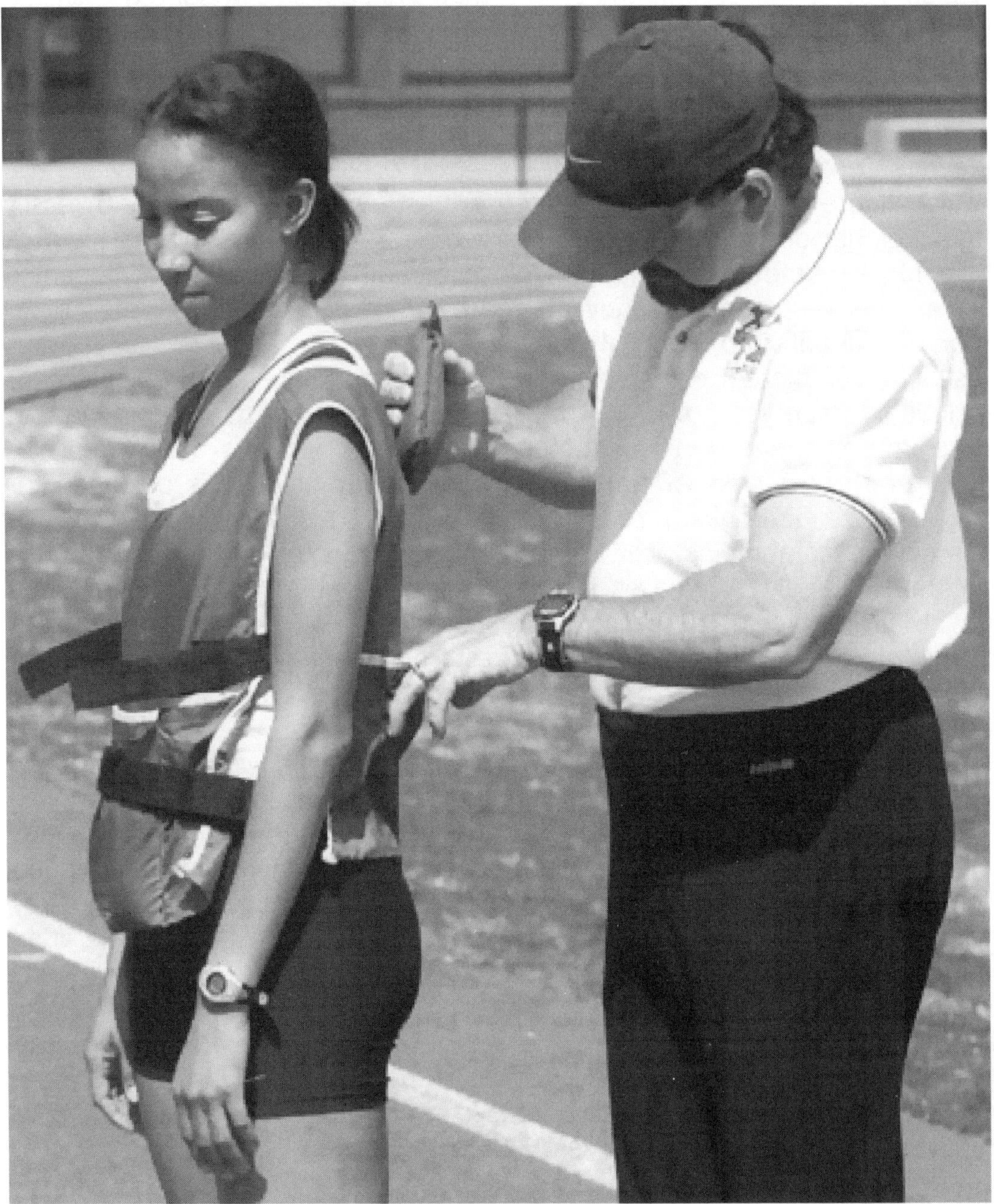

Figure 8.34. Weighted vest

Table 8.12 Sample Sports Speed Vests and Body Suit Programs

Vest	Name	General Purpose	Weight range*
I	Basic training vest	Speed-strength, Increased ground contact force	1 to 20 lb. maximum
II	Speed-endurance vest	Strength-endurance	1 to 15 lb. maximum
III	Speed vest	Speed and quickness	1 to 8 lb. maximum

*For the body suit, use comparable weights.

A sample sport loading program using Vest I is shown in table 8.13. The program progresses from heavy weights (20 pounds) to lighter weights (2 pounds) over a 10-week period. Athletes slowly progress to high-speed training with a weight that permits rapid, explosive turnover in sprinting.

Vests can also be used during various parts of a practice session in almost any sport. In general, it is wise to avoid using a vest during highly technical drills or other aspects of a sport that require considerable precision. The majority of precision practice should be done in a training zone that uses the same high-speed work levels that are expected during competition. The loads selected should depend on the objectives set up for the practice period. If the vest is used intelligently, skill development and conditioning will occur simultaneously.

Coaches can handicap elite players during training sessions to stimulate competition and force the more talented players to work harder. Table 8.14 lists several key practice elements and provides suggested vest loads and durations for each. Table 8.15 lists six training zones and their suggested loads and durations for organizing a training program. Be aware that Vest II and III can be used for all of Vest I weights. The big advantage for using Vests I and II is that they are designed to fit better, allow greater freedom of movement, and are less likely to cause athletes to deviate from correct sprinting form and technique.

Table 8.13 **Sport Loading Program for Hypergravity Vest and Body Suit Training**

Week	Repetitions	Vest	Distance	Rest	Progression
1	3 to 5	20 lb.*	120 yd.	Walk back HR> 120	40-yd. building to 75% speed gradually 40 yd. at 75% speed 40 yd. easing off
2	4 to 6	18 lb.	120 yd.	Walk back HR > 120	40 yd. building to 75% speed gradually 40 yd. at 75% speed 40 yd. easing off
3	6 to 8 3 to 5	20 lb. 16 lb.	20 yd. 120 yd.	Full recovery Walk back HR >120	Power starts at 85% 40 yd building to 80% speed gradually 40 yd at 80% speed 40 yd easing off Complete two sets
4	6 to 8 3 to 5	18 lb. 14 lb.	20 yd. 120 yd.	Full recovery Walk back HR > 120	Power starts at 90% 40-yd. building to 80% speed gradually 40 yd at 85% speed 40 yd easing off Complete two sets
5	6 to 8 3 to 5	16 lb. 12 lb.	20 yd. 120 yd.	Full recovery Walk back HR > 120	Power starts at 95% 40 yd building to 88% speed gradually 40 yd at 88% speed 40 yd easing off Complete three sets
6	6 to 8 3 to 5	14 lb. 10 lb.	20 yd. 120 yd.	Full recovery Walk back HR > 120	Power starts at 95% 40 yd. building to 90% speed gradually 40 yd. at 90% speed 40 yd. easing off Complete three sets

Table 8.13 **(continued)**

Week	Repeti-	Vest	Distance	Rest	Progression
7	6 to 8 3 to 5	12 lb. 8 lb.	20 yd. 120 yd.	Full recovery Walk back HR > 120	Power starts at 95% 40 yd. building to 90% speed gradually 40 yd. at 980% speed 40 yd. easing off Complete three sets
8	6 to 8 3 to 5	10 lb. 6 lb.	20 yd. 120 yd.	Full recovery Walk back HR > 120	Power starts at 95% 40 yd. building to 95% speed gradually 40 yd. at 95% speed 40 yd. easing off Complete three sets
9	6 to 8 3 to 5	8 lb. 6 lb.	20 yd. 120 yd.	Full recovery Walk back HR > 120	Power starts at 95% 40 yd. building to 95% speed gradually 40 yd. at 95% speed 40 yd. easing off Complete 3 sets
10	6 to 8 3 to 5	6 lb. 6 lb.	20 yd. 120 yd.	Full recovery Walk back HR > 120	Power starts at 95% 40 yd. building to 98% speed gradually 40 yd. at 98% speed 40 yd. easing off Complete three sets

Note: Vests I and II can can be used for all loads; Vest III can be used for loads of 8 pounds or less. For the body suits, use comparable weights.

Table 8.14 **Sports Specific Training Using a Weighted Vest and Body Suit**

Practice Period	Suggested Load and Duration
Warm-up and drills	Vest I, II, III; 1 to 20 lb.* for 10 to 15 min.
Scrimmage sessions	Speed vest; 1 to 4 lb. until the end of scrimmage
Drills	Speed vest; 1 to 8 lb. throughout practice
Conditioning sessions (end of practice)	Vest I, II, III; 1 to 20 lb. for 10 to 30 min.

* For the body suit, use comparable weights.

How can this be integrated into a training program?

The first step toward using weighted garments in a training program is to master the mechanics. For 20-30 minutes at the beginning of a training session, athletes focus on executing the mechanics required to complete a sport-specific skill (e.g., a basketball player performing a crossover dribble into a two-step jump shot or a volleyball player going up to block an opponent's shot).

The second step is skill drill mastery. First, slow the movements down and focus on the rhythm (flow) and power necessary to most effectively execute the movements within the skill. As confidence builds. increase the intensity to game-like conditions. Remember, the goal is for the mind to automate these skills so the athlete no longer need to focus on them. This frees the mind to focus on other aspects of the game.

In the third step, strengthening and reinforcing movements, weighted vest and shorts are used. By adding weight in 1-2 pound increments, athletes are able to mastery these movements more quickly.

Where can weighted vests be purchased??

Vest information is available by contacting Training Zone Concepts, Inc. through the internet-http://www.sportsscience.com. Smart Vest and shorts are the best on the market. The key features are a distraction free fit, adjustable half and one pound weights, and a men and women's model. By simply providing your height, weight and true waist size, you will receive a guaranteed body glove fit. The Smart Vest is sold with 12 pounds and shorts with 8 pounds.

Table 8.15 **Sports Specific Training Zones Using a Weighted Vest and Body Suit**

Practice Period	Distance (meters)	Suggested Load and Duration
Starting zone	0 to 20	Vest I, II, III; 1-20 lb.* for 15 to 30 min.
Acceleration zone	0 to 30	Vest I, II, III; 1-20 lb. for 15 to 30 min.
Flying zone	20 to 40	Speed vest; 1-4 lb. for 15 to 30 min.
90 percent zone	100 to 300	Speed vest; 1-4 lb. for 15 to 30 min.
Speed-endurance zone	30 to 200	Speed vest; 1-8 lb. for 15 to 30 min.
Aerobic zone	400	Speed vest; 1 to 8 lb. for 30 to 60 min.

*For the body suit, use comparable weights.

The Austin Leg-drive Machine

Although expensive, this heavy duty machine is one of the best sport loading equipment items on the market for increasing ground contact force during the starting, acceleration, and maximum speed phases of sprinting. Athletes sprint up adjustable inclines against preset resistance ranging from low to very heavy weight. The action closely mimics the start and early acceleration phase of the sprinting. The leg drive machine is capable of placing the very high weight loads necessary for improving ground contact force in a sprint-specific movement.

For detailed information and a video demonstration, go to *legdrive.com.*

Harnesses and Parachutes

How are harnesses and parachutes used?

The two-person harness is an affordable and effective tool for increasing ground contact force and improving sprinting technique. Two athletes of similar body weight and power use the same harness (figure 8.35). One provides the resistance, the other provides the power.

Parachutes of various sizes provide some degree of resistance; however, the additional benefits that can be gained from other methods outweigh the cost and inconvenience associated with the use of parachutes. Younger athletes tend to enjoy parachutes as a sport loading technique (figure 8.36).

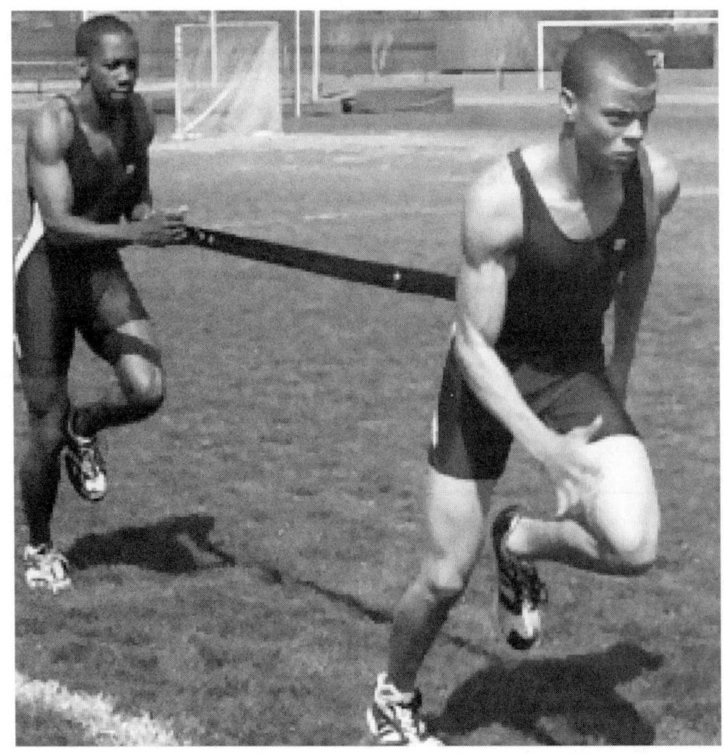

a

Figure 8-35 a, b Harness resistance (a) release and sprint (b).

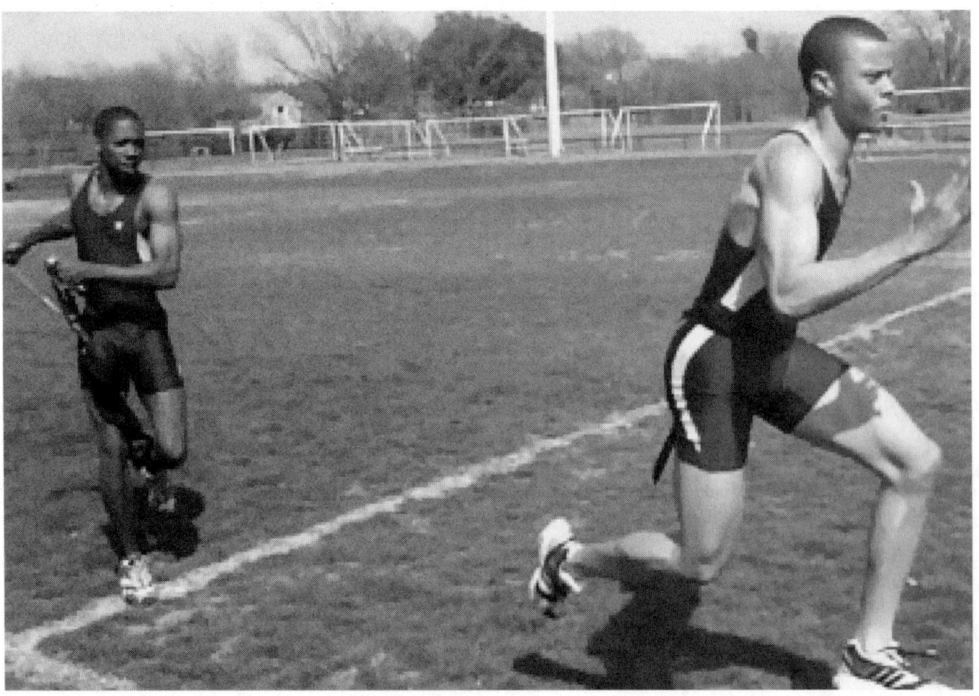

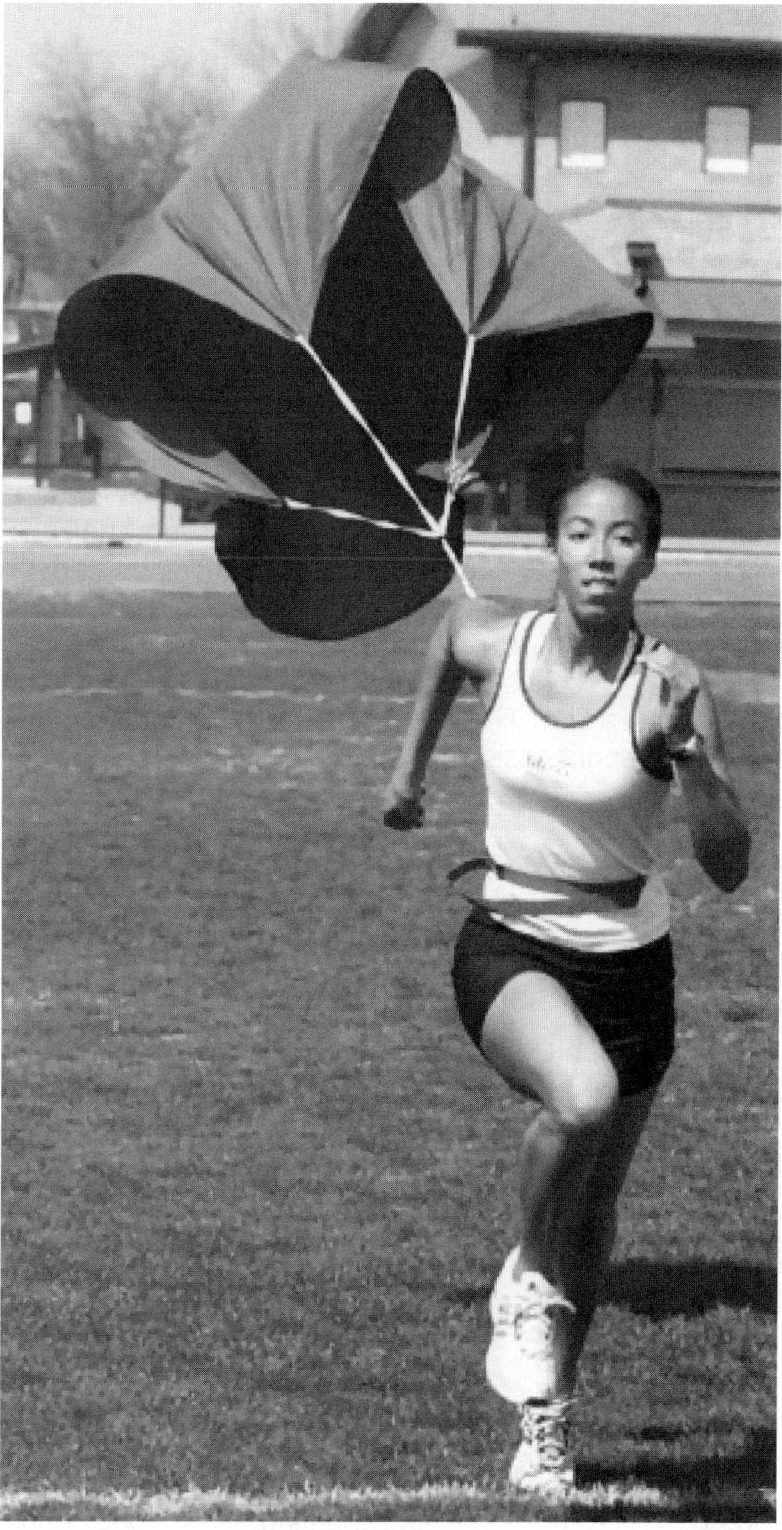

Figure 8.36 Wind resistance using a parachute

Uphill Sprinting, Stadium Stair Sprinting, Sand Sprinting, and Weighted Sleds

How are incline and sand resistance sprinting programs used?

Uphill sprinting can be used in most parts of the country. Although a wide range of grades can be used, it is recommended that the degree of incline allow proper starting and sprinting form. When Bob Ward designed the course for the Dallas Cowboys in the 1980s, he included the best features for uphill training. The angles and distances were selected from extensive research, consultation with experts from around the world, and practical coaching experience (see table 8.16). In general, steep angles (8.0 degrees) were used only for the start and acceleration loading, and angles of 1.0 degree, 2.5 degrees, or 3.0 degrees were used for the start and speed endurance workouts. A 10- to 30-yard incline of 8 to 10 degrees should be covered in 2.5 to 3.5 seconds, followed by a near full-speed sprint of 20 to 80 yards at the same incline. These inclines are considerable higher that what is recommended for sprint-assisted training designed to increase stride rate and speed.

Stadium or other stairs can be used in the same manner as hill sprinting. Locate stairs that have the same approximate angle and make certain the steps provide a safe environment for training.

Table 8.16 **Dallas Cowboy Incline/Decline Course**

Total Distance (Yards)	Distance (Yards)	Distance (Meters)	Featured Angles	Uphill Use
0.00	0.00	0.00	Start	
27.25	27.25	25.00	Flat	Recovery
33.81	6.56	6.00	8.0 degree angle	Starts
34.90	1.09	1.00	Flat	Recovery
67.70	32.80	30.00	3.5 degree angle	Acceleration
89.57	21.87	20.00	Flat	Recovery
122.37	32.80	30.00	3.0 degree angle	Acceleration
131.12	8.75	8.00	Flat	Recovery
196.72	66.60	60.00	2.5 degree angle	Speed-endurance
278.72	82.00	75.00	1.0 degree angle	Speed-endurance
328.72	50.00	46.00	Sand sprinting	Body control Speed-endurance

Sand running is an excellent way to stress the total body, especially the lower extremities. The foot, knee, and hip muscles and joints are required to adjust to the unstable sandy running surface. This adjustment develops and toughens the body's ability to handle unexpected stability changes. Very few activities can work all joint actions like sand running.

Herschel Walker said that his father had him running over plowed fields in Georgia when he was a youngster. While running in a sand session with the Cowboys, Walker looked as if he were running on the top of the sand, while most other players labored or dug deep holes with each step. His early training must have given him that kind of control.

Weighted Sleds are available in all price ranges. Metal and plastic models can also be found that allow quick and easy weight changes. For very little cost, a spare tire with a rope and weighted belt can be used. Regardless of the device chosen, use a load that allows proper form and high-speed sprinting when focusing on speed. Heavier weight is used to increase ground contact force and involves starting and early acceleration repetitions for 5 - 15 yards.

When should Sport Loading be used?

The ideal point to include sport loading training in a workout regime is at the latter part of Wednesday's workout.

There are two training phases to consider: *The power start and explosive close-range movement phase (Phase I, acceleration)* helps overcome inertia to get started in any sport-task. This is extremely important in sports that deal in close ranges. *Phase II acceleration* marks the end of an an athlete's maximum speed and an attempt is made to "hold" maximum speed as long as possible before slowing occurs.

Unique studies conducted on the Dallas Cowboys by strength and conditioning coach, Bob Ward, showed that maximum acceleration takes place very close to the start (one to three feet) and rapidly diminishes to zero or to very low amounts somewhere around 50 to 60 yards. The end of the acceleration phase obviously occurs somewhat sooner in team sport athletes than in elite sprinters. The rate of drop-off is a very good indicator of running skills and conditioning levels. The timeline of an all-out sprint shows that the length of an athlete's ability to accelerate and apply full anaerobic power continues for about six to eight seconds. It has also been demonstrated that world-class 100-meter sprinters reach maximum speed at the 60-70 meter mark and can hold that speed for another 20 meters before some minor slowing occurs.

In most sports, usable acceleration is attained within approximately 10-15 yards (0.6 to 1.5 seconds). Athletes should train multidirectional peak power by playing handball, basketball, and racket sports. Ten to fifteen starts that cover 5 to 20 yards will help train linear velocity or straight ahead sprinting.

The power sprint phase trains athletes to develop power at high speeds. The speed curves of sprinters show that deliverable power drops off as they move faster. The best way to train maximum mph sprinting speed is to work from a flying start, using light weight vests and holding full speed for up to 20 yards. Six to ten repetitions for 10 to 80 yards should be used with weights or resistance that does not reduce performance speed by more than one to five percent.

A sample sport loading program for hill sprinting, stadium stair sprinting, harnesses, sand, parachute, and weighted sleds is shown in table 8.17.

Table 8.17 Sport Loading Program Using Hill Sprinting, Stadium Stairs, Harnesses, Sand Sprinting, Parachutes, or Weighted Sleds

Week	Repetitions	Pulling Distance*	Rest	Progression
1	3 to 5	15 yd.	Walk back** HR > 120	Use power starts at 75% speed for hill sprinting, sand running, stadium sprinting or with no weight on the sled. Two sets are completed.
2	3 to 5	20 yd.	Walk back HR > 120	Repeat at maximum speed.
3	6 to 8 3 to 5	25 yd. 30 yd.	Full recovery Walk Back HR > 120	Repeat power starts at maximum speed. Power starts at 75% speed for hill sprinting, sand running, and stadium sprinting or with no weight on the sled. Two sets are completed.
4	7 to 9 3 to 5	 50 yd.	Full recovery Walk back HR > 120	Use power starts at 90%. Repeat power starts and sprints. Add sled weight that allows you to sprint with good form. Two sets are completed.
5	7 to 9	50 yd.	Full recovery	Repeat workout. add more weight. Complete three sets.
6 to 9	7 to 9	60 yd.	Full recovery	Repeat workout. Add more weight each week. Three sets. Include one final run to exhaustion by continuing your sprint for as long as possible. Record the distance and try to improve each week.

* Adjust distance you are pulling the sled, sprinting uphill, or up stadium steps.

** No walk back if you ae using a weighted sled.

Sport Loading Training Variables

How do I utilize overload training to maximize performance results?

To optimize training results, consider these guidelines:

• *Progression and amount of weight.* The rule is to master the mechanics of movement before weight is added. The strategy of adding weight depends on the training phase (off-season, pre-season or in-season). In the off-season, athletes may begin with 2.5 percent of their body weight. A 160-pound football player, for example, would start with four pounds in the vest or shorts. Usually, every 2/3 weeks the athlete is ready for additional weight such as two pounds for the vest and one pound for the shorts. While performing high speed movements the key is to avoid dropping below 5 percent of an athlete's maximum speed. Most athletes will fall below this threshold when the weight load reaches 5-7.5 percent of body weight, depending on their level of strength and conditioning. Progression involves the gradual adding of weight to provide a safe, effective means for building strength and speed.

Separate workouts are scheduled involving heavier resistance (weights, Austin Leg Drive Machine) to move away from maximum speed and switch the focus to increasing ground contact force during the start and acceleration phases of sprinting.

• *Tapering.* The athlete begins with a heavy load (10 percent of body weight) and performs the drills at 75 percent of maximum speed. The key is to determine a target date to peak (e.g., a tournament at the end of the season). Tapering is a gradual process of decreasing the amount of weight while increasing speed intensity. The goal is to stop weight load training one to two weeks before the target date. An athlete wants to gradually add weight in the off- and pre-season, with intent to begin tapering at the start of the season to peak for the play-offs.

• *Volume, duration and intensity.* Volume focuses on the number of drills, duration or length of the drill, and intensity or degree of maximum effort while performing the drill. In the off/pre-season 60-75 percent of the drills should be performed with the vest or shorts; during the season 20-40 percent. Duration is longer in the off- and pre-season then gradually shortened as the in-season period approaches.

Chapter 9

SUSTAINED POWER OUTPUT TRAINING

A high level of anaerobic endurance (speed endurance) is critical to athletes in power sports to make certain repeated short sprints take place throughout the entire game at the same high speed with little slowing due to fatigue, to increase anaerobic threshold (point at which lactic acid buildup begins to produce a slowing effect), and to reduce slowing to a minimum at the end of a long sprint of 60 yards or more. Each training program discussed in this chapter can be altered to meet the specific needs of a sport and player position.

SPEED ENDURANCE TRAINING PROGRAMS

What training programs are most effective for team sports?

Team sport coaches use several programs originally developed by track coaches to train 60-meter, 100-meter, 200-meter and 400-meter sprinters. Programs are altered depending upon the common distances sprinted during competition in a particular team sport.

Pickup sprints involve a gradual increase from a jog to a striding pace, and then to a maximum effort sprint. A 1:1 ratio of the distance and recovery walk that follows each repetition is recommended. For example, an athlete jogs 25 yards, strides 25, sprints 25, and ends that repetition with a 25-yard walk or slow jog. The walk or slow jog allows some recovery prior to the next repetition. This jog-stride-sprint-recovery cycle is an example of early season training. As improvement occurs, the distance is lengthened, with late-season pickup sprints reaching segments of 50 yards or more.

New Zealand athletes use a routine similar to pickup sprints that involves a series of four 50-meter sprints at near-maximum speed (6 to 7 seconds) per 400-meter lap, jogging for 10 to 12 seconds after each sprint and completing the 400-meter run in 64 to 76 seconds. Athletes have performed as many as 50 sprints with little reduction in speed on any repetition.

Hollow sprints involve the use of two sprints interrupted by a hollow period of recovery such as walking or jogging. One repetition may include a 40-yard sprint, 40-yard jog, 40-yard sprint, and a 40-yard walk for recovery. Similar segments of 80, 120, 150, 220, and 300 yards are used.

Interval Sprint Training is also easily adapted to improve each metabolic system (two anaerobic pathways and the aerobic system). Since more work can be performed at high intensity when repetitions and sets are interrupted by recovery techniques (walking, jogging, complete rest) than through continuous exercise, interval sprint training is effective in improving the energy system that dominates a specific sport. The intensity and duration of exercise and the rest interval can be altered to achieve maximum results. "Wind sprints," alternates, and other similar programs have commonly been used in most team sports. The key difference is that such programs often have had little formal structure, poor record keeping, and only a limited ability to control the variables responsible for producing optimum results: frequency of training sessions, length and intensity of each repetition, and the length and intensity of the rest interval. Modern day team sport coaches keep careful records to make certain athletes do progressively more work each training session.

Frequency of Training Sessions. Adequate resting time is necessary prior to the next scheduled exercise session if the body is to fully recover and benefit from the previous workout. Most athletes train daily, alternate light and heavy workout days, and use at least one day of rest at the end of the week and just prior to competition during the season. For team sport athletes, 2-3 speed endurance sessions weekly is sufficient.

Length and Intensity of the Work Interval. The number and length of repetitions vary from one team sport to another and depend upon the average distance sprinted and the number of times sprints occur. It is not unreasonable for an athlete to complete 10-50 repetitions of a distance mixed with walk-jog recovery periods. The intensity of training (speed of each repetition) is more important than the length of the workout. After an initial 2 weeks of progressing from one-half speed sprints to three-quarter to nine-tenths speed for untrained athletes, repetitions should be completed at maximum speed, except for the initial 2-3 used as part of a warm-up routine. To train both anaerobic pathways, the time of each sprinting repetition will range from 5-10 seconds, to 15-30 seconds, to 1-3 minutes, and occasionally, in excess of three minutes

Length and Intensity of the Rest Interval. Although complete recovery does not occur during the rest interval, partial return to pre-exercise heart rate and breathing rate levels does take place. The recovery interval between repetitions is based on the estimated time of recovery between sprints during competition in each sport.

Speed of Each Repetition. Sprints take place at maximum speed for distances of up to 120 yards and at near maximum speed for longer distances.

Is a stationary cycle effective in improving speed endurance?

Cycling workouts can also be designed to mimic the length of the sprint (time in seconds), the rest period between repetitions (10-40 yard sprints at 25-30 second intervals for football), and alter resistance or load. The objective is to make high speed cycling as close to actual game conditions as possible. Stationary cycling can be adapted to any sport since it allows repeated high speed, low to high resistance, and repetitions that simulate the distance or time and rest intervals of most activities. Used as a supplement to, and not a replacement for, traditional speed endurance programs, cycling has considerable potential for improving and maintaining speed endurance.

How do each of the speed endurance training programs impact the anaerobic and aerobic energy systems?

Table 9.1 compares the effects of speed endurance programs on the anaerobic and aerobic energy system. This information allows athletes and coaches to select the method that best matches the energy demands of their sport and position.

Table 9.1 Estimated Effect on Energy Systems

Training Method	Definition	ATP-CP and -LA (%)	LA-02 (%)	02 (%)
Pickup Sprints	Gradual increases in speed from jogging-to-striding-to sprinting in 25 to 120-yd. segments.	85	10	5
Hollow Sprints	Two sprints interrupted by "hollow" periods of jogging or walking.	80	10	10
Interval Sprints	Alternate sprints of 20 to 300 yards, jogging and walking for recovery.	80	10	10
Jogging	Continuous running at a slow pace over a distance of 2 or more miles	0	0	100

It is important to point out at this time that although sprint-assisted training does involve the anaerobic energy system, it is NOT an effective speed endurance training program. Overspeed programs require 4-5 minutes of rest between repetitions to allow full recovery and are designed to train the neuromuscular system and allow faster steps per second; therefore, it should not be confused with anaerobic training.

What would an 8-week speed endurance program look like for team sport athletes preparing for the first game?

Speed endurance training programs are designed to train both the ATP/CP system and the ATP/Lactic acid system since both systems play a major role in your ability to continuously sprint at maximum speed for 5-8 seconds (ATP/PC system) and up to 60 seconds (Lactic Acid System). The eight-week program described in Table 9-2 combines the use of the three main programs presented in this section: Pickup Sprints, Hollow Sprints, and Interval Sprint Training and is based on the estimated percent of anaerobic and aerobic involvement discussed in Chapter 6 and shown in Table 9.2. The improvement of each energy system occurs by manipulating the training variables: frequency of training, number of repetitions, intensity of each repetition, distance covered or time required to complete each repetition, and recovery time and action between each repetition. The program is designed to improve the speed endurance of athletes in baseball, basketball, field hockey, football, lacrosse, rugby, soccer, and other power sports.

Can programs be customized even further to fit any sport?

Sprint distances and rest periods can easily be altered to mimic game conditions in any sport. Table 9.3 provides some assistance in estimating the average distance covered and the typical rest period that occurs. Depending on player position, further adaptation may be needed.

What is maximum effort training and how is it used to improve speed endurance?

Maximum effort training is designed to completely exhaust athletes through all-out efforts at the end of a workout. It is one of the few good methods of equalizing exercise effort among athletes at different conditioning levels. Training is geared to the individual with each working against his own previous distance or time, each coping with his own stress and psychological barriers, until only exhaustion stops exercise.

The program in Table 9-3 is used no more than 1-2 times weekly. Records are kept and periodic testing is scheduled to measure individual progress.

TABLE 9.2 Eight-week Speed Endurance Program

Week	Workout	Distance	Repetitions	Rest Interval
1	1	Jog 15 yards, stride 15 (3/4 speed) jog 15, walk 15	5	The walk is the recovery each set.
1	2	Same as previous workout	7	Same
1	3	Jog 20 yards, stride 20 (9/10 speed), jog 20, walk 20	5	Same
2	4	Same as previous workout	7	Same
2	5	Jog 15 yards, stride 15 (3/4 speed) sprint 15 (maximum speed), walk 15	5	Same
2	6	Same as previous workout	7	Same.
3	7	Jog 20 yards, stride 20, sprint 20, walk 20	7	Same
3	8	Same as previous workout	9	Same
3	9	Jog 25 yards, stride 25, sprint 25 walk 25	7	Same
4	10	Sprint 15 yards, jog 15, sprint 15, walk 15	7	The walk is the recovery
		Distance hop to exhaustion	1	Each leg
4	11	Sprint 20 yards, jog 20, sprint 20, walk 20	7	Same
4	12	Sprint 20 yards, jog 10, sprint 20, walk 20	9	Same
		Bench Jump to exhaustion	2	1 minute
5	13	Sprint 25 yards, jog 25, sprint 25, walk 25	9	Same
5	14	Sprint 20 yards	10	Walk 10-30 seconds
		300-yard sprint	1	3-4 minutes
		Run in-place to exhaustion	2	1 minute
5	15	Sprint 30 yards	10	Walk 10-30 seconds

TABLE 9.2 **(continued)**

Week	Work out	Distance	Repetitions	Rest Interval
6	16	Sprint 40 yards	8	Same
		300-yard sprint	2	3 minutes
		Distance hop to exhaustion	1	each leg
6	17	Sprint 40 yards	10	Walk 10-30 seconds
		440-yard dash	1	
6	18	Sprint 20 yards, jog 20, sprint 20, walk 20	12	Walk is the recovery period
		440 yard sprint	2	4-5 minutes
		Bench Jump to exhaustion	1	
7	19	Sprint 20 yards, jog 20, sprint 20, walk 20	15	20 yard walk is the recovery period
		300 yard sprint	3	2 1/2 Min.
7	20	On a 400-meter track, sprint 50, jog for 10 to 12 sec., sprint 50, jog for 10-12 seconds and so on.	20	Jog is the rest period.
		Sprinting in place with high knee to exhaustion	2	1 minute
8	21	440 yard sprint	4	4-5 minutes
8	22	On a 400-meter track, sprint 50, jog for 10-12 seconds sprint 50, jog for 10-12 seconds and so on.	25	Jog is the rest period
		Bench Jump to exhaustion	4	1 minute

Note: The cycle begins eight weeks from competition. The program assumes that each athlete begins with a solid aerobic fitness foundation based on the scores in the 1.5 mile run test described in Chapter 2.

Table 9.3 **Maximum Effort Training**

Program	Training Action
BASIC:	
All-out sprint	Sprint up and back the length of an athletic field until you are no longer able to continue. Record the distance.
Distance hop	Perform a one-legged hop at maximum speed until no longer able to continue. Record the distance and time. Repeat using the opposite leg.
Squat jumps	Perform a maximum number of squat jumps, falling to a right angle only and avoiding the full squat position, in a period of 90 seconds. Slowly increase the time limit as you progress.
CONCENTRATION I:	Supplement your basic workout with concentrations I and II to add variety to the lower torso muscles involved in the sprinting action. Sprint in-place to exhaustion. Record the time.
Treadmill pacing	Set the treadmill for 15 mph and run until no longer able to continue.
300-yard run	Record your time in a 300-yard sprint.
Two-legged hop	Record the distance covered in 45 seconds. Slowly increase the time limit.
CONCENTRATION II	
400-meter dash +	Surprise runners at the finish of the 400-meter dash with the command to continue sprinting as far as possible.
Bench jump	Stand parallel to a bench, jump to the other side using a two-foot takeoff, immediately jumping back to the starting position. Repeat until you are no longer able to continue. Record the total number of jumps.
Isometric charge	With the legs moving continuously and shoulder and hands placed against an immovable object (sled, wall, post), continue to drive forward until no longer able to continue.

How do athletes maintain their speed endurance during the competitive season?

Coaches include speed endurance training a minimum of twice weekly during the in-season period using a maintenance workout based on the average distance sprinted in various sports shown below in Table 9-4. Athletes sprint 12-15 repetitions at the distance specified for their sport and rest the number of seconds indicated in the right-hand column between each repetition, and end the workout with two 300-meter sprints using a two minute rest period between repetitions.

Table 9.4 **Speed Endurance In-season Maintenance Loads**

Sport	Average Distance Covered (sec.)	rest Interval (sec.)
Baseball. Softball	30	30 to 60
Basketball	30	5 to 20
Football	10 to 40	25 to 30 (huddle time)
Soccer, Lacrosse, Rugby, Field Hockey	10 to 40	5 to 15
Tennis	5 to 10	3 to 5 (same sport) 20 to 30 (between points) 60 (between games)

What can be done to make sure athletes get the most out of their speed endurance training program?

The following tips represent a summary of recommendations for speed endurance training that can be applied to all programs:

• The speed endurance training programs discussed in this chapter allows athletes to choose the specific energy systems critical to their team sport. Most team sports require energy use similar to repeated high intensity sprints interspersed with walking, jogging or complete rest. The combination of pick-up sprints, hollow sprints, and interval sprint training can easily duplicate competitive conditions to engage athletes in sports-specific speed endurance training. This type of training, combined with a solid aerobic foundation, will prepare athletes for all levels of team sport competition.

• As Vince Lombardi once said, "Fatigue makes cowards of us all." Speed is hindered by fatigue and fatigue keeps athletes from exerting their maximum effort. Athletes do need to learn to tolerate "discomfort" and not allow the general feeling of fatigue to dictate effort. Obviously, failure to control the mind to allow maximum effort during each repetition is counterproductive.

• The majority of speed endurance work for athletes in football, basketball, soccer, baseball, field hockey, rugby and lacrosse should involve segments of 20- to 80-yard sprints or 5-10 second all-out sprints with a recovery interval of slightly less than the time that occurs between sprints during competition. Longer, intermediate distances (100, 150, 200, 250, 300-yards) requiring a 15-30 second sprint are also important in the training of the ATP Lactic Acid System. Runs of 400-1200 yards and maximum effort training are used occasionally as the final 1-3 repetitions of a workout.

• Repetitions of "maximum effort sprinting" for 30-60 seconds should be a part of every program. At least one maximum effort exercise to complete exhaustion should be included at the end of each speed endurance workout.

• All-out sprints covering approximately the same or greater distances than those normally sprinted in your sport should be used.

• Coaches must keep careful records of each workout to apply the concept of progressive resistance exercise and ensure gains throughout the season. Distances covered, number of repetitions, speed of each repetition, and the length (time) and type (standing, walking, jogging) of the rest interval are recorded to make certain that training loads are increased each workout.

• Coaches should check the current level of speed endurance of each athlete several times during the in-season period by retesting in the NASE repeated 20, 30 or 40-yard distances. Ten consecutive dashes at one of the above distances is completed using a 10-30-second rest interval between each repetition. Ideally, none of the ten timed repetitions should be more than 0.2 second slower than the best time.

Chapter 10

NEUROMUSCULAR TRAINING

A neurosurgeon, speaking on the topic of neuromuscular training at an NASE National Convention said, "After several weeks of sprint-assisted training such as towing, the nervous system allows you to continue these assisted higher rates of stride frequency without any help. As a result, you can now take those faster steps without any assistance." Although this statement is only theory, research shows that the number of steps you take per second does improve following 8-12 weeks of training. Part of this improvement is due to to neuromuscular adaptation to the forced higher speeds (the neuron recruitment level increases) and, after several months of continued training, from conversion of the intermediate fast twitch red fibers (type IIa) to fast twitch white (type IIb). As indicated in Chapter 8: Power Output Training (speed-strength) that increases ground contact force or the pushing force against the ground with each step is also a major contributor to stride rate increases.

Researchers at Lisle confirm the value of sprint-assisted training (Jakalski, 2000):

> "At Lisle we have done quite a bit of research on the effects of sprint-assisted training and are convinced that two things occur when athletes are sprint-assisted: first, the towing procedure "lights up" the central nervous system, bringing into play great numbers of neurons; second, it makes the legs more responsive to ground reaction. By lighting up the central nervous system, I mean that towing alters the timing of the nervous system to the effecter muscles. In other words, towing creates some anticipatory firing, and this kind of firing enhances intramuscular coordination. In terms of ground reaction response, we theorize that the increase in horizontal momentum resulting from towing alters the capacity of joint stabilization at the ankle and knee, thereby allowing for a greater transmission of force."

Although still considered somewhat controversial, numerous other studies, including the Virginia Commonwealth University studies conducted in the early 1980s (Dintiman, 1980, 1982, 1984), revealed similar findings.

How much can athletes expect to improve?

Athletes have improved their 40-yard-dash times by as much as 6/10 second following an 8-12 week period. Track athletes in the 100-meter dash have improved their times by more than 8/10 second. Keep in mind that such improvement won't happen overnight. Training the neuromuscular system takes time, so you need to stay with the program a minimum of eight weeks. Eventually, an ongoing maintenance program involving one to two workouts per week is used to avoid losing the acquired gains.

Does engaging in sprint-assisted training minutes before a race improve performance?

Yes. Using electronic timing, researchers found that sprinters who performed repeated 30 and 60-meter flying or block starts, after two or three repetitions of 30-60-meter assisted sprints, ran their "unassisted sprints" noticeably faster. This enhanced performance "window" remains open for a short time only with levels dropping back to normal in 5-10 minutes. Using 2-3 towing repetitions immediately prior to the 40-yard dash test as a warm-up technique may also improve times for team sport athletes.

SPRINT-ASSISTED TRAINING PROGRAMS

What training programs effectively increase stride rate?

The two main training programs are Power Output Training (speed-strength training in the weight room, plyometrics, and sprint-resisted training) and the sprint-assisted training programs described in this chapter.

The purpose of sprint-assisted training is to "reset the speed clock" and it is one of the most demanding phases of a sports speed improvement program. This phase is also the most fun. Athletes experience the feeling of raw power and are amazed at the results as they sprint at high speeds often as fast or faster than NFL halfbacks, MLB leading base stealers, or pro soccer and NBA speedsters.

What training tips should athletes follow with this program?

Athletes should adhere to the following guidelines for each of the sprint-assisted training methods discussed in this chapter:

- Build a solid conditioning base of speed endurance and speed-strength before beginning a sprint-assisted program.

- Warm up thoroughly. Begin every workout with a general warm-up routine to increase core temperature. Use the large muscle groups first with a slow jog for 400 to 800 meters, followed by a faster jog for an additional 400 meters or more. When perspiring freely, stop and complete the dynamic stretching routine described in Chapter 7 for 8 to 10 minutes. Now complete a walk-jog-stride-sprint cycle (walk 15 steps, slow jog 15 steps, stride 15 steps at three-quarters speed, and sprint 15 steps). Continue this cycle for 400 meters or until you feel prepared to execute all-out assisted training sprints.

- Sprint-assisted training is an advanced program designed for athletes who have a stable motor pattern of correct sprinting technique. Form errors by those with poor sprinting mechanics are likely to become exaggerated with sprint-assisted training. Take training very seriously and pay attention to the specific suggestions for each method to avoid muscle or equipment-related injuries that may occur due to horseplay or carelessness.

- Use sprint-assisted training only on a soft, grassy area. Inspect the surface for broken glass and other objects.

- Apply the concept of "work fast to be fast." Since fast-twitch muscle fibers have a high firing threshold, training must include work at high intensity levels.

- Expect to experience muscle soreness one to two days after the first training session. This type of training will recruit motor units and muscle fibers that most athletes are not accustomed to using. Expect muscle soreness even if you have been involved in some form of sprint training for several weeks. This soreness is a sign that training is going beyond your normal workout routine.

- Always use sprint-assisted training in the beginning of a workout, immediately after completing the general warm-up and stretching session.

Athletes can only take ultra-fast natural strides when free from fatigue. Avoid any type of sprint-assisted training after being fatigued from drills, calisthenics, scrimmages, speed endurance training, weight training, or plyometrics.

• Remember, the objective is to force faster steps than ever before, not to improve speed endurance. Utilize the entire recommended rest period between each repetition and make certain full recovery occurs before completing the next assisted sprint.

• Emphasize quality form in all repetitions. If you are sprinting out of control, the force of the pull must be reduced on subsequent repetitions to allow perfect sprinting form. *For maximum results, stay within the 10% zone on all repetitions.* The most effective training of the neuromuscular system for speed improvement occurs when a sprint-assisted training program forces athletes to run no more than 10 percent faster than their unaided maximum speed. If an unassisted 40-yard dash can be completed in 4.8 seconds, for example, the sprint-assisted towing time must be in the 4.3 - 4.5 (5 to 10%) range Faster pulls produce a braking action to avoid falling, longer ground-contact time, less ground contact force, and develop habits that have a negative impact on forward movement.

• After sprinting with the assistance of a pull or decline, try to maintain the high speed for another ten meters without assistance.

• In early workouts, be patient, use correct form, and progress slowly from one-half to three-quarter to maximum speed runs over a period of 2-3 weeks.

How does sprint-assisted training differ from speed endurance training?

The difference is not always clear, although the training objectives are not the same. The mere fact that a sprint-assisted technique is being used, for example, does not guarantee that a speed workout is taking place. Speed work is designed to train the neuromuscular system by helping the body adapt to extremely fast muscular contraction and high stride rates (steps per second). Improvement occurs through neuromuscular adaptation to forced higher speeds. Since everyone can improve their stride rate, speed work focuses on helping athletes get as close as possible to 5.0 (males) or 4.5 (females) steps per second without reducing the natural length of the stride. These high speeds can only be obtained when athletes are fatigue free.

What distinguishes speed work from speed endurance work (anaerobic training) is not the program but the way it is conducted. *If a sprint-assisted activity occurs with less than full recovery between repetitions, only the first repetition is considered speed work. The remaining repetitions fall in the category of speed endurance training.* For speed work, complete recovery must occur between each repetition. Depending on the distance covered in each sprint, a 4-6 minute rest period may be needed. This allows each repetition to be completed with correct form at super high speeds without the slowing effect of fatigue. The recommended distance of the assist or pull phase is 10-30 yards. .

The key to effective speed endurance training for team sports is to prevent full recovery between repetitions by progressively reducing the rest interval, increasing the distance covered, and working at high intensity (maximum sprinting effort). The key to effective sprint-assisted training is to make certain full recovery does occur before completing the next assisted repetition.

TYPES OF SPRINT-ASSISTED TRAINING

What sprint-assisted training methods are effective?

There are four basic methods of sprint-assisted training: downhill sprinting; high-speed cycling; towing with surgical tubing, pulley devices, and the Sprint Master; and high-speed treadmill sprint training. Not every method is equally effective. Some are also less expensive, more practical and more effective than others.

Downhill Sprinting

How is downhill or incline sprint training used?

Downhill sprinting is one of the most practical forms of sprint-assisted training and requires no special equipment. Stronger, more experienced athletes are less likely to be injured and more likely to benefit from this training technique.

The trick is to locate the proper slope and distance for a training session. A general guideline is to find a 50-meter area with a slope no greater than one percent. Consult your coach for suggestions. A one percent slope will keep athletes under the 10% zone, avoid a braking effect, incorrect form, increased ground contact time, and falling which is much more likely to occur with higher slopes. The ideal area will allow a 20 yard sprint on a flat surface (to reach near top speed), a 15-yard sprint down a one degree slope (to force higher stride rates and speed), and end with a 15 yard sprint on a flat area as athletes attempt to maintain the higher speed rates without the assistance of gravity

The "crown" on a football field is close to a 1% grade and can be used by sprinting from one sideline of the field to the crown, up the slope, and down the other side at high speed to the opposite sideline.

Carefully examine the grounds in your school, university, park, and neighborhood, looking in the surrounding areas of soccer and football fields and other grassy areas, or ask your coach to consider building an area specifically for downhill sprint training. Once a suitable place is found, follow the program shown in table 10.1 and pay attention to the rest or recovery period between each repetition.

Combining downhill (resisted) and uphill (assisted) sprinting in the same workout has been shown to significantly increase stride rate.

Towing

Is towing an effective sprint-assisted method?

Yes. Towing or pulling athletes at high rates of speed is not a new approach. Before surgical tubing and two-person pulley arrangements, currently outdated methods such as motor scooters, motorcycles, and even automobiles were used (Dintiman, 1968 and other researchers). In 1956, towing was used to train Olympic medal winner Al Lawrence, who held on to a rigid bar attached to a car four times per week for distances of 100 to 600 yards. In the 1960s, towing was successfully used in Australia to reduce the 100-meter time of one subject who held on to the side of a tram car. Young sprinters increased their stride length considerably (an average of six inches) and improved their 100-yard dash time from an average of 10.5 to 9.9 seconds. In 1976, a four-station tow bar attached to an automobile was used to improve 40-yard dash times with a flying start. Towing has also been a regular part of the NASE annual speed camps since 1970, and sprint-assisted training has been an important part of the training programs to improve 40-yard dash times for team sports.

Towing produces higher stride rates and is more effective than downhill sprinting and high-speed cycling. It also will improve 20, 30, 40 or 60-yard dash time more than most other sprint-assisted training techniques. Athletes can choose from three unique methods: towing with surgical tubing, towing with the Ultra Speed Pacer, or towing with the Sprint Master.

Towing With Surgical Tubing

How is surgical tubing used in a towing program?

Surgical tubing with the bullet belt release and other specialized items from Power Systems can force athletes to take faster and longer steps and complete a 40-yard dash at world-record speed simply by providing a slight pull throughout the sprint. A 20 to 25 foot piece of elastic tubing is attached to the waist by a belt. The opposite end can be attached to another athlete or to a stationary object such as a tree or a goal post to allow individuals to work out alone. Athletes now back up approximately 25 yards before running at three-quarters speed with the pull for 4-5 repetitions using proper sprinting form. After the practice runs, athletes usually become acclimated and are capable of all out sprints without breaking form.

Surgical tubing will safely stretch to six times its unstretched length (20 feet X 6 = 120 feet or 40 yards). *It is important to avoid stretching the tubing beyond this recommended limit and to apply the 10 percent rule described previously.* Repetitions can be completed from a stationary position using a standing, 3-point or 4-point track start.

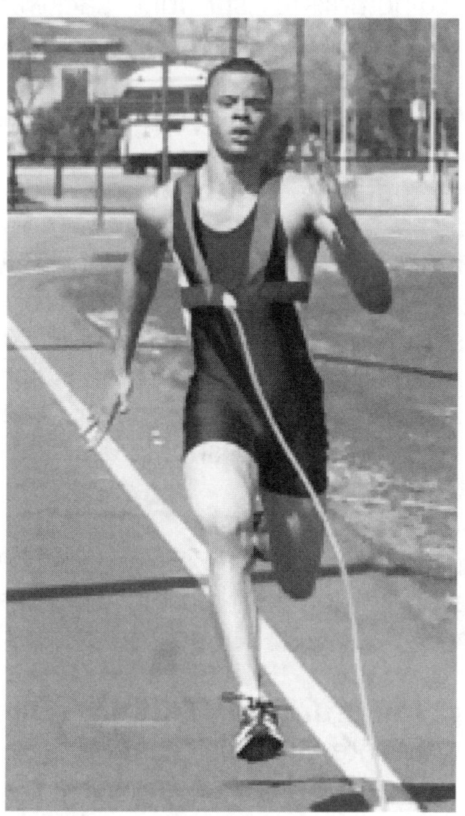

Figure 10. 1 Towing with Surgical Tubing using the chest harness.

A variety of general and sports-specific drills can be used:

• Acclimation--Attach one end of the tubing to a goal post and the other to your waist with the tubing tied in front. Stretch the tubing by walking backward about 15 yards. Jog forward toward the goal post with the pull. Repeat this drill four times, two with a three-quarter speed run and two a full-speed sprint. Within the next three sprints, back up an extra five to eight yards each time to increase the pull and the speed of the sprint.

• Repeat the last part of the preceding drill, emphasizing a high knee lift.

• Complete 4-5 all-out sprints using the exact rest interval recommended in table 10.1. Allow the tubing to pull at no more than one-half second faster than your best 40-yard dash time. It takes only a slight pull to produce this effect and pulls that produce more than a 10% improvement in your 40-yard time are dangerous and counterproductive. Place two cones 40 yards apart and have someone time one of the assisted sprints.

• For athletes who are required to do so in their sport (defensive backs in football; basketball, baseball, field hockey, lacrosse, rugby, soccer, and tennis players), repeat the preceding drills by sprinting backward and in a side ward motion. Turn the belt around to the center of your back or to the hip.

• Choose a faster athlete and race him or her while being towed.

• Complete the two-person drill by attaching one end of the tubing to your waist and the other to a partner's back. Have a partner sprint 25 to 30 yards ahead against the resistance, and then stop. You now sprint toward your partner in a sprint-assisted training run. Continue for two to three more repetitions before reversing the position of the belt. You are now sprinting against resistance (sport loading), and the partner is sprinting with assistance (sprint-assisted training). A 5-6 minute rest period is needed if more than one set is used. This contrast training drill should be the last drill in a sprint-assisted training workout.

Follow the sprint-assisted training training program in table 10.1 two to three times per week (every other day) during the preseason period in your sport and one to two times per week during the in-season period.

Safety Precautions for Surgical Tubing. Surgical tubing can be dangerous and requires adequate supervision at all times. Tubing can break if stretched too far, belts can come loose if they are carelessly fastened, too much pull can produce falls, soft tissue injuries, braking, increased ground-contract time, inappropriate loading of the nervous system, and runners can get tangled at the end of the run as the tubing returns to its pre-stretched length. The risk of injury and other undesirable effects can be reduced by applying the following guidelines:

• Make certain the tubing is tied securely to the belt. After tubing is used a few times, the knots will tighten. Newly tied belts must be inspected before each run. After putting on the belt, there will be an extra length of leftover belt (the "tail"). It is important to wrap the tail around the stomach, then thread it again through the loop formed before pulling securely to form a knot. This process should be repeated until most of the leftover belt is used.

• Inspect the tubing on the first run by letting it slide through your hand as you back up to locate a nick or rough mark. If a nick is detected, discard and replace with a new tubing.

• Avoid stretching the tubing more than six times its unstretched length.

• Inspect the knots on both belts and retie them if they are not tight or appear to be coming loose.

• Avoid standing with the tubing fully stretched for more than a few seconds. It is during this stretched phase that knots come loose and tubing breaks.

• When using a 3-point stance with the tubing fully stretched for a quick test, protect your face and avoid staying in the "set" position for more than 5/10 of a second. If the opposite end comes lose, it could recoil to the face and eyes.

• Use tubing that attaches to a belt around your waist rather than to a harness. With only slight differences in height between partners, a broken tubing or a loose belt could snap upward and strike the eyes. Tubing attached to the waist that comes loose when stretched is unlikely to produce any serious injury.

• Use shoes without spikes for the first several workouts until fully acclimated to the high speed sprints.

• Use surgical tubing on soft grassy areas only.

• Adhere to the 10% rule at all times, deny requests to use more than one tubing on athletes under 200 pounds, and never allow the use of three pieces of surgical tubing.

Towing With the Sprint Master®

How did the Sprint Master® evolve and and how does it work?

Following a summer speed camp in the late 1970s at Virginia Commonwealth University (VCU) in Richmond, Virginia, there was frustration over problems with the use of a motor scooter to tow athletes at high speeds. It was then that Dr. Dintiman indicated the need for a motorized device that could be attached to a wall and used indoors or outdoors that was also capable of towing athletes at high, regulated speeds. John Dolan, who assisted in the speed camp and is also one of the early pioneers in experimenting with sprint-assisted training, was immediately enthusiastic. He and a highly mechanical friend, Michael Watkins, constructed more than 20 prototypes before the Sprint Master was perfected. The machine is engineered to pull athletes at speeds faster than any human can sprint. It attaches to the goal posts of a football or soccer field or to the wall in a gymnasium and provides controlled, variable speed for each athlete. It is also a safe device that eliminates the cumbersome, dangerous use of a vehicle and allows the athlete to merely release his or her grip if balance is lost. The Sprint Master® also permits full use of the arms while being towed at high speed. The athlete grasps the two handles and is literally reeled in by the Sprint Master®.

To initiate a sprint-assisted program with the Sprint Master®, consider the following suggestions:

• Use the workout schedule shown in table 10.1 two to three times per week (ever other day).

• Have a coach or friend pull you at approximately one-half second faster than your best flying 40-yard dash time. The operator quickly learns how to judge pace and can group athletes of similar speed together. It is also quite simple to place two marks 40 yards apart and time athletes as they are being pulled. The set screw on the machine can then be fixed at the proper speed.

• During the pull, grasp the tow-rope handles and accelerate slowly for 10 to 15 yards. The Sprint Master will then exert its proper pull as full speed is obtained for the recommended 10 to 30 yards. Pump the arms correctly using normal sprinting form instead of placing the hands and arms in front of the body and being pulled in water-ski like fashion.

• Practice the art of letting go of the rope handles if balance is lost. On an athletic field, especially in a full football uniform, a high-speed fall and a roll is generally safe. Very few runners fall at any towing speed once they are acclimated. Operating the Sprint Master® is easily learned and speeds can be individually determined for each athlete to help the operator make the pull safely. Most of the towing drills described previously for surgical tubing can also be used with the Sprint Master.

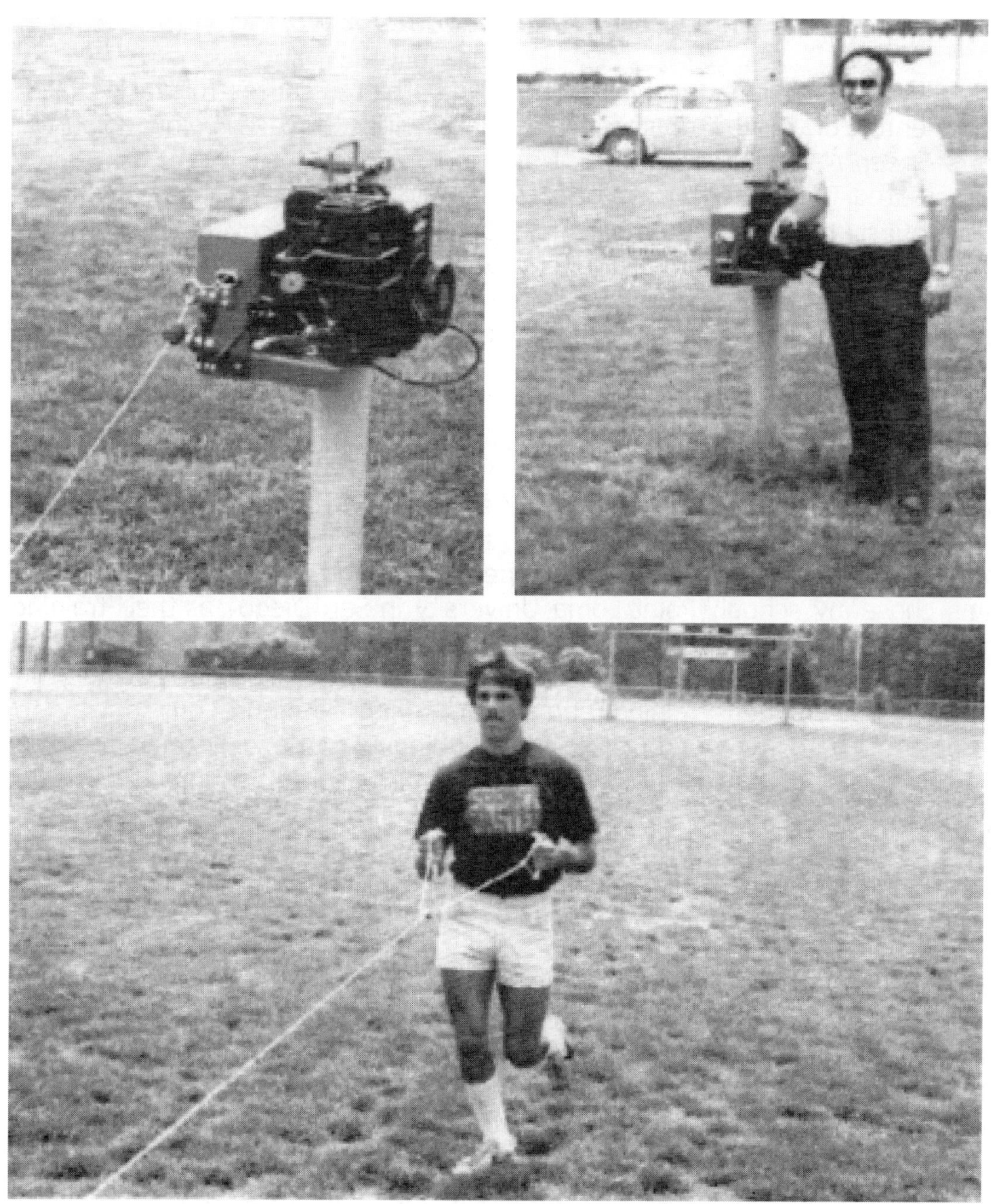

Figure 10.2 Towing with the Sprint Master

Towing With the Ultra Speed Pacer

What is the Ultra Speed Pacer and how does it work?

Marty Honea, former national level decathlon athlete, successful track coach, and inventor of the Ultra speed Pacer describes its use below (Source: *Sports Speed News Bulletin,* NASE, November, 2008 Issue).

"I created the Speed Pacer because of my own deficiencies in this area. In my quest to become an Olympic Decathlete I discovered that what seemed fast in high school was quite slow in college and was a snail's pace in the elite world of track and field. I did everything my coaches asked but after four years of college track and three years of post collegiate training, I saw very little speed improvements."

The Speed Pacer Story

I began reading everything I could find about speed training and ran across some articles on overspeed training, (some were written by Dr. George Dintiman). Around that same time, the British and Italian track and field teams chose my school (Point Loma University in San Diego) as their training grounds for the 1984 Olympics in Los Angeles. They were training with a very expensive motorized towing device. I became intrigued with the concept of overspeed training and began trying to figure out a way to incorporate it into my workouts. Surgical tubing was the only thing available on the market but that did not offer the control I desired. Running with the wind was hit and miss, so I tried hills, but couldn't find the right slope or surface. The motorized unit was way out of my budget, and running behind a car didn't seem wise. I even tried rigging up a device using bicycle gears, but nothing worked.

The Concept

Near the end of my career I discovered what a pulley as a *third class lever* was and created the first crude version of the *Ultra Speed Pacer*. Although I never set out to market it, several elite coaches discovered the item and asked me to make one for them. Although it was too late for me to use this tool to further my athletic career, I am very happy that the Speed Pacer has helped many other athletes. Within a few years every indoor and outdoor national championship track and field team was using the Speed Pacer. **The reason? It works**. At the age of 32. I began training with the high school track team I was coaching and, within 12 weeks, my personal best in the 100m dropped from 11.37 to 10.88. I was not as strong, couldn't jump as well, and wasn't near as fit, but my time dropped half of a second.

How the Speed Pacer works

The "Sprinter" attaches one end of the rope to the "automatic release hook" on his/her Speed Belt. The rope goes from the Sprinter to the Pacer and through a pulley that gives the Pacer a 2:1 mechanical advantage over the Sprinter. This advantage allows the Pacer to only have to go half as far and half as fast as the Sprinter. The key to overspeed training success is not too much, not too little, and, in one word, **CONTROL**. Running mechanics can never be compromised and the Speed Pacer is the only viable way to train within what I call the "Ultra Speed Zone" which is a zone just beyond the athletes' top speed and just below where mechanics suffer.

Why training in the "ULTRA SPEED ZONE" works

It is common knowledge that sprinting speed is the product of stride length and stride rate. The real issue is how to improve these two components. Some coaches focus on sprinting mechanics while others say that better sprint mechanics are the result of increased strength. An unbiased look at the research suggests that both are right and both should be trained. A proper testing protocol to determine the needs and deficiencies of each athlete will help coaches determine the correct primary and secondary focus of training. Regardless of the focus, all training should be geared toward:

- Increasing the force applied into the ground during both the acceleration phase and the maximum velocity phase in order to increase stride length. (The Speed Pacer allows the athlete to run against a steady resistance during both of these phases *without sacrificing mechanics*).

- Decreasing ground contact time each step (The Speed Pacer allows the athlete to run with a steady, controlled assistance from the acceleration phase to just beyond maximum velocity *without sacrificing mechanics*).

- Increasing the distance the athlete can maintain maximum velocity. (The Ultra Speed Pacer allows the athlete to increase this, often overlooked, factor by exerting less energy during acceleration).

Each must be improved and not to the detriment of the others. The Ultra Speed Pacer is the ONLY way you can consistently train these components because it puts the control in your hands.

A personal note

I believe that the greatest benefit to using the Speed Pacer is that it causes the neuromuscular system to "learn" to fire at a more rapid rate. I know that is what happened to me. The athletes I have trained absolutely love it. They love feeling fast. High school athletics got almost addicted to it, especially just before their race. (I have since read research that shows a "window" of about 5-10 minutes where overspeed carries over immediately to performance). Several overspeed sprints just prior to a race has shown to improve race times.

Have you heard the saying; "You have to run fast to run fast?" Well let me leave you with this, "YOU HAVE TO RUN FASTER TO RUN FASTER!"

Can you describe a complete sprint-assisted for team sport athletes?

An eight-week sprint-assisted training program using downhill slopes, surgical tubing, the Ultra Speed Pacer and the Sprint Master® is shown in Table 10-1. Unless athletes possess a solid conditioning foundation, sprint-assisted training should be avoided until completing the first three weeks of the Speed Endurance Training Program presented in Chapter 9 which prepares the body for the extremely high stride rates experienced in this program.

The first two weeks (four workouts) are designed to acclimate athletes to the use of surgical tubing and other towing devices, downhill sprinting and the pulling action while maintaining proper sprinting form. It wise to avoid exceeding a 3/4 speed striding action in any of the first four workouts. The sprint-assisted distance represents the area towed or the actual downhill distance covered and does not include the 20-25 yards used to accelerate to maximum speed, or the final 10-meters covered without assistance at the end of each repetition.

High-Speed Stationary Cycling

What type of stationary cycling program is recommended?

High-speed cycling is one of the least popular sprint-assisted programs in spite of the potential to improve several factors associated with sprinting speed. Very few studies, however, have examined the effect of this method on stride rate, maximum speed, and speed endurance even though stationary cycles are readily available and easily adaptable to most speed training programs. In addition, wind resistance, gravity, and body weight are eliminated to allow athletes to complete more revolutions per second (similar to steps in sprinting) than they are capable of completing during the sprinting action. Although the muscular movements of cycling and sprinting are not the same, the possibility of neuromuscular transfer does exists and it is theorized that high speed cycling involving low-to-moderate resistance for maximum revolutions and high resistance for improving speed endurance and speed-strength would improve speed in short sprints.

Table 10.1 Eight Week Program Using Downhill Slopes, Surgical Tubing, The Ultra-speed Pacer and the Sprint Master®

Week	Work-out	Overspeed Distance	Repeti-tions	Rest Interval
1	1	1/2 speed runs toward the pull for 15 yd. using correct sprinting, 1/2 speed (backward) toward the pull for 20-yds.	5 3	1 min. 1 min.
1	2	3/4 speed runs for 20 yd. with proper form 3/4-speed (backward) toward the pull for 20 yds.	5 3	2 min. 2 min.
2	3	3/4 speed runs for 25 yd. 3/4 speed (backward) toward pull for 20 yds. 3/4 speed turn-and-runs at a 45-degree angle for 25 yds. (left and right)	5 3 3	2 min. 2 min. 2 min.
2	4	Same as workout 3		
3	5	3/4 speed runs toward the pull for 15 yds. Maximum-speed sprints toward the pull for 15 yds.	3 5	2 min. 2 min.
3	6	3/4 speed runs for 25 yd. Maximum-speed sprints for 25 yd.	3 6	2 min. 2.5 min.
4	7	3/4 maximum speed runs for 25 yds. Maximum-speed pulls for 30 yds.	3 3	1 min. 2 min.
4	8	3/4 speed sprints for 30-yds. Maximum-speed sprints for 30 yds.	3 6	2 min. 3 min.
5	9	3/4 speed runs toward the pull for 15 yds. Quick feet, short step, low knee lift sprint for 15 yds. with rapid arm-pumping action Quick feet, short step, high knee lift sprint for 15 yds. with rapid arm-pumping action Maximum-speed pulls for 30 yds.	3 3 3 3	1 min 2 min. 3 min. min.

Table 10.1 **(continued)**

Week	Work-out	Overspeed Distance	Repeti-tions	Rest Interval
5	10	Same as workout 9		
6	11	High speed stationary cycling. With the resistance on low to average, warm-up for 5 to 7 min. until you perspire freely. Pedal at 3/4 speed for 30 sec.	3	1 min.
		Pedal at maximum speed for 2 sec. as you say "one thousand and one, one thousand and two"	7	2
		Pedal at maximum speed for 3 sec. as you say "one thousand and one, one thousand and two, one thousand and three"	3	2
		Pedal at maximum-speed for 5 sec.	6	2.5 min.
6	12	Same as workout 11		
7	13	Repeat workout 11		
		Two-man pull and resist drill for 100 yds.	2	5-6 min.
		Maximum speed sprints for 25 yds.	6	3 min.
7	14	Same as workout 11		
8	15	3/4 speed runs toward the pull for 15 yds.	3	1 min.
		Quick feet, short step, low knee lift sprint for 15 yds. with rapid arm-pumping action	5	2 min.
		Quick feet, short step, low knee lift sprint for 15 yd. with rapid arm-pumping action	5	2 min.
		Maximum-speed pulls for 30-yd.	5	3 min.
8	16	Maintenance Program		
		3/4 speed runs towards the pull for 15 yds.	2	2 min.
		Quick feet, short step, high knee lift sprint for 15 yds. with rapid arm-pumping action	2	2 min.
		Maximum-speed pull forward for 20-yd., planting the left foot and sprinting diagonally right for 20 yds.	3	2 min.
		Maximum speed pulls forward for 30 yds.	3	2 min.

Although evidence was revealed by Hudson (1968) that cycling and running depend on different neural firing rates due to the specific cyclic frequencies of each movement, preliminary evidence from our studies at Virginia Commonwealth University (VCU) indicated that such a program may carry over to increased stride rate in sprinting. In addition to increasing stride rate, cycling has the potential to improve speed endurance, expedite recovery from injury, and return athletes to competition with minimal loss of conditioning.

Are there any immediate after effects of using high speed cycling minutes before a race or 40-yard dash?

Studies have demonstrated that athletes performing a rhythmic activity for an extended period of time involuntary continue the movement pattern. An example of this phenomenon, referred to as *perseveration*, examined the rate of leg turnover (stride rate) in triathlon runners immediately following the cycling portion of the race. Faster cadences with low resistance in cycling substantially increased the subsequent average running speed and stride rate of runners during the race, according to a study by Gottschall and Palmer (2002). Participants ran faster primarily by increasing stride frequency. Immediately after each cycling bout, the participants ran with a stride frequency that reflected the prior cycling cadence. There is no evidence to date that high speed cycling just prior to a 40-yard dash improves race times. However, studies using towing with surgical tubing 10-15 minutes before a competitive 100-meter dash did result in an increase in stride rate and speed.

What are the long-term effects of high speed cycling?

High speed cycling has the potential to improve two areas: *ground contact forces* and *swing time* or time in the air as the feet switch position. Of the two, *ground contact* time is the most important and training is designed to increase the force of the push-off and reduce the time the foot spends on the ground. Gains in speed-strength that also involve a significant change in the athlete's strength-weight ratio is critical to faster leg turnover. The better the strength-weight ratio, the faster the leg turnover (stride rate). Although ground contact forces have long been the target of training to improve stride length, the same type of training has also been shown to improve stride rate.

Findings by a Harvard research team revealed the importance of strength-weight ratios, referred to as Mass-specific force applied to the ground, as the key contributor to improvement in stride length and rate. Strength-weight ratios are changed by altering current training methods slightly to increase speed-strength and reduce body fat to minimum levels. Leg strength/weight and other strength-weight ratios described in the test battery in Chapter 2 can be used to measure changes produced by a properly prepared speed-strength program. The second area of stride rate, *swing time*, or the recovery phase when the leg swings from the hip while the foot clears the ground, does not appear to be as important as ground contact forces with world class sprinters differing only slightly from other sprinters in the time required to reposition the legs in the air.

Although the VCU studies did show carry-over to flat surface unaided sprinting when stride rates were measured and compared during a flying 40-yard dash, only a small number of subjects were used and training protocols involved a combination of high speed cycling at a low-to-moderate resistance that allowed maximum revolutions per minute and heavy resistance settings for short bursts designed to improve speed-strength. The study did not isolate the two protocols. The changes in stride rate could have occurred from changes in speed-strength from the high resistance portion of the program.

Can you describe a cycling protocol?

High speed cycling programs, such as the program in table 10.2, should be used with one additional sprint-assisted method, such as towing or downhill sprinting. Resistance is adjusted to find the optimum load that allows the athlete to reach maximum pedaling speed. A load that is too light or too heavy will not accomplish this goal. A tapering off period of 5-10 seconds occurs after each pedaling repetition to return athletes to a slow cadence in preparation for the next repetition. Athletes are told to continue pedaling at this slow cadence of 25-30 revolutions per minute while in the two minute recovery period.

After an acclimation period, each repetition of maximum speed pedaling continues for one to two and one half seconds followed by a rest period that allows full recovery.

Cycling can be performed indoors using a stationary cycle or outdoors using a racing bicycle that allows use of the gears to regulate low and high resistance pedaling. During high-speed cycling, wind resistance, gravity, and body weight are eliminated to allow athletes to complete more revolutions (similar to steps in sprinting) per second than they are capable of completing during the sprinting action.

Treadmill Sprinting

What type of treadmill do I need to begin a program? How it is used?

It is actually difficult to find a high-speed treadmill without a special order and very high cost. In the VCU Laboratory, the A.R. Young high speed

Table 10.2 **Eight-week High Speed Cycling Program**

Week	Work-out	Repeti-tions	Acceleration Time (sec.)	Pedaling Speed	Overspeed time* (sec.)	Rest (min.)
1	1 2	2 3	1.5 to 2.0 Same	1/2 Same	1.0 to 1.5 Same	2 2
2	3 4	3 3	1.5 to 2.0 Same	3/4 Same	1.0 to 1.5 Same	2 2
3	5 6	4 4	2.0 to 2.5 Same	9/10 Same	1.5 to 2.0 Same	2.5 2.5
4	7 8	5 5	2.5 to 3.0 Same	Maximum Same	1.5 to 2.0 Same	2.5 2.5
5	9 10	6 6	2.5 to 3.0 Same	Maximum Same	1.5 to 2.0 Same	3 3
6	11 12	7 7	2.5 to 3.0 Same	Maximum Same	2.0 Same	3.5 3.5
7	13 14	8 8	2.5 to 3.0 Same	Maximum Same	2.0 Same	4 4
8	15 16	9 9	2.5 to 3.0 Same	Maximum Same	2.0 to 2.5 Same	4.5

* Overspeed time is the actual time you are pedaling at high speeds. A tapering off period of approximately 5-10 seconds occurs after each sprint-assisted pedaling sprint to return to a slow rhythm in preparation for the next repetition. Do not stop pedaling. Continue in the slow cadence of approximately 25-30 revolutions per minute while in the recovery period. Cycling can be performed indoors using a stationary cycle or outdoors using a racing bicycle that allows the use of lower gears and low resistance pedaling. As mph speed increases, a higher gear will be needed to complete the sprint-assisted phase.

treadmill, with a speed adapter kit (capable of speeds of 0 to 26+ miles per hour and a 100-meter dash under 10 seconds) was used to improve stride length, stride rate, form, speed endurance, and sprinting speed. Cinematography identified differences in stride length and rate at various speeds in both treadmill and unaided, flat-surface sprinting. Form was corrected by an expert standing on a stool facing and looking downward at the subject during high-speed sprinting.

The following guidelines were developed for use on the treadmill as an sprint-assisted training technique:

- Athletes use a standard warm-up procedure and stretching prior to entry on the treadmill.

• A harness that attaches to the support rails and allows free arm movement, balance, and safety is used. One spotter is placed on each side of the tread belt.

• A one-week acclimation period is used to allow sprinters to adjust to entry on the tread belt at high speeds and to treadmill sprinting.

• Since the tread belt accelerates slowly and would introduce a fatigue factor if sprinters were required to jog and stride until higher speeds were reached, belt speeds are preset prior to entry. After 6-8 practice attempts, sprinters can easily enter at high speeds. The "greyhound" effect allows athletes to reach maximum speed in approximately two seconds.

The sample program shown in table 10.3 has been used in a number of experiments at Virginia Commonwealth University.

Treadmill sprinting is not without its special problems. The sprinting action produces a slight slowing effect each time the foot strikes the tread belt; however, aiding factors predominate and allow a faster rate for most individuals even without training. This braking or slowing effect is greater for heavier athletes (over 200 pounds) and for athletes of all sizes in the initial stages of training and tends to be eliminated as acclimation occurs and form instruction is given. At high speeds beyond one's maximum speed (in early training sessions), the braking effect almost reduces tread belt speed to a sprinter's maximum speed. This problem is soon overcome.

There are additional problems. It is difficult to determine true tread belt speed with and without a sprinter on the treadmill. In one study (Dintiman 1984), a highly accurate surface speed indicator was used to determine belt speed variations with a sprinter (a 159-pound individual and a 197-pound individual) and without a sprinter. Several findings deserve attention:

• A heavier sprinter has a greater braking effect.

• The percent of braking increases as tread belt speed increases for both light and heavy subjects.

• As training progresses in several weeks, the amount of braking is reduced in both light and heavy sprinters at the higher speeds.

• At speeds in which the sprinter is being supported by the belt and is unable to maintain belt speed, only a normal expected braking occurs.

Most of the problems of treadmill sprint training can be overcome for athletes of all sizes by using an ample number of practice sessions at various speeds (acclimation), seeing that athletes master proper sprinting form, and avoiding a tread belt speed too far beyond the subject's maximum speed

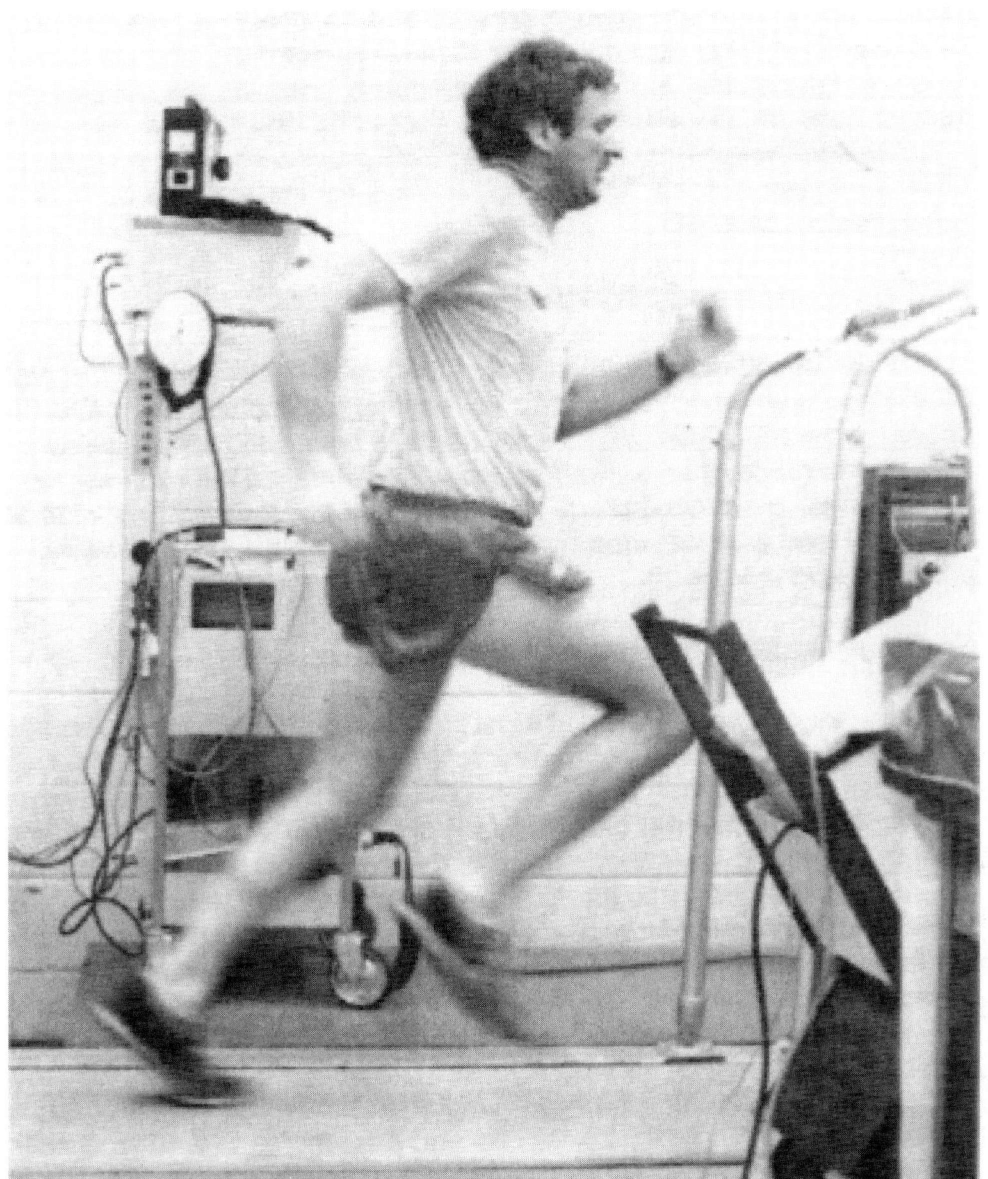

Super high stride rates can be produced on the high speed treadmill.

Figurer 10.3 High Speed Treadmill Sprinting

(the point at which proper sprinting form cannot be maintained). Ongoing research with high-speed treadmill sprinting continues to show improvements in speed with this effect carried over to unassisted sprinting.

Table 10.3 **High Speed Treadmill Sprint Program**

Purpose	Speed	Repetitions
Acclimation	90% of maximum	6-20 at 2-minute intervals for 10 seconds.
Entry practice	75% under maximum 90% under maximum At maximum speed	10-30 for two seconds
Improved stride rate and stride length	1-2 mph and 3-4 mph above maximum speed	2-6 for 3-5 seconds with full recovery after each repetition

The program described in table 10.2 for cycling can also be used in treadmill sprint training. Overspeed distances are converted to seconds on the treadmill (10 yards = 1 second; a 25-yard sprint requires 2.5 seconds on the treadmill). The number of repetitions, length of the rest interval, and progression are similar for both techniques.

ADVANCED SPRINT-ASSISTED TRAINING

Are there any other sprint-assisted programs that have proven effective?

Several sprint-assisted variations have been tested by researchers with athletes at the middle school, high school, university, and professional levels. However, these advanced methods are designed only for older, mature athletes who meet the leg strength standard (2.5 times body weight) described in Chapter 2 and have completed at least a four week preconditioning program that included speed endurance training.

What is Contrast Training and how is it used?

The main purpose of "contrast training" is to alter motor patterns associated with sprinting by using programs that impose demands *easier* (sprint-assisted training) or *harder* (sprint-resisted training) than the normal sprinting action. Contrast training "lights up" the central nervous system, brings into play a greater number of neurons, and makes the legs more responsive to ground reaction. This serves to force the neuromuscular system to perform at a higher level. Both assisted and resisted programs are used to improve each phases of a short sprint for team sports, including the start, early and late acceleration, and maximum speed. Research findings, including the Virginia Commonwealth University studies conducted in the 1980s (Dintiman, 1980, 1982, 1984), reveal improvements in the start, acceleration and maximum speed following the use of several forms of contrast training.

The most important aspect of the sprint for football players is the start and early acceleration (0-20 yards). For *interior defensive lineman* involved in penetration against the run (the first 3-steps) or the pass rush (first 3-steps followed by a 5-8 yard sprint), early acceleration speed is the key to success. This is also true for *offensive linemen* in executing pass protection blocking and blocking (including down field) for the run. *Wide receivers, tight ends, and defensive backs and linebackers* are more likely to sprint over 20 yards and to reach maximum velocity than players in other positions. The majority of running plays fail to cover 20 yards. Most of the game of football involves the start and early acceleration and this should receive the major training effort. Basic speed tests should focus on improving times in the First Three-Step test, and the 5, 10, and 20-yard dash.

Athletes in all positions in football should devote the majority of their training efforts to the programs that are most effective in improving starting and acceleration speed. Maximum velocity training can also be included for receivers, defensive backs, running backs and some linebackers.

The following concepts are recommended in utilizing contrast training in football and other team sports during the off-season period.

- Build a solid conditioning base of speed endurance and speed-strength before beginning a contrast training program.

- Schedule contrast training shortly after the general warm-up period when athletes are fatigue free.

- Emphasize quality form in all repetitions. If an athlete is sprinting out of control, reduce the force of the pull (assisted or resisted) on subsequent repetitions to allow perfect form and technique.

- For maximum results, stay within the 10% zone on all repetitions. The most effective training of the neuromuscular system for speed improvement occurs when a sprint-assisted training program forces athletes to run no more than 10 percent faster than their unaided maximum speed or 10% slower when resisted training is used. If an unassisted 40-yard dash can be completed in 4.8 seconds, for example, the sprint-assisted towing time must be in the 4.3 - 4.5 (5 to 10%) range. Faster pulls produce a braking action to avoid falling, longer ground-contact time, less ground contact force, and develop habits that have a negative impact on forward movement. The same concept is applied to resisted training. Heavier resistance is generally relegated to the start, the first three steps, and a total of 10 yards.

- The neuromuscular system fires at a specific motor pattern at maximum levels for only 2-3 seconds. Training distances (all out effort) and repetitions are therefore kept to 20-30 yards.

- The rest period between each repetition and set must allow complete recovery before another repetition is completed. Failure to do so changes the session into a speed endurance (anaerobic) training workout and eliminates its effectiveness

- During training to improve maximum velocity, resistance or assistance training still must avoid reducing or increasing an athlete's speed by more than 10 percent.

- Periodic timing is used to make certain the 10% rule is followed. If an athlete has been timed in 2.0 seconds for a "flying" 20 yard dash, the assisted repetitions should be no faster than 1.8 seconds. The same rule applies to resistance training. Inexpensive electronic timing systems are available that can be set up and used during resistance and assistance sessions to regulate speed and avoid violating this concept.

- Slopes for uphill and downhill sprinting should not exceed one percent when the training objective is to increase maximum velocity.

- Slightly steeper slopes than 1% and slightly heavier resistance is used only for acceleration training from the start to the end of early acceleration (about 0-20 yards).

- Resistance from behind using a automobile tire or sled requires a smooth surface such as grass to control friction and stabilize the resistance. Rough surfaces may provide too much resistance to aid maximum velocity training.

- Towing with surgical tubing is most effective during the start and early acceleration phase of sprinting (0-20 yards). Although tubing provides excellent initial pull or tension, after early acceleration, the assistance dissipates rapidly and contributes little to maximum velocity. The length of the pull can be extended another 10 yards or more if the partner begins by backing up 30 yards, then sprints in the same direction of the pull as soon as the repetition begins.

- For maximum velocity training, a pulley system such as the Ultra Speed Pacer® is superior to surgical tubing. The "Sprinter" attaches one end of a rope to an "automatic release hook" on his/her Speed Belt. The rope goes from the Sprinter to the Pacer and through a pulley that gives the Pacer a 2:1 mechanical advantage over the Sprinter. This advantage allows the Pacer to only have to run half as far and half as fast as the Sprinter to produce a significant "assist" or pull. The key to success with the pacer is CONTROL. Running mechanics are not compromised and the Speed Pacer allows athletes to train within the "Ultra Speed Zone" which is a zone just beyond the athletes' top speed and just below where mechanics suffer. (For more information on the Ultra Speed Pacer, e-mail its inventor, Marty Honea, at *M.L.Honea@maranausd.org).*

Table 1 lists specific training programs (assisted and resisted) and the phase of a short sprint in team sports that is most affected. The specifics of each method have been discussed in previous issues of *Sports Speed News Bulletin: (SSNB).*

Off-season Contrast Training Program

Athletes complete a general warm-up session to elevate core temperature, a dynamic stretching routine, and a series of walk-jog-stride-sprint cycles for 2-3 laps before beginning the Contrast Training Program. The start and acceleration parameters are then set at 0-20 yards and the maximum velocity parameter is set at 30 yards.

What are Ins and Outs and how are they used in team sports?

Ins and Outs is a training technique designed to improve an athlete's linear maximum velocity capacity. The drill is used to change what Manfred Steinbach, former international sprinter, refers to as the "Dynamic Stereotype." For speed improvement, this terms involves a rather fixed movement pattern of neural firing and timing that is difficult to alter. To improve linear velocity, training programs must be used that break down the dynamic stereotype and change and improve the parameters to allow faster movement. The In Phase is reached after a 3 second flying start when athletes attempt to sprint as fast as possible for 10 yards with or without assistance. The Out Phase immediately follows for 20 yards as an athlete reaches the point where an increase in velocity is impossible due to limitations of the nervous system and the body to further increase ground contact force and move the limbs through the full range of motion at a faster rate. At this point the athlete continues to hold proper form, maintain only a slightly reduced stride rate and stay relaxed in "overdrive."

After the "Out" phase ends, a second "In" is initiated with the athlete again making an attempt to sprint faster with greater stride frequency than ever before. As the technique is mastered, 20 yards can be used for the Ins and 10 yards for the Out phase. Adding a third and forth In and Out to the same repetition is not recommended since it moves training away from maximum velocity and becomes a speed endurance training program.

Table 10.4 Contrast Training and Most effective Use

TRAINING PROGRAM	MOST EFFECTIVE USE	SSNB ISSUE
SPRINT-RESISTED TRAINING Parachutes	Start and Acceleration	Nov. 2007
Sprinting Against Head Wind	Maximum Velocity	July, 2008
Uphill Sprinting	Start and Acceleration	July, 2008
Weighted Vests	Start and Acceleration	July, 2008
Weighted Sleds, Tires	Start and Acceleration	Nov. 2007
SPRINT-ASSISTED TRAINING: High Speed Cycling	Maximum Velocity	Sept. 2007
Sprinting with a Tail Wind	Maximum Velocity	July, 2008
Towing with Surgical Tubing	Start and Early Acceleration	Nov. 2007
Towing with the Ultra Speed Pacer	Maximum Velocity	Nov. 2008
Treadmill Sprinting	Start and Early Acceleration Maximum velocity	July, 2008

Table 10.5 Basic and Alternate Contrast Training Program

TRAINING PROGRAM	SETS	REPETI-TIONS*	REST BETWEEN REPS (Min.)	TECHNIQUE CHOICE	DISTANCE(YARDS) **
BASIC PROGRAM:					
1. Resisted Sprints	1	3	2-5	Uphill Sprinting Weighted Vests/Sleds	0-20
2. Assisted Sprints	1	3	5-8	Towing, High Speed Treadmill Sprinting Ultra Speed Pacer, High Speed Cycling,	0-20 After a 3 sec. flying start, 20-30 at max. speed
3. Unaided Sprints	1	3	4-5		
ALTERNATE:					
1. Resisted Sprints	1	1	3-4	Same as above	Same
2. Assisted Sprints	1	1	3-4	Same as above	Same
3. Unaided Sprints	1	1	4-3	Same as above	Same
Repeat second and third time after a 6-8 minute rest interval.					

* Repetitions are timed for each athlete. Adjustments are made to adhere to the 10% rule

** Olympic sprinters reach maximum velocity after approximately 60 meters. Team sport athletes use shorter steps in the start and early acceleration phase and reach maximum velocity sooner. With the right type of sprint assisted training, maximum velocity can be achieved quickly. In treadmill sprinting, for example, studies at Virginia Commonwealth University showed subjects were reaching maximum velocity in 3 seconds. Subjects stepped onto the tread belt while it was already at or slightly above their maximum velocity. Labeled the "greyhound effect, subjects caught up with the belt speed quickly. If the speed was set too high, a braking effect occurred that reduced belt speeds.

Which sprint-assisted training program is most effective and least expensive?

Table 10.6 describes the advantages and disadvantages of each sprint-assisted method and compares their cost and effectiveness. In team sports, several training techniques, such as high-speed treadmill sprinting, high-speed cycling, and towing with the Sprint Master® and the Ultra Speed Pacer are unsuited for group training. Practice and training time restraints make them impractical during the in-season period. These methods are better suited to off-season one-on-one training and use by personal trainers.

Table 10.6 Comparison of Sprint-assisted Training Programs

Method	Advantages	Disadvantages	Effectiveness
Downhill Sprinting	Practical, suited for large groups	Chance of injury, less assistance, less increase in stride rate and length	Good, will improve stride rate and speed.
High speed cycling	Used in home, gym, or outside. No wind or gravity.	Unproved.	Fair, more research needed. Use with one other method.
Towing (Tubing)	Inexpensive, can train alone safely indoors, excellent pull.	Falls may occur, no bailout, tubing can break or come loose.	Excellent, improves stride rate and speed in short sprints.
Sprint Master	Operator controls pull, elicits high stride rates, athletes can bailout by releasing the grip.	Expensive, impractical for group work.	Excellent, same as above.
Treadmill Sprinting	Performed inside, high stride rates, guard rails, harness and spotters protect the sprinter.	Expensive, requires spotters.	Excellent, improves stride rate, acceleration, and speed.
Ultra Speed Pacer	Performed inside or outside, produces high stride rates, athletes can bailout.	Difficult to use with groups, cannot combine with sport-specific drills.	Excellent, improves stride rate and speed.

Chapter 11

FORM AND TECHNIQUE TRAINING

Although training to improve form and technique in the start, acceleration and maximum speed phase of sprinting varies slightly from one sport to another, basic mechanics remain the same regardless of the type of start used in various sports and positions (3-point, 4-point, standing, moving).

Coaches have become adept in developing drills that mimic game situations and in combining drills with speed training to focus on the primary goal of improving "playing speed" for their sport. In the area of form and technique, coaches break down the running action and use drills involving exact movement patterns that occur during competition. Defensive backs, for example, are taught the exact footwork involved in backpedaling, turning and sprinting diagonally or straight ahead to cover a receiver. Athletes in basketball, soccer, rugby, field hockey, lacrosse are taught the correct footwork and sprinting form in executing the various fakes, feints, and cuts used in their sport. The theory is that this approach will transfer to team sports and allow athletes to perform sport-specific tasks at higher speeds when correct sprinting form is used.

What techniques are used by elite sprinters to develop proper form?

Form drills help establish correct neuromuscular movement patterns. Establishing as near error-free movement as possible will improve stride rate and stride length and eliminate wasted energy that does not contribute to forward movement.

Four muscle groups highly associated with fast sprinting are the quadriceps, plantar flexors, hamstrings, and dorsiflexors. The flexor muscles overcome limb weight and inertia; the extensors overcome their own weight and gravity. Form training and speed-strength training focus on these four groups. Since speed improvement occurs through well developed, efficient reflex patterns of action, correct repetitions using proper form are essential in every drill.

Other factors that are a part of the total speed improvement program described in this book also improve form and technique. Increasing the strength of the knee extensors and plantar flexor muscles of the feet, for example, helps the legs handle the workload during the drive phase, or push-off at ground contact. When these muscles are stronger, the less distance the center of mass drops and the faster the muscles contract with each stride. A strong upper body and trunk also help maintain good sprinting posture. All key muscle groups involved in sprinting, such as the hip flexors, are strengthened through power output training (weight room exercises, plyometrics, and sprint-resisted training). While some training programs focus on specific areas, others have a positive effect on many different aspects of speed improvement.

Sprinting form is evaluated in a number of ways. Slow motion taping and analysis of the entire sprint by the coach and athlete is one of the best methods of detecting and correcting problem areas. Athletes have an opportunity to see the incorrect technique before initiating hours of practice to establish the correct movement pattern in an area, then re-taping to make certain the correction has been made. This method is also used by the speed coach in team sports as part of off-season workouts. With the availability of the modern digital camera and flip video cameras, this simple technology is available to every athlete to analyze the start, acceleration and maximum speed phases of sprinting.

Drills vs. Observation of the complete act of sprinting. Coach Tom Tellez, famed University of Houston Track Coach and coach of numerous olympic sprinters such as Carl Lewis, Leroy Burrell, and Maurice Green, favors the method of observing and correcting sprinting errors using the entire action or 100-meter sprint rather specific drills that break sprinting down into separate components. Coach Tellez is of the opinion that drills dealing with component parts of sprinting technique are not performed in exactly the same manner as actual sprinting and therefore have little transfer value. Few coaches have the trained eye of Coach Tellez who is excellent at this technique with or without video analysis.

Ralph Mann, former Olympic silver medalist in the 400-meter hurdles and current speed improvement specialist, recommends both the "whole-part" method of Coach Tellez and the "part-hole" use of specific form drills. Dr. Mann evaluated more than 1,000 drills for downtime, proper technique, and duplication of skills. His sprinting drills have been successfully used by track and team sport coaches throughout the world o correct form errors. These drills have also been a key part of the NASE form and technique training program since the early 1970s and are still used to correct errors identified through observation and video analysis.

DRILLS TO IMPROVE STARTING SPEED

What drills are used to improve the start for team sport athletes?

Two-foot Push-off and Dive

Assume a crouched starting position and move to the "set" position. Now exert as much thrust as possible off both feet and dive forward onto a grass or matted area. Complete 15-20 repetitions. Pushing off both feet is the most difficult and most important habit to form for team sport athletes.

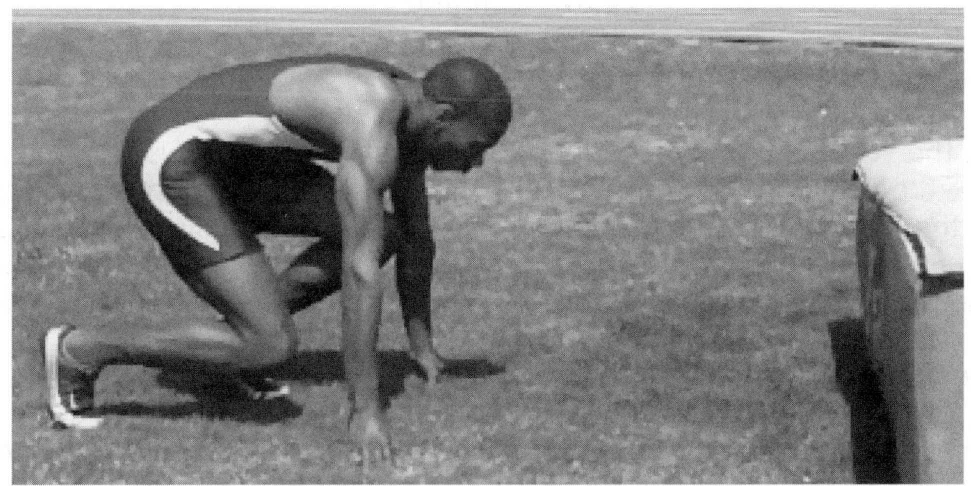

11.1a Two foot push-off

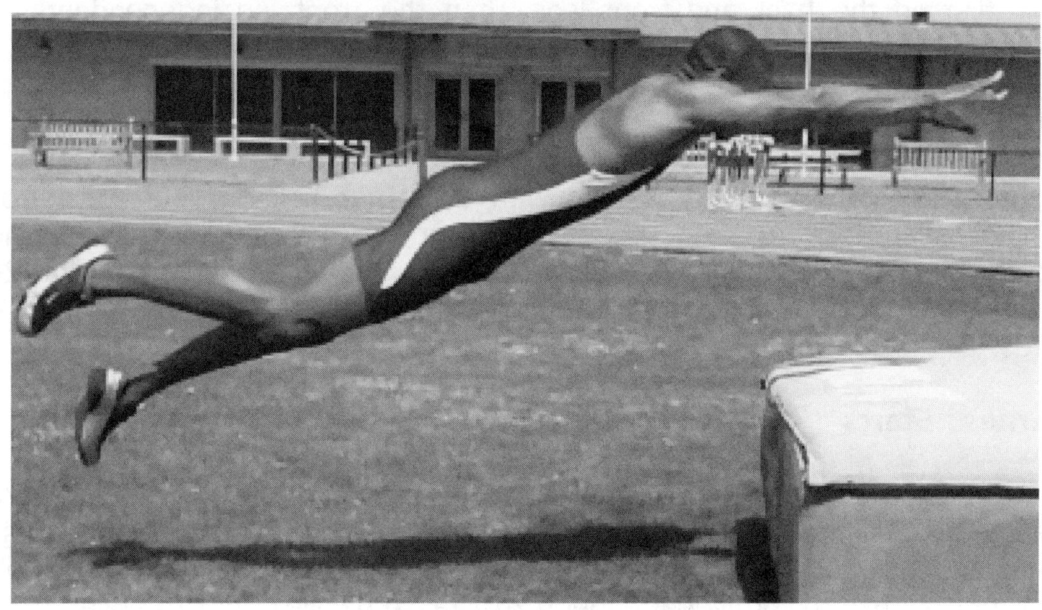

11.2b Dive

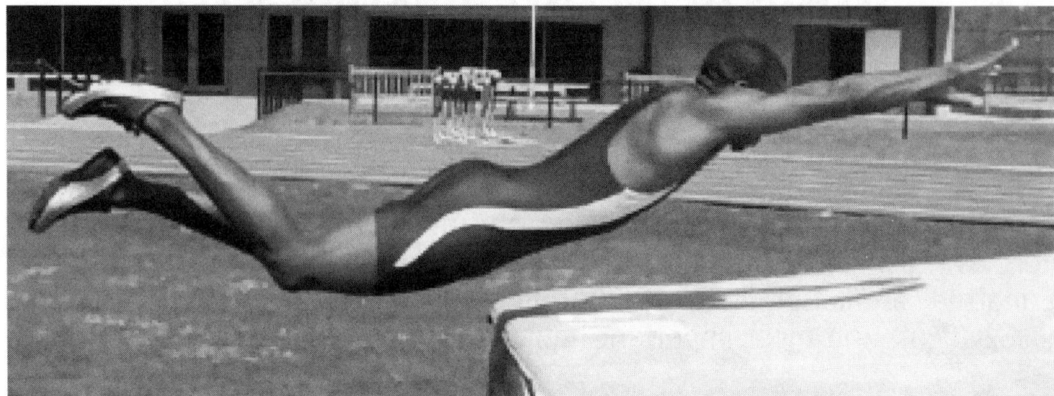

11.1c Landing

Two-foot Push-off and Drive

From the crouched start, "set" position, exert maximum thrust off both feet to get the body in motion. Now make the transition by continuing the thrust with the lead foot as the rear foot moves forward to begin the sprint cycle. The purpose of this drill is to help athletes develop the "feel" for thrusting off both feet and moving into the acceleration phase.

Falling Starts

From a stationary starting position, move your body weight forward on the command "set" by falling to about 90 degrees without moving the feet. On the command "go" swing the forward arm back and back arm forward as you drive first off the back and front legs, then the front leg independently to initiate the first stride.

Partner-Assisted Starts

Assume the standing start position with a partner holding your waist from behind. Lean forward 45-degrees and complete 4-5 strides as a partner provides enough resistance to allow only slow forward movement for 2-3 seconds before releasing the hold and permitting and all out sprint for 8-10 yards.

Harness Starts

Using a shoulder harness held by a partner, assume the crouched and/or standing start position. Move into the "set" position, use a short holding time, and the command "go" before executing a powerful push-off both feet with a partner providing enough resistance to allow you to cover 10-15 yards in 2-3 seconds.

Harness and Release Starts

Repeat the same drill with a partner using a quick release harness or bullet belt after the count of one-thousand-and one, one-thousand-and two to permit 1-2 seconds of heavy resistance, followed by a 8-10 yard sprint.

Arm Movement

As proper arm action is performed in a seated position, coaches observe from both a front and side view to make corrections. Observation and form correction is also effective while an athlete jogs-in-place.

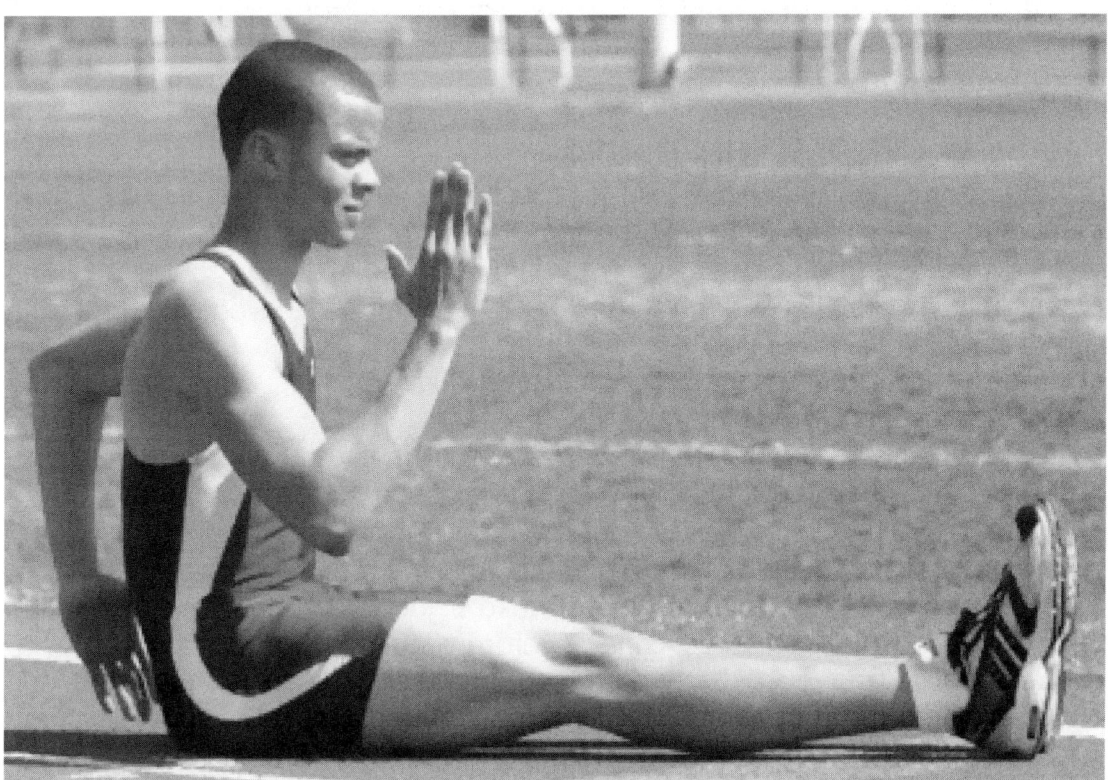

Figure 11.2 Practicing correct arm action

Sprint-assisted Start Using Tubing

Attach one end of the surgical tubing to your waist and other end to the front of a partner's waist and walk back to stretch the tubing about 25 yards. Assume the proper *standing start* position and execute a high speed 10-15 yard start and sprint with the pull. Repeat using a *crouched start* taking special care to make certain knots and belts are securely fastened and the tubing is free of nicks and cuts. Have a spotter stand just in front of you who is prepared to protect your head and face should the tubing snap from the partner's side. The crouched position is immediately assumed after the tubing is stretched and the start is quickly executed to shorten the time you are in this vulnerable position.

Sprint-Assisted Start Using a Downhill Area

Assume the crouched or standing start position in the center mound (50-yard line) of a football field and complete 3-5 starts for 10-15 yards using the force of gravity to aid your movement.

TRANSITION DRILLS TO IMPROVE ACCELERATION
(Walk or Jog to a Sprint)

What acceleration or transition drills are recommended?

Start and Sprint

From a stationary crouched or standing position, start quickly, and feel the power being applied behind your body. Ten yards out, quickly shift from running in back of the body to sprinting in front of the body. This drill should helps athletes tune in to the the difference between the start and acceleration phase (backside sprinting) and maximum speed phase (front side sprinting).

Gears

Place 5 cones 20 yards apart. Each cone represents gears 1-5. The task is to run in first gear (starting speed-strength) between cones 1 and 3, third gear between cones 2 and 3, and fourth gear (maximum speed) between cones 4 and 5. Now use an easy standing start to a jog by cone 1, one-half speed at cone 2, maximum speed by cone 3 before reducing intensity and trying to maintain stride frequency through cones 4 and 5.

Ins and Outs

Place 5 cones 20 yards apart. Progress from a slow walk to a jog by the first cone, accelerate to near maximum speed by the second cone, then to maximum speed by the third cone. At the third cone, attempt to sprint faster than ever before. At cone four, reduce the intensity and try to maintain stride frequency to cone five.

Pickup Sprints

Complete 15-20 repetitions of the walk-jog-stride-sprint cycle (10 yards at each pace) around a track concentrating on the rapid transition from a jog to a sprint.

SPRINTING FORM DRILLS

The information in this section emphasizes correct form after the starting and transition phases of sprinting. The mechanics of sprinting are broken into smaller segments and reinforced through specific drills.

What drills are recommended for team sport athletes?

Elite athletes use most of the drills described below that are designed to develop perfect mechanics and maximize strength and power. The length of each sprint can be altered to any desired distance to mimic play in team sports. Each drill focuses on 1 to 2 components of the total sprinting action which allows coaches to emphasize specific areas of difficulty.

The drills described below can be used as a separate workout or as part of a workout. Typically three sets of each drill is performed.

Butt Kickers

From a jog, the lower leg is allowed to swing back and move toward, rather than kick the buttocks. The upper leg moves very little. Emphasis is placed on allowing, not forcing, the heel to come up to the butt.

Wall Slide

From a jog, the action is the same as for butt kickers except that the heel of the recovery leg must not travel behind the body. Imagine a wall of glass running down your back and do not allow the heel to break the glass. This action will produce knee lift without forcing the action. When this drill is done properly, the heel moves close to the buttocks.

Quick Feet Drill

From a jog, increase stride rate and take as many steps as possible in a 10-yard interval. Jog for 10 yards and repeat. Emphasize quick turnover with the legs moving in front of, not behind or under, the body.

Cycling

Leaning against a wall, bar, or any support, one leg is cycled through in a sprinting manner. Emphasize keeping the leg from extending behind the body, allowing the foot to approach the butt during recovery, and pawing the ground to complete the action. Ten cycles with each leg make up one set.

Down and Offs

From a high knee position, the emphasis is on decreasing foot/ground contact by hitting the ground with the ball of the foot and getting off as quickly as possible. In turn, the effort on the ground should bounce your leg up into the high knee position. Ten down and offs make up one set.

Pull-Throughs

Extending the leg in front of the body (like a hurdler), the leg is then brought down and through ground contact in a power motion. Ten pull-throughs with each leg make up one set.

Stick Drill

Twenty sticks (18 to 24 inches in length) are placed 18′ apart on a grass surface. Athletes sprint through the sticks as fast as possible, touching one foot down between each emphasizing high knee lift and quick ground contact. Coaches can time athletes by starting a stopwatch when the foot contacts the ground between the first and the second stick and by stopping the watch when a foot contacts the ground after passing the final stick.

African Dance

While running forward, raise each leg to the side of the body as in hurdling, and tap each heel with the hand. A 10-yard run equals one set. Start this drill easily and gradually build up the intensity.

Drum Major

While running forward, rotate the leg inward to the mid line of the body and tap the heel at the mid line. A 10-yard run equals one set.

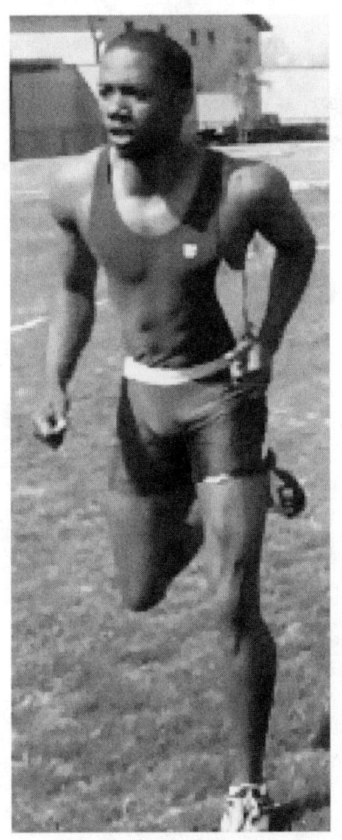

11.3 Butt kickers

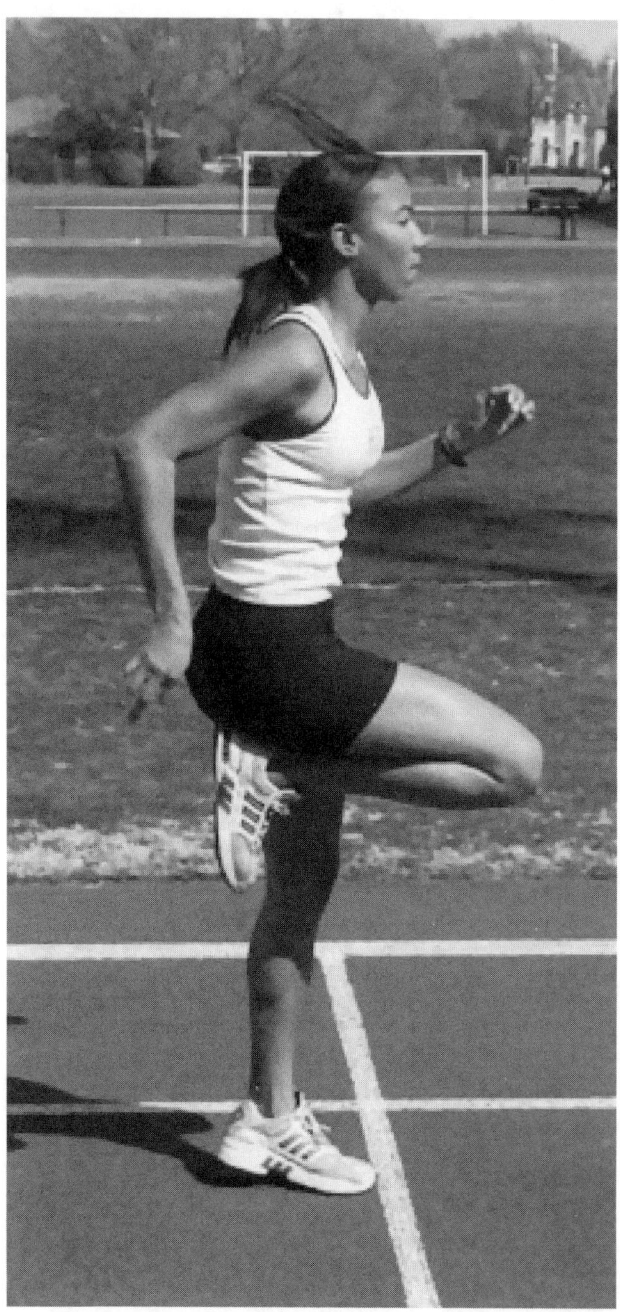

11.4 Wall slide

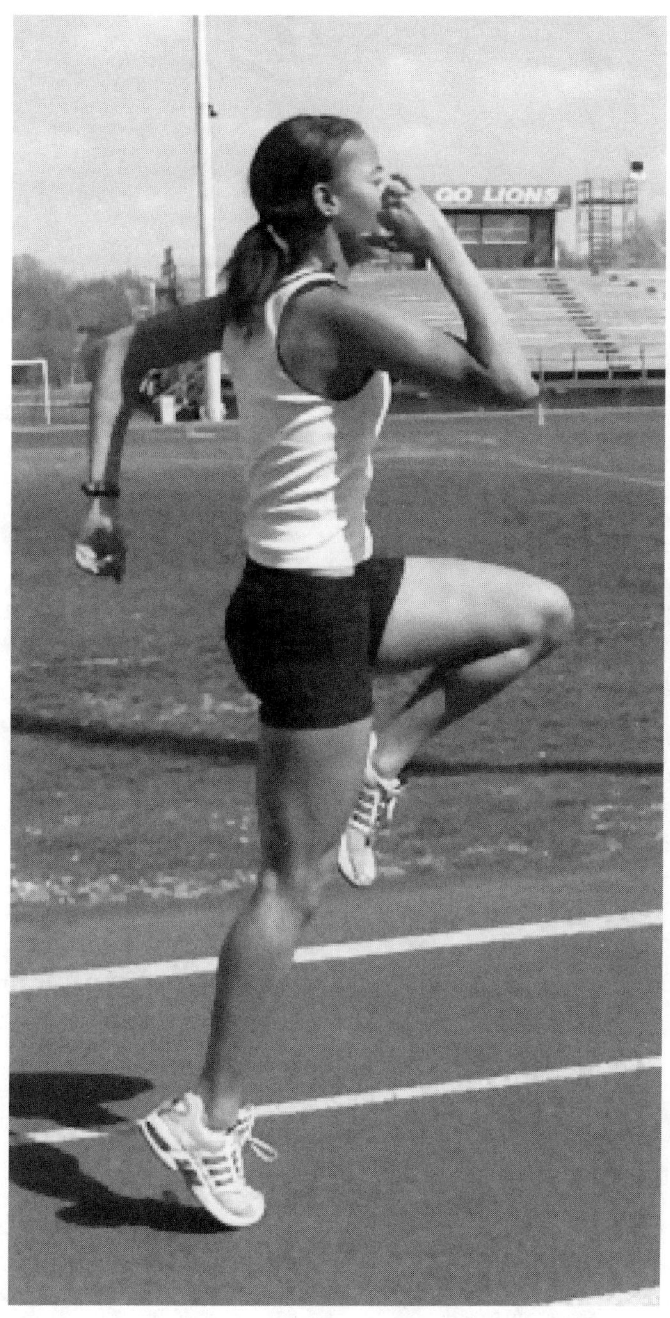

11.5 Down and offs

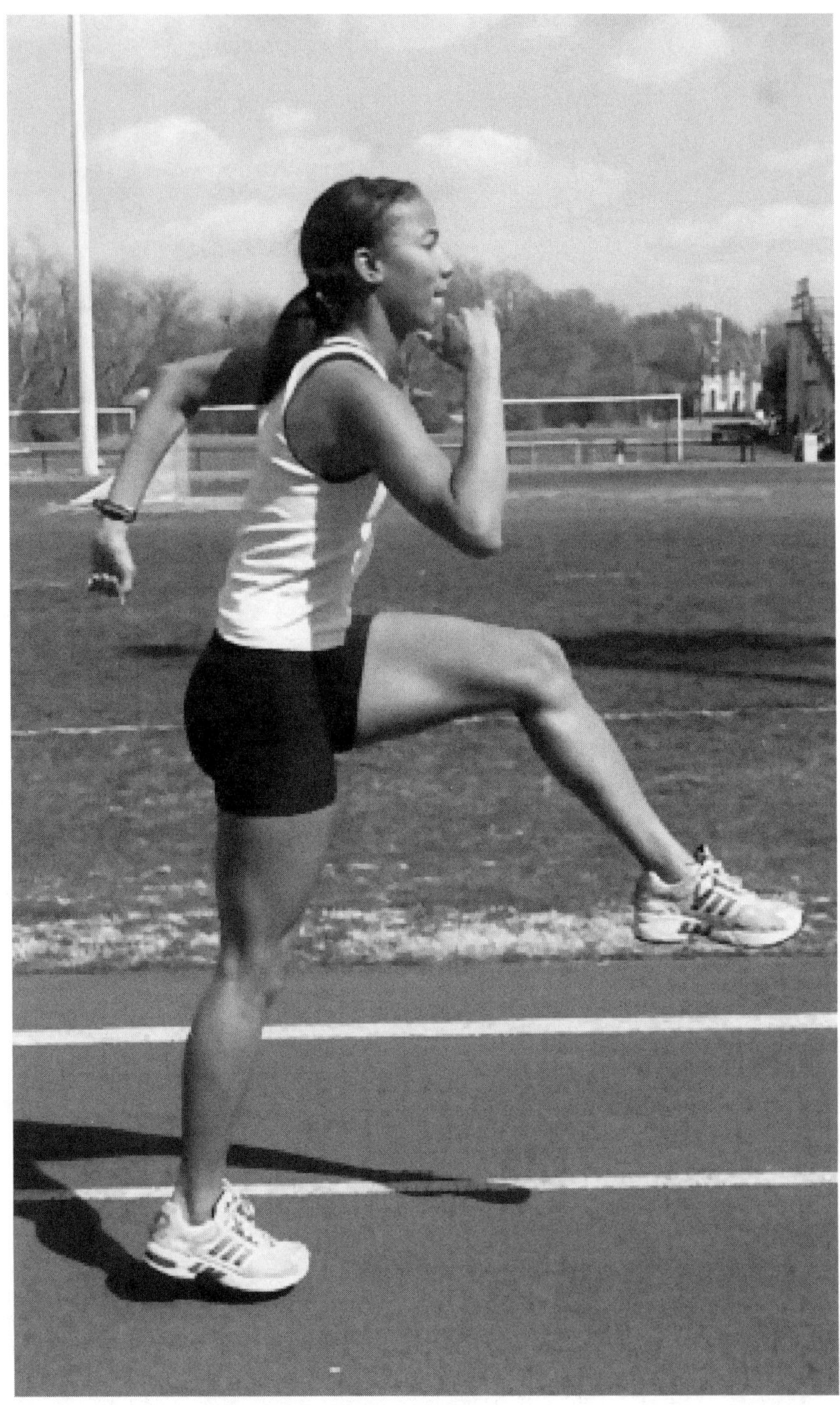

Figure 11.6 Pull throughs

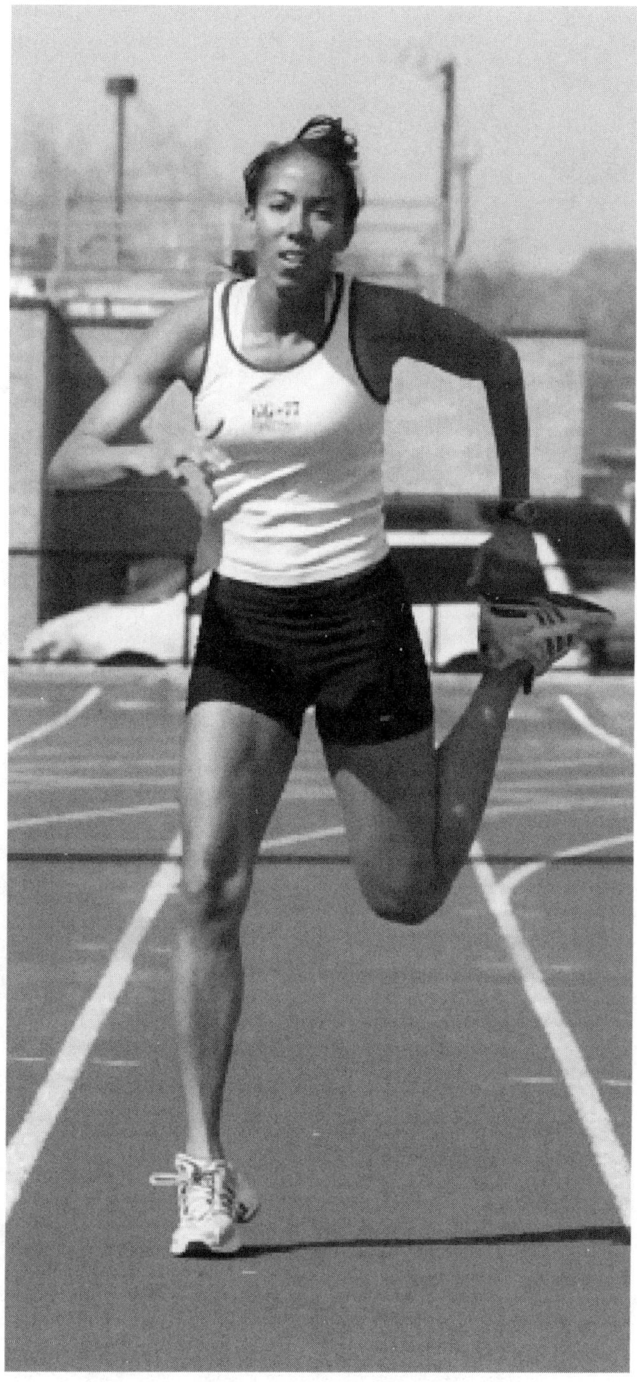

Figure 11.7 African dance

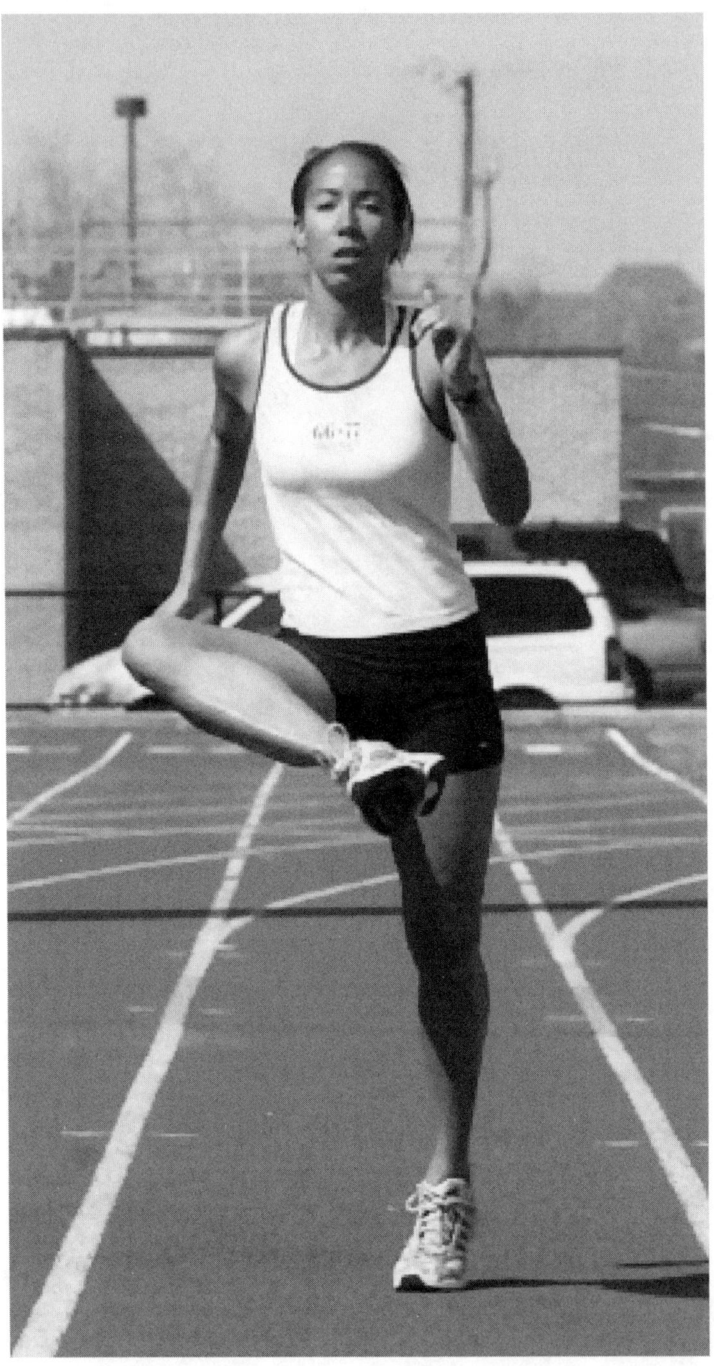

Figure 11.8 Drum major

Relaxation Drills

Coach White recommends the use of sprinting relaxation drills when athletes are fresh, in the early part of the workout. His basic relaxation drill designed to improve key arm movement patterns, remove tension, and balance the leg action can be done without moving forward:

Athletes square up in front with the feet slightly apart.

Proper arm movement is used to drive the arms in a sprinting action: elbows back beyond the hips, forward, and up level with the chin.

Hands remain open with no clenching of the fist permitted since this moves tensions through the arms to the shoulders and into the neck.

Athletes are told not to lift their shoulders

The head and neck are kept naturally aligned and not pulled back.

The jaw is relaxed by avoiding tightening the lips or gritting the teeth.

Additional drills used by track and team sports coaches to develop tension-free sprinting in their sport follow.

Treadmill Sprinting--In our Virginia commonwealth University Laboratory, athletes engaged in 3/4 to full speed treadmill sprinting with intermittent acceleration changes while the coach stood on a chair directly in front, behind, and to the side of sprinters to observe, correct form and encourage relaxation. This is one of the few settings in sports that permit an exchange between the coach and athlete with time to make and observe corrections during the sprinting action.

*Transition Sprints (*10-40 yards)--Acceleration/deceleration sprints are performed with minimum changes in speed. A smooth, relaxed transition from a jog to fast sprinting and deceleration back to a jog are emphasized using correct form.

Segment Sprints--The total distance to be covered is divided into thirds. For team sport athletes, a 40-45-yard distance uses three equal segments of 15 yards. The second and third segments are completed as relaxed as possible with little effort; and with no loss of mph speed. Coaches should time both segments with and without the emphasize to compare results and show the benefits of relaxed sprinting.

Switch-Off Starts---A smooth transition from a 3-point or 4-point football stance to near maximum speed is stressed making certain forward lean occurs with little or no bending at the waist, in a straight line from the ankle through the head. After a 30-40-yard sprint, 5-6 relaxed strides are taken before accelerating to maximum speed.

Falling Starts--Athletes use a falling start, followed by a 20-yard sprint and 5-6 relaxed strides to complete one of 5-6 repetitions. Four to five repetitions are completed around the track. A 10-15 yard recovery walk is used between each repetition.

Change the Leader--This common sprinting drill is performed in a group of 6 or more athletes who jog in single file around a track or field at a slow, pre- determined pace. The drill begins with the last runner accelerating and sprinting to the front of the line emphasizing a smooth, relaxed transition from a jog to rapid acceleration to the front of the line. The new individual who is now last in line immediately accelerates and sprints to the front to become the leader.

Drills do require the careful observation of a coach with a trained eye for relaxed sprinting. The track coach at the middle school, high school, and college levels can be a tremendous help to team sport coaches in this critical area for team sports.

STOPPING DRILLS

Is it unusual for coaches to work on stopping? What type of drills are these?

As discussed in Chapter 3, stopping and starting are common actions in most team sports and need to be executed with maximum efficiency. Stopping requires specific footwork that needs to be learned if this skill is to be done as quickly as possible and in a manner that allows the greatest ground contact force to propel the body into the new direction.

Each drill in this section must involve a rapid countermovement and minimum "pause" between the stop and starting action to produce quickness. According to Twist (Foran, Ed., 2001), a simple test can be used to determine whether an athlete is ready for this type of training. "When the player performs a lateral stop-and-start drill, does he or she land evenly with both feet at the same time? Is the footprint consistent, or does the athlete land at different places throughout the drill?" Athletes who do not meet these criteria may need to improve their quickness foundation through the use of additional speed endurance training, weight training, balanced flexibility training, and plyometrics.

Keep in mind that quickness is improved by learning, practicing, and mastering correct form and technique in sport-specific stopping and starting drills that emphasize quality, not quantity. Like sprint-assisted training, the emphasis is on training the neuromuscular system and requires all-out maximum effort in each drill and repetition followed by near complete recovery. Inadequate recovery time between repetitions and drills will produce fatigue, slow movement time and lead to incorrect form and technique. Athletes without excess body fat who possess adequate strength and power in the legs and abdominals, lower back, adductors, abductors, hip rotators, hip flexors, hip extensors, and gluteul muscles will benefit the most from this type of training

Start, Stop and Cut Drill

The Pro Agility Test described in Chapter 2 is also an excellent drill to develop the ability to accelerate and decelerate quickly, execute high speed stops, high speed cuts, and multidirectional sprints. Each repetition should be timed to compare performance as improvement in technique takes place. Proper form is emphasized on each separate maneuver in the test.

Box Jump Drop and Cut

Beginning with a height of 12-15 inches, an athlete steps off the box, absorbs the landing on both feet and cuts and sprints to the left or right for 4-5 strides, depending on the signal given by a partner (movement to guard, tackle, or block must be avoided with a plant and cut in the opposite direction). The drill is repeated with the athlete stepping off the box backwards, rotating one leg outward and sprinting 4-5 strides.

Backward to Lateral and Forward Movement

Athletes are directed to sprint backwards using the proper arm action. At the command, "left," athletes plant the right foot to initiate the stopping action, rotate the left foot outward, and execute a right foot crossover step and sprint 5-8 yards laterally. Five to eight repetitions to the left and the right are completed.

Athletes are directed to sprint backwards. At the command, "forward," either the right or left foot is planted behind the body to create the stopping action, followed by a powerful push-off and forward sprint for 5-8 yards.

High-Speed Stops using Surgical Tubing

Surgical tubing is attached to an athlete and a partner's waist and stretched for 20-25 yards. One athlete sprints toward the pull to a cone placed 20 yards from the starting line, executes a high speed stopping action by shifting his center of gravity before planting either the right or left foot, then the opposite foot to push-off and execute a 5-8 yard backward sprint, lateral sprint, and 90 degree angle sprint in three separate repetitions.

Side, Front and Back Shuffle (see Figure 8.33 in Chapter 8)

The *side* shuffle begins by standing with the left foot on an angle board and the right foot on the flat run. A short lateral step is taken with the right foot, then the left foot before hitting the opposite angle board with the right foot. A short lateral step is taken with the left foot, then the right foot before hitting the opposite angle board with the left foot. The drill continues for 8-10 repetitions and requires a hard plant foot on the angle board to initiate the stopping action and a strong push-off to change direction.

The *front* shuffle begins by standing with both feet on the flat run facing one of the angles. A short forward step is taken onto the angle board with the left foot, then a shuffle with the right foot onto the angle. The left foot now steps back to the flat run before repeating the action on the same angle board beginning with the opposite (right) foot.

The *back* shuffle begins with the athlete standing with both feet on the flat run facing away from one of the angle boards. A short step is taken back to the angle board with the left foot, then a shuffle with the right foot onto the angle board. The left foot now steps on the flat run before repeating the action on the same angle board beginning with the right foot.

Four Corner Drill

A 10-yard square is marked off on a field or gymnasium floor using four cones. Beginning in the top left corner using a standing start, a sprint is made for 10 yards to the right. At the first cone, a pivot is made inward to begin a crossing-leg movement (carrioca) for 10 yards to the bottom right corner and location of the second cone. The athlete pivots again and sprints backwards to the third cone, where another pivot is made and a sprint to the top left-hand corner of the square past the fourth cone completes the test.

FAKING AND CUTTING DRILLS

Chapter 3 discussed 17 different fakes and cuts used in football and other team sports. The task now is to practice each fake over and over at varying speeds until each maneuver can be used automatically during competition. This only occurs after thousands of correct repetitions. It is important to add this phase to the off-season practice schedule for a minimum of 30 minutes each workout.

Approximately how many times do I have to practice each faking and cutting maneuver?

We recommend braking down the repetitions into workouts and progressing to reach a cumulative total of 4,000 - 5,000 correct repetitions. This total is in the range of repetitions needed before such a skill will be used automatically under the right conditions during competition.

- 100 repetitions of walking fakes to master the footwork and body movement.
- 100 repetitions of jogging fakes.
- 100 repetitions of 3/4 speed fakes
- 100 repetitions of maximum speed fakes

What type of drills can I use?

Drills to improve faking and cutting skills can be completed in a backyard, gymnasium, track, or any practice area. The task is to begin by mastering the footwork described in Chapter 3 for each fake by executing walking fakes, progressing to jogging fakes and finally, high speed competition fakes.

Initial Four weeks (Walk - 2 weeks, Jog - 1 week, Full speed - 1 week) - 45 - 60 Min.

- Begin with the following six faking actions: single and double leg plants (right and left), open field banana left and right, and ball change. Stress perfect footwork on each repetition.

- Place 5 cones 20 yards apart with the first cone 20 yards from a starting line. Walk toward each cone and perform the same faking and cutting move on each cone. Be certain to plant the foot 3′ or so from the cone, sell the fake using the head, face, and upper torso before accelerating.

- Place a sign on the five cones, each with a different fake. Walk through the cones executing proper footwork for each fake.

- Repeat the above at home using trees or other obstacles. Accumulate 1,000 repetitions.

• Work with a teammate with each alternatively becoming the defender; each evaluates the effectiveness of their teammates' moves.

• Live action--Players sprint at the defender and execute any of the above fakes while the defender attempts to make contract with both hands around the waist.

Second Four weeks (Walk--2 weeks, Jog--1 week, Full speed--1 week) 45-60 Minutes)

• Begin with the following six faking actions: triple sideline plants - cut right and left, dancing in your shoes, overpower move, shoulder drive-contact-and-spin (left and right),

• Repeat the sequence described for the initial four-week period.

• Once each practice session, complete 10 repetitions of each of the moves mastered during the initial four-week period.

Third Four weeks (Walk--2 weeks, Jog--1 week, Full speed--1 week) 45-60 Minutes)

• Begin with the following six faking actions: full spin (left and right), Hit and side step (left and right), stop and back (cut at 8, catch at 10), Stop, Back and Go.

• Repeat the sequence described for the second four-week period.

• Once each practice session, complete 10 repetitions of each of the moves mastered during the second four-week period.

Maintenance (Full Speed)

• Continue to complete a minimum of two 15-minute faking and cutting sessions weekly during the in-season period.

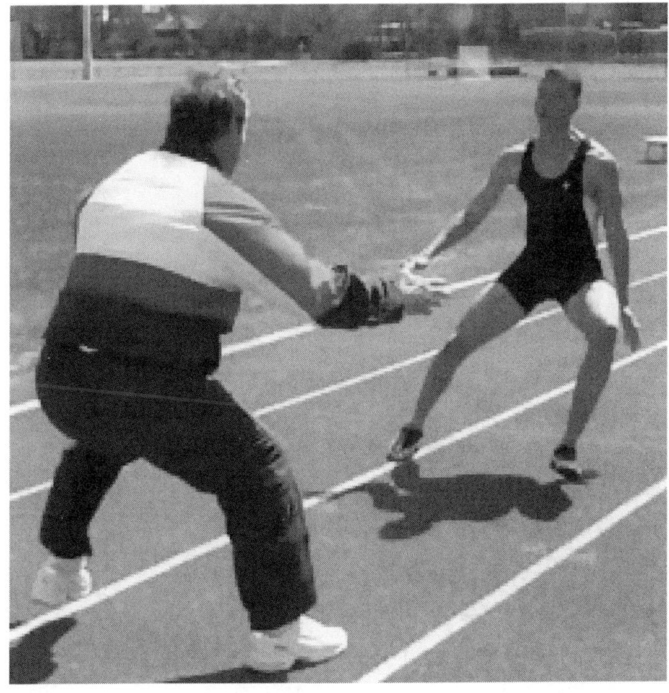

a

Figure 11.9 a, b Coach Bob Ward observing faking and cutting maneuvers based on his action as a defender.

PART IV

PUTTING IT ALL TOGETHER

Chapter 12

SPORT-SPECIFIC TRAINING

This chapter begins by providing a summary of current findings in the area of improving playing speed for sports competition described in the previous eleven chapters. The initial section, "What We Know and Don't Know," provides valuable insight about how to develop a speed improvement program for specific sports using the most effective techniques and training programs available.

The chapter then discusses off-season training, establishes a research-based order of use for each training program in a workout, provides sample off-season training programs for football, baseball, basketball and soccer, presents an in-season maintenance program to prevent detraining or loss of the gains acquired in the off-season, discusses in-season speed training in team sports, presents Eastern and Western periodization styles, and ends with a specific plan to track the progress of each athlete.

As a final note, a brief tribute is included to the late Lloyd "Bud" Winter whose sprint training methods as a track coach over 50 years ago are still meaningful today.

WHAT WE KNOW AND DON'T KNOW

The information that follows summarizes what we actually know for sure about improving playing speed and what is still to be learned. It also highlights areas where additional research is still needed. Much of this needed study is underway thanks to the efforts of Dr. Ralph Mann, Tom Tellez and other coaches and researchers throughout the world.

Playing Speed

1. "Heredity deals the cards, environment plays the hand." Every athlete can improve speed in short sprints regardless of genetic make-up and the preponderance and distribution of slow and fast twitch muscle fiber.

2. No athlete will reach their maximum speed potential without proper training.

3. One hundred meter dash times of elite sprinters and the speed of athletes in all sports have steadily improved each decade. The 40-yard dash times of team sport athletes have also improved by as much as 7/10 of a second following 8 to 12 weeks of training.

4. Improvement in playing speed occurs through changes in power output (speed-strength), stride rate, stride length, starting and sprinting form, cutting, faking, and acceleration, and diagnosis, recognition, and reaction to game situations.

5. For team sports, the attack areas designed to increase playing speed should focus on training programs that improve the start and acceleration.

6. The importance of each attack area varies depending upon the sport and player position.

7. Coaches in all sports expect a number of speed performance related aspects from each athlete: a fast start from a standing or crouched position; fast acceleration after the start to near maximum speed from a 3-point, 4-point or standing position, a jog, 3/4 sprint, or a fake and cut and a stop and start; high top end speed; quick recognition of game situations and the ability to apply rapid multidirectional forces; and a high enough level of speed endurance to complete the above skills throughout the entire game with minimum slowing due to fatigue.

Muscle Fiber Types and Speed

1. The percent and location of ST (slow twitch) and FT (fast twitch) fibers in the body varies for each athlete, with the majority of human muscle containing a mixture of both.

2. Percentages depend mainly on heredity and, to a small extent, on training adaptations.

3. Training promotes changes within the population of fast-twitch fibers (type IIb to IIa) and, to a much lesser extent, from fast- to slow-twitch fibers (Gollnick and co-researchers).

4. With training, FTIIa fibers take on some of the strength and power qualities of FTIIb fibers.

5. Regardless of intensity, ST motor units are recruited first. If the intensity is low, these may be the only units recruited. If intensity is high, such as when lifting weights or engaging in interval sprint training, ST motor units are still recruited first, followed by FTIIa and FTIIb.

6. In order to recruit the Type IIb FT fibers (the fiber to train), exercise must involve heavy loading and high output.

7. New information on the function, biochemical properties, and enzyme profile of fast and slow twitch fiber has helped coaches adapt and improve the effectiveness of their speed training programs.

Test Battery

1. The main purpose of testing is to identify the key factors limiting the speed of each athlete to provide focus for off-season speed improvement training.

2. The 40-yard and 60-yard dash are the most used and misused tests in sports. A 40-60 yard linear velocity sprint during competition in sports other than track and field is a rare occurrence.

3. Although this still cannot be achieved with one test, the ideal single test should measure starting time, first-three step time, split times, acceleration, mph speed, speed endurance, ground force production, stride rate and stride length.

4. The best single speed test available at this time is the NASE 120-yard dash with 5, 10, 20, 40, and 80-yard split times. This test provides results for the first -three steps, 10-yard dash, 20-yard dash, 40-yard dash, flying 40-yard sprint (mph or maximum speed), and speed-endurance. It also provides one-half of the information needed to determine the stride rate (number of steps per second) of each athlete.

5. The First 3-Step Test (time and distance covered) and the 10 and 20-yard dash are key speed tests that are critical to performance to any sport.

6. The most important speed-strength tests are those that measure power output or the pushing force against the ground with each step (dead lift, single and double leg press), kickback (single and double leg), and tests that reveal muscle imbalance or differences between the ground contact force of one leg and the other (stride length with right and left foot takeoff, right and left leg kick back and leg press), and hamstring-quadriceps imbalance.

7. Since linear velocity and playing speed is maximized in athletes who apply the greatest ground contract force in the leanest body, tests that determine body composition and the percent of body fat are also an important part of the test battery.

8. When possible, tests should be sport-specific and used during an actual game such as the "crack of the bat to first test" and the base running test (first to second, second to third for the steal) in the sports of baseball and softball.

Starting, Stopping, Acceleration, Faking and Cutting

1. The proper technique in the 3- and 4-point start should be mastered by all team sport athletes to obtain the best time possible in linear velocity tests that are a part of almost every program.

2. In the crouched start, too much weight forward in the set position decreases ground thrust force, too little provides too much resistance. Both errors negatively affect starting speed. The use of shorter initial steps to begin a short sprint in power sports tends to produce a faster 20-yard sprint.

3. Two-leg drive. The first action in starting from a standing, three or four-point stance is the simultaneous push-off both the lead and rear feet with near equal thrust. This behavior needs to be taught to team sport athletes who commonly utilize only the lead foot, sacrificing as much as 400 pounds of thrust. Placing the strongest foot in the forward position and learning to apply near equal pushing force against the ground with both feet immediately improves an athlete's start and acceleration time.

Sequence of action after the initial thrust off both feet:

One-Leg Drive. The back foot now leaves the ground to initiate the first step with the lead foot continuing to push-off the ground.

First step. The rear foot moves forward to complete the first step.

Second-step. The lead foot leaves the ground to initiate the second step. The only thing keeping the ground portion of the start from equaling the stride rate attained in the rest of the race is the speed-strength of the athlete.

Transition (steps 3-12). In the first three steps, ground contact is on the ball of the foot without the heel striking the ground. Throughout the remaining steps in the acceleration and maximum speed stage, ground contact is almost flat with contact made first on the outside front of the ball of the foot, then with the heel. This places the body in perfect position for the hip flexors and extensors to maximize the push off the ground.

4. Although ground contact force (amount and speed of application) is critical in all phases of sprinting, it is the single most important factor in acquiring a fast start, fast stop or cut, and fast acceleration to full speed.

5. Young preadolescent athletes often do not possess the speed-strength to execute an efficient 3- or 4-point start and may have better times with the standing start.

6. The best method of improving acceleration is to increase power output in the form of ground contact force through the use of speed-strength training in the weight room and sprint-resisted training (plyometrics and sport loading) on the court or field.

7. Mastering basic and advanced faking and cutting moves that are performed automatically at high speeds during competition requires thousands of repetitions and hours of practice time.

Mechanics of Sprinting

1. Sprinting with proper form and technique reduces speed-strength and energy requirements, delays fatigue, and ensures that all forces are being applied in the right direction at the right time.

2. Sprinting takes place with the body perpendicular to the ground with the neck and rear naturally in line. Proper body lean occurs from the center of the foot through the head in a straight line with little or no bending at the waist.

3. Sprinters do not run on their toes. The ball of the foot is the only part capable of creating an efficient, powerful push off the ground. The foot first makes contact with the ground on the outside edge of the ball of the foot. The faster the speed, the higher the contact point on the ball of the foot. This support phase begins with a slight load on the support foot, then rides onto the full sole. As the body passes over the foot, the heel touches the ground slightly and the ankle extends naturally as the hip joint is stretched.

4. The improperly named "butt kick" is a natural movement that occurs in sprinting. During the recovery of the leg, the foot leaves the ground with the knee leading the foot forward. With the heel tucked close to the gluteul muscles (butt), the leg is allowed to make a natural swing forward to increase the angular velocity of the leg. The heel does not kick up behind, it moves toward the butt after ground contact is broken.

5. After the acceleration phase, a sprinter must shift contact efforts to the front of the body (front side mechanics) for optimum speed of movement.

6. The "push" off the ground with each step, originates at the hip joint, and is the most important part of each stride.

7. The arms do not remain at 90 degrees throughout the sprint. As the arm swings down, the elbow extends slightly. At the bottom of the swing, the hand is next to the thigh.

8. To sprint faster, athletes must concentrate on pushing off the ground, landing with the proper foot placement, using correct arm action, and staying relaxed.

Stride Rate and Stride Length

1. Ground contact time + air time (exchange in the positioning of the legs in the air) equals stride rate.

2. Male athletes should strive to develop a stride rate of close to 5.0 steps per second. Female athletes strive for 4.5 steps per second or more.

3. Both stride rate and stride length can be improved with training.

4. Good sprinters find their optimum stride length, then focus on maximizing stride rate.

5 After proper form is established, stride length can only be increased by improving ground contact force.

6. As ground contact forces are increased, stride rate is increased and stride length increases naturally.

7. Although stride rate is more dependent on ground contact forces than air time (exchange of the legs in the air), improvement in both areas is needed. Even small improvements of one to two tenths of a second in a short sprint have a significant impact on performance.

Speed-Endurance

1. Improving speed-endurance allows athletes to make repeated sprints during competition with minimum slowing due to fatigue.

2. Excellent speed-endurance increases the anaerobic threshold, the onset of blood lactate accumulation (OBLA), and allows athletes to sprint further before a slowing effect occurs.

3. A high level of speed endurance also reduces the amount of slowing that occurs during a long sprint of 60-80 yards or more.

4. Maximum speed can only be maintained for 1 to 2 seconds. Athletes who reach top speed too quickly will slow down more over a longer portion of the distance sprinted.

Aerobic Fitness and Speed

1. Attaining a higher level of aerobic fitness also favorably impacts the anaerobic energy system (speed-endurance) by improving recovery time between short sprints and by extending the anaerobic threshold.

2. Although aerobic training is often a neglected phase in power sports, an above average level is necessary for optimum performance.

Foundation Training

1. Athletes warm-up to stretch, they do not stretch to warm-up. General warm-up that produces perspiration is needed prior to the dynamic stretching session.

2. Dynamic stretching exercises are used at the beginning of each workout or practice session to prepare athletes for vigorous movement.

3. Static stretching exercises are used at the close of a workout or practice session to improve range of motion.

4. Excess body fat has a negative affect on playing speed. Athletes in positions of speed should strive to obtain the leanest, strongest body possible to provide the best body weight/ground contact force ratio. Removing only five pounds of excess body fat, for example, improves this ratio and requires about 10 pounds less ground contact force with each step to maintain an athlete's current speed.

5. Athletes in all sports execute certain moves such as a fake, plant and cut to the right, a double fake and cut to the right, and movement with the ball in one direction faster and more efficiently to their dominant side. Lack of recessive hand and leg skill in sports contributes to differences in directional speed and the speed with which the basic, intermediate and advanced fakes, feints and cuts are made in sports.

Power Output Training (speed-strength)

1. A sprinter needs enough vertical force to stop downward velocity and overcome gravity, produce vertical velocity, project the body into the next air phase, eliminate unwanted breaking, and also support body weight.

2. An athlete who adds 20 pounds of muscle mass will need to increase ground contact force on each step by more than twice that amount (approximately 44 pounds) just to maintain current speed. In sports where such additional muscle mass is critical to performance, athletes and coaches must make certain that this extra weight is offset by increased ground contact force.

3. Training to increase ground contact force occurs in the weight room and on the field with plyometrics, heavy sleds, resistance cords and harnesses using sprint-specific movements and exercises.

4. A solid foundation strength training program and a phasing in period is needed prior to the use of the low repetition, heavy weight, and lengthy rest interval program designed to increase ground contact force with little muscle mass weight gain. In the *early* stages of speed-strength training, low resistance, high repetitions (8-12), and moderate intensity (50-70% of 1 RM) is used. This gradually changes to the minimum hypertrophy program involving high resistance (90-100%), low repetitions (1-5), multiple sets (2-5) and a 5 minute rest period between sets.

5. To improve starting speed and acceleration, weights, plyometrics and other sprint-resistance training methods are used. The amount of weight and resistance must be carefully adjusted to allow near maximum speed of contraction and proper sprinting form.

6. Ballistic training, plyometrics and sport loading are capable of increasing power output. Plyometric hops and bounds and sprint-resisted training focuses on the exercises and muscles that simulate the pushing action against the ground in sprinting.

7. Sprint-resisted training with sleds, harnesses, and uphill sprinting, is designed to improve the drive phase (start and acceleration).

8. No speed-strength training technique used outside the weight room should change the dynamics of the sprinters movements.

9. Sport loading resistance should not slow the athlete by more to 10% to avoid altering ground dynamics.

10. When using the sled, a shoulder harness is preferred since a waist harness tends to alter a sprinter's normal movement pattern.

11. Harness lines should be shortened and held 6-8 yards behind the runner when training during the drive phase, 0-15 yards when training maximum velocity.

12. Ankle weights are best avoided as a sprint-resisted technique, even with low weights under 1,000 grams. Studies indicate that the possibility of injury is increased, sprinting form is altered, and the technique is not effective.

14. Speed and quickness drills must simulate game conditions closely if transfer is to occur to performance in a specific sport or specific action in a sport. Such drills aid playing speed by improving recognition and reaction time to sport-specific situations.

Sustained Power Output (speed endurance training)

1. A high level of speed endurance increases the anaerobic threshold allowing athletes to sprint a longer distances before lactic acid build-up begins, decreases recovery time between repeated sprints, and decreases the amount of slowing at end of a long sprint.

2. Athletes who possess a moderately high level of aerobic endurance recover faster between repeated sprints during competition.

3. Sports-specific speed-endurance training for team sports aligns key variables such as the starting position of the sprint (3 or 4-point stance, standing start, moving start), speed of the sprint (maximum velocity), distance covered, and recovery interval with what actually occurs in the sport.

3. Pickup sprints, hollow sprints, and interval sprint training can improve the speed endurance of athletes in 4 to 6 weeks.

4. Coaches and athletes must keep careful records each workout to ensure progression. The number of sprint repetitions, sets, distance covered, speed, and rest interval between repetitions should be recorded each workout.

5. One to two maximum effort sprints should be used at the end of each speed-endurance session.

Neuromuscular Training

1. Conditioning the neuromuscular system requires near full recovery (2-6 minutes of rest, depending on the number of repetitions) between each repetition of sprint-assisted training, regardless of the method used.

2. The concept of "speed before fatigue" is used. Sprint-assisted training is conducted early in the workout following general warm-up and stretching when athletes are fatigue-free and capable of taking fast steps.

3. Sprint-assisted training has been shown to be a factor in the improvement of stride rate, stride length and times in the 40-yard dash.

4. Sprint-assisted training is designed to increase stride rate and improve maximum sprinting velocity by decreasing ground contact time and the time in the air for the leg exchange. The goal is to activate motor units more quickly and produce a better neuromuscular adaptation. Stride rate is increased through power output training (speed-strength) to maximize the pushing force against the ground with each step and through sprint-assisted training to reduce air time and train the neuromuscular system to permit faster steps.

5. Some types of sprint-assisted training are more effective and more practical than others. Towing with surgical tubing is better suited to team sports than other methods since it allows group training, meets the standards for the force and length of the pull, allows free sprinting at the end of the pull, and is safe when supervised properly.

6. Sport-specific drills and sprint-assisted training (towing) are combined when possible to train the neuromuscular system in sports-specific movements.

Form and Technique Training

1. If a sprinting form drill does not mimic the exact correct movement pattern of the arms, legs, and torso in the start, acceleration, and maximum speed phase, it will not improve technique.

2. Form and technique training in the start, acceleration and maximum effort phases of sprinting also contribute to increased ground contact force.

3. Specific drills to master stopping and starting, cutting and faking eventually lead to improved sports performance.

THE 100-METER DASH: Summary Training Recommendations

Developing a training program for the 100-meter dash is a complicated task. At first glance, it appears that it is merely an all-out sprint as athletes attempt to reach maximum speed as fast as possible and maintain that speed throughout the race. In reality, the race involves five different phases, each requiring special training techniques:

1. Reaction Time (RT)
2. Block Clearance
3. Speed of efficient Acceleration
4. Maintenance of Maximum Velocity
5. Lessened Degree of Deceleration

Based on a 10.0 second 100-meter dash time, famed sprint coach, Tom Tellez provides a breakdown of these factors in Figure 12.1 with an estimated percentage of their contribution to the race.

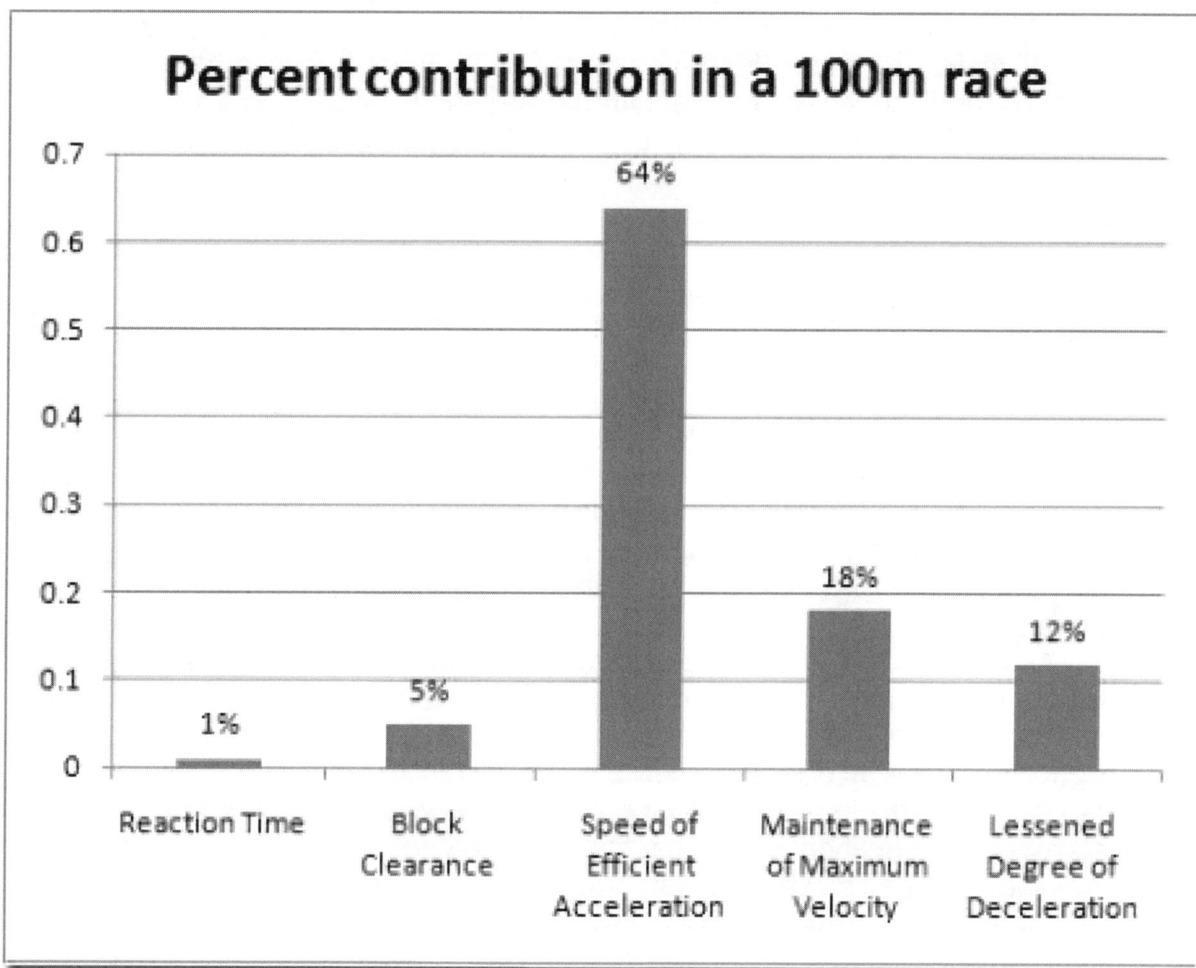

Figure 12.1. Percent Contribution in a 100-meter race

A complete training programs for sprinters evolves around these five factors.

Proper *Block Clearance* allows the desired *Speed of Efficient Acceleration* to maximum speed over the longest possible distance. As Coach Tellez indicates, "the block clearance sets up the acceleration pattern of the race and really contributes much more than only 5 percent of the race."

Efficient acceleration continues at a decreasing rate until it reaches zero. The fastest rate occurs at the start and slowly decreases as maximum speed is attained.

Acceleration is held at zero for 20 meters or so (*Maintenance of Maximum Velocity*) before shifting to negative and producing slight slowing as fatigue occurs. Only a minimal amount of slowing affect may occur in highly trained sprinters such as was the case during Usain Bolt's world record 9.58 100-meter dash. Bolt's reached 99% of his maximum velocity at 48.18 meters and 100% of maximum velocity at the 65-meter mark (12.27 mps). Very little slowing took place after reaching maximum speed. After completing the 60-70 meter segment in 0.81 seconds, Bolt completed the 70-80 meter segment in 0.82 seconds, 80-90-meter segment in 0.83 seconds and the final 10-meters in 0.83 seconds. This was a phenomenal example of anaerobic fitness by the Olympic sprinter. Such minimum *Lessened Degree of Deceleration* (slowing) would be impossible for team sport athletes whose anaerobic or speed endurance training focuses on much shorter distances.

Coach Tellez adds further clarification to understanding the forces needed to complete the five phases of a 100-meter dash. A combination of vertical and horizontal force is applied. As the race begins, vertical and horizontal forces are equal due to the 45 degree angle of projection. Horizontal forces are big at the start of the race and get progressively smaller as speed increases, reaching zero at maximum speed. Vertical forces continue for the entire race. As stated previously, research indicates that it requires approximately 2.1 lb. of vertical force per lb. of body weight to overcome the force of gravity, clear the ground, and propel the body forward.

Clearly, a comprehensive program is needed to help sprinters reach their maximum potential. *Form training* in the start, acceleration, maximum speed, and finish phases is critical and allows athletes to apply forces at the right time and accelerate over a long distance. *Power output training* (speed-strength) increases ground contact force and not only improves the start and acceleration phase but maximum speed as well. *Speed endurance training* minimizes slowing at the end of the race. And, finally, *Neuromuscular training* contributes to fast stride rates to aid top speed.

PRESEASON SPEED IMPROVEMENT

Athletes and coaches now have enough information to begin a personal program and are aware of how important each area is to a specific sport, are aware of individual weaknesses based on test results, and know how to properly utilize each training program to eliminate weaknesses and improve playing speed through a holistic approach.

The speed improvement attack areas for each sport and the specific training programs designed to strengthen these areas were presented in Chapter 1, tables 1.2 and 1.3. Take a moment now to write the areas for your sport in a column on the left side of a piece of paper. Now list the specific training programs shown to improve the attack areas. There is no need to concentrate on any of the training programs specified unless test results revealed a weakness. It is important, however, for each athlete to maintain the level of conditioning they already possess in each area. It is also important for every athlete to focus on improving stride rate and stride length during the start, acceleration, and maximum speed phase of sprinting by increasing power output (ground contact force) even when a weakness has not been revealed since further improvement in speed will occur with training. Unless a weakness is revealed in other areas, such as body composition, speed endurance, muscle imbalance, form and technique, training is valuable but should not be the major focus of the program.

Placement of Training Programs in a Practice Session

In what order should athletes and coaches complete the different training programs used in a practice session?

Although there are differences of opinion among conditioning coaches, there is a logical and research-supported sequence for the placement of different training programs in a workout session (see table 12.1).

Following a *general warm-up* routine that produces perspiration, involves large muscle activity, and progresses from walking-to-jogging to striding-to-sprinting, *dynamic stretching exercises* are completed. These exercises include jogging in place, butt kickers, high knee lifts and other movement exercises that progress from low to medium to high speed action. This type of stretching is designed to prepare athletes for vigorous high speed drills and sprinting, not to increase range of motion.

Form training is third in and involves the basic drills to master correct starting and sprinting technique described in Chapter 4. Fourth on this sequence is *Sprint-assisted training,* used every other workout, that must be done when the body is still fatigue free and capable of very high speed. High speed sport-specific *drills* follow while athletes are still fatigue free and can exert maximum effort to work on timing under game conditions. *Scrimmage,* including full contact in football and rugby, is sixth when athletes remain relatively free of fatigue and can execute skills at full speed.

Conditioning activities such as *speed endurance training, sport loading, plyometrics, and weight training,* are completed near the end of the workout schedule. Not all conditioning sessions are included in every workout. A 5-10 minute *cool-down* period is followed by *static stretching* which is designed to increase range of motion at the end of the workout.

There are variations of the above order in a practice session or workout. Depending on the emphasis for the day, James Radcliffe, Strength coach at the University of Oregon, places plyometrics at the end of the session prior to the cool-down as suggested above, or after the warm-up and before the sprint or strength work. Coach Radcliffe uses sprint-type plyometrics, which are "complexed" with the lifts performed in the weight room or used with actual sprint work on the field the day of explosive, dynamic, intense work, not the day after or the recovery day. He also favors using plyometrics (depth and box jumps, sprint movement hops and bounds) in conjunction with weight room training providing it is completed near the end of the workout during the conditioning phase of a practice session. Plyometrics are also recommended for use in the weight room following each set of the dead lift and other speed-strength exercises designed to increase ground contact force.

Research also supports a system introduced by Italian coach, Carlo Vittori, for the proper order of use for conditioning activities in the latter part of a workout: weight training, followed by plyometrics, and ending with a series of short all-out sprints. Study the logic behind each suggested order and adapt it to your practice philosophy and special needs.

Eight-Week Sports-Specific Pre-season Programs

The preseason period begins two months from the first scheduled practice day in a sport. For best results, count back 8 weeks from the start of the in-season period (first day of regularly scheduled practice). It is assumed that athletes have maintained a solid aerobic, strength and power foundation prior to beginning this eight-week period.

Sample pre-season program for team sports?

Tables 12.2 - 12.5 describe a sample weekly pre-season workout schedule for football, baseball, basketball, and soccer. Specific 8-week programs for Foundation Training, Power Output Training (speed-strength, plyometrics, and sport loading), Sustained Power Output Training (speed-endurance), Neuromuscular Training (stride rate), and Form and Technique Training are presented in Part III: The 5-Step Model in Chapters 7, 8, 9, 10, and 11.

Table 12.1 Order or Training Program Use in the Off-Season Period

Training Program *	Length (Min.)	Order	Fre-quency	Explanation
General Warm-up	8-12	1	Before each workout	Warm-up continues until you are perspiring freely.
Dynamic Stretching	10-15	2	Each workout	Use dynamic stretching to prepare the the body for sprinting.
Form Training	15-20	3	Each workout	Practice both starting, acceleration, and sprinting form using the Olympic form drills.
Sprint-assisted Training	10-15	4	2-3 weekly	Used before athletes are fatigued. Rest between repetitions should result in near full recovery. The purpose is to exert sub maximal stride rates and train the neuromuscular system.
Speed Endurance Training	15-20	7	2-3 weekly	The main objective is to improve your ability to make repeated short or long sprints in your sport without slowing due to fatigue.
Sport Loading	10-15	8	2 weekly	Include uphill sprinting, sleds or light-weighted vests when emphasizing speed; and heavier resistance when emphasizing speed-strength and ground contact force.
Speed-strength Training	30-60	9	3 weekly	Conditioning items 7, 8, and 9 and 10 are used near the end of the workout.
Ballistics	10	10	1 weekly	Ballistic training can be both a fun and conditioning session for athletes. Sport-specific exercises are used.
Plyometrics	15-20	10	1-2 weekly	Exercises closely mimic the starting, acceleration and sprinting action. Used separately or combined with speed-strength training in the weight room to improve ground contact force.

Table 12.1 **(continued)**

Short Sprints	10-12	11	2-3 weekly	A series of 4-10, 15-40 yard sprints.
Cool Down	10	12	Each work	Light jogging and walking.
Static stretching	10-15	Last	2-3 weekly	Designed to maintain and increase range of motion in joints specific to the sport. Important for all athletes, particularly following speed-strength training.

* Obviously, not all programs are used in every workout or practice session.

These programs are designed so athletes will develop a GOOD level of conditioning by the first official practice day. At that point, the coaching staff will strive for peak performance by mid-season without losing any of the gains acquired through the preseason speed improvement program.

This 8-week period allows athletes to concentrate specifically on the critical areas (power output, sustained power output, neuromuscular training and sprinting technique) that may be preventing them from sprinting faster and moving quicker in their sport. It is important to take each training program seriously, focusing only on improving speed in short distances. Other than this off-season period, there is no other period of time that permits athletes to totally devote their efforts to this one objective.

Pre-season Testing

Plan to retake the speed tests described in Chapter 2 at the end of the first 4-week period and again at the start of the season to plot progress.

IN-SEASON SPEED IMPROVEMENT

Normal practice sessions during the in-season period in most sports are not long enough to bring about great improvement in most basic training areas. Coaches may also have difficulty finding enough time and deciding where to place the key *maintenance* programs that will prevent athletes from losing much of their off-season gains. This section provides some guidelines for the proper placement of various training programs during the in-season period and a reasonable time frame that does not significantly detract from the practice schedule and still maintains off-season gains in power output (speed-strength and speed-endurance) flexibility, stride rate and length, starting speed, acceleration and maximum mph speed. Without a well-designed in-season program, it is quite common in most sports for athletes to lose a percentage of the gains acquired in the off-season period. Although additional improvement can also occur in an attempt to peak for a specific game or tournament at the latter part of the season, the primary objective of an in-season program is to maintain the gains acquired in the off-season.

Order of Use During the In-Season or Competitive Period

Fortunately, there is also a logical order for coaches and athletes to follow during the in-season period:

1. *General warm-up* (jogging, striding, and light sprinting) is used until athletes are perspiring freely.

2. *Dynamic stretching* exercises help prevent injuries, and prepare the body for the more vigorous training to follow in a practice session.

3. *Sprint-assisted training* maintains and improves stride rate and stride length. Scheduled third in the workout, immediately following the stretching session, this program is most effective when athletes are fatigue-free and capable of sub-maximal stride rates.

4. *High speed sports-specific drills* are used early in a practice session to improve game skills and develop proper timing when athletes are unfatigued.

5. *Scrimmage* follows sprint-assisted training when the body is still unfatigued, less apt to be injured, and athletes are more likely to execute skills at high speed under game conditions.

6. *Calisthenics* are used to improve general conditioning, develop strength and muscular endurance, and improve aerobic fitness. They are conditioning-oriented and should not be at the beginning of a workout. Thirty minutes of calisthenics will only change a fresh athlete into a fatigued athlete. This interferes with skill and timing and makes an athlete more susceptible to injury.

7. *Speed endurance* training such as interval sprint training as commonly used in football, baseball, basketball, and soccer, and other tram sports is also a conditioning activity. Because such training brings about a high level of fatigue and makes it difficult to continue a workout much longer, speed-endurance training is completed near the end of the workout.

8. *Power output training* (speed-strength, plyometrics, and sport loading) is the most fatiguing of any program. It leaves athletes weak and vulnerable to injury. These activities are therefore placed close to the end of the workout.

9. A *cool-down* period is desirable as the last item in a workout and may involve a slow jog or walk.

10. *Static stretching* is important for all athletes as the final in-season practice item and is performed in a relaxed manner, emphasizing key joints involved in the sport.

Table 12.2 Weekly Preseason Schedule for Football Players

Day	Training programs	Guidelines
Daily	General warm-up Dynamic stretching Sprinting form drills Static stretching	Slow jog 1/2 to 3/4 mile increasing the pace the final 100 yards of each 1/4 mile. Use dynamic stretching before completing the form drills. End the workout with static stretching.
Mon.	Sprint-assisted training	Follow the program in Chapter 10, table 10.1.
	Starting/Stopping	Follow the program in Chapter 11. Use the stance required by your position for the start.
	Football speed-endurance	Use repeated high-speed sprints following the program described in Chapter 9. Use some backward high-speed sprints on both a level surface and a slight incline to develop the hamstring muscle group.
	Speed-strength	Follow the programs in Chapter 8.
Tue.	Aerobics	15-30 minutes of continuous work at your target heart rate.
	Football skill	Integrate speed into football drills with sprinting as the major objective. Include drills using a 3-pt and 4-pt. stance and a two-foot push-off for offensive backs and lineman and the standing start for defensive backs and linebackers.

Table 12.2 **(continued)**

	Football cutting and acceleration drills	Complete the drills in Chapter 11. Master 7-8 different cuts and fakes if you are a running back, defensive back, or receiver.
	Sprint-resisted training	Follow the program in Chapter 8, tables 8.13. and 8.14. Use a weighted vest, harness, or parachute to execute power starts from the 3-pt, 4-pt. or standing start, depending upon your position.
	Plyometrics	Follow the program in chapter 8, table 8.10.
	Short-all out sprints	4-10 repetitions of 10-20 yard sprints with a 30 second rest interval.
Wed.	Starting/Stopping Drills	Follow the program in Chapter 11. Use the starting stance required by your position.
	Football speed-endurance	Use repeated high-speed sprints following the program described in Chapter 9, tables 9.2 and 9.3. Use some backward high-speed sprints on both a level surface and a slight incline to develop the hamstring muscle group.
	Speed-strength	Follow the upper body program in Chapter 8.
Thur.	Aerobics	15-30 minutes of continuous work at your target heart rate
	Football skill session	Integrate speed into your football drills. High-speed sprinting is the major objective; think speed and quickness as you work out. Include drills using the 3-pt and 4-pt stance emphasizing a two-foot push-off for offensive backs and lineman and the standing start for defensive backs and linebackers.
	Sprint-resisted training (Sport loading)	Follow the program in Chapter 8, tables 8.13 and 8.14. "Hill bursts" (2.5 to 7-degree stadium steps or hill) for 10 to 60 yards. Use a weighted vest, harness, or parachute to execute power starts from the 3-pt, 4-pt. or standing standing start.

Table 12.2 **(continued)**

	Speed-strength training (lower body)	Follow the program in Chapter 8.
Fri.	Sprint-assisted training	Follow the program in Chapter 10, table 10.1.
	Football speed-endurance training	Use repeated high-speed sprints following the program described in Table 9.2 Use some backward high-speed sprints on a level surface and a slight incline to develop the hamstring muscle group.
	Speed-strength	Follow the program in Chapter 8.
	Short-all out sprints	4-10 repetitions of 10-20 yard sprints with a 30 second rest interval.
Sat.	Aerobics	15-30 minutes of continuous work at your target heart rate.
	Starting/Stopping Drills	Follow the program in Chapter 11. Use the starting stance required by your position.
	Football cutting and acceleration drills	Complete the drills in Chapter 11. Master at least eight different cuts and fakes if you are a running back, defensive back, or receiver.
	Football skill session	Integrate speed into your football drills. High-speed sprinting is the major objective; think speed and quickness. Include drills using the 3-pt and 4-pt stance emphasizing a two-foot push-off for offensive backs and lineman and standing start for defensive backs and linebackers.
	Plyometrics	Follow the program in chapter 8, table 8.10.
	Muscle endurance	Circuit weight training; complete three sets at 50-85% of your 1 RM, 8-12 repetitions, resting 15-40 seconds between exercises.

Table 12.3 Weekly Preseason Schedule for Baseball Players

Day	Training programs	Guidelines
Daily:	General warm-up Dynamic stretching Sprinting form drills Static stretching	Slow jogging 1/2 to 3/4 mile increasing the pace the final 100 yards of each 1/4 mile. Use dynamic stretching before completing the form drills. End each workout with a static stretching session.
Mon.	Sprint-assisted training	Follow the program in Chapter 10, table 10.1.
	Starting/Stopping Drills	Follow the program in Chapter 11. Use the standing start and crouched position of a base runner or fielder.
	Baseball speed-endurance	Use repeated high-speed sprints following the program described in chapter 9. Use some backward high-speed sprints on both a level surface and a slight incline to develop the hamstring muscle group.
	Speed-strength Training	Follow the program in chapter 8.
Tue.	Aerobics	15-30 minutes of continuous work at your target heart rate.
	Baseball skill session	Integrate speed into the baseball drills with sprinting as the major objective. Include drills that involve the standing start with a two-foot push-off for base runners and explosive lateral starting movement for all players.
	Baseball cutting and acceleration drills	Complete the drills in Chapter 11. Master base running and high speed changes of direction.
	Sprint-resisted training	Follow the program in Chapter 8, table 8.13. Use a weighted vest, harness, or parachute to execute power starts from a standing start and from the batter's box, first and second base, and infield and outfield positions.

Day	Training programs	Guidelines
	Plyometrics	Follow the program in chapter 8, table 8.10.
	Short-all out sprints	4-10 repetitions of 30-40 yard sprints with a 30 second rest interval.
Wed.	Starting/Stopping Drills	Follow the program in Chapter 11. Use the standing start and crouched position of a base runner or fielder.
	Baseball speed-endurance	Use repeated high-speed sprints following the program described in Chapter 9, tables 9.2 and 9.3. Use some backward high-speed sprints on both a level surface and a slight incline to develop the hamstring muscle group.
	Speed-strength (Upper Body)	Follow the program in Chapter 8.
Thur.	Aerobics	15-30 minutes of continuous work at your target heart rate
	Baseball skill session	Integrate speed into your baseball drills. High-speed sprinting is the major objective; think speed and quickness as you work out. Include drills using the standing start emphasizing a two-foot push-off for base runners and explosive lateral starting movement for all players.
	Sprint-resisted training (Sport loading)	Follow the program in Chapter 8, tables 8.13 and 8.14, "Hill bursts" (2.5- to 7-degree stadium steps or hill) for 10 to 60 yards. Use a weighted vest, harness, or parachute to execute power starts from a standing position.
	Speed-strength (Lower Body)	Follow the program in Chapter 8.
Fri.	Sprint-assisted Training	Follow the program in Chapter 10, table 10.

Day	Training programs	Guidelines
	Baseball speed-endurance	Use repeated high-speed sprints following the program described in chapter 9. Use some backward high-speed sprints on both a level surface and a slight incline to develop the hamstring muscle group.
	Speed-strength Training	Follow the program in Chapter 8.
	Short-all out sprints	4-10 repetitions of 30-40 yard sprints with a 30 second rest interval.
Sat.	Aerobics	15-30 minutes of continuous work at your target heart rate.
	Starting/Stopping	Follow the program in Chapter 11. Use the standing start and crouched position of a base runner or fielder.
	Baseball cutting and acceleration drills	Complete the drills in Chapter 11. Master base running technique and high speed changes of direction.
	Baseball skill session	Integrate speed into your baseball drills with sprinting as the major objective. Include drills that involve a standing start emphasizing a two-foot push-off for base runners and explosive lateral starting movement for all players.
	Plyometrics	Follow the program in Chapter 8, table 8.10.
	Muscle endurance	Circuit weight training; complete three sets at 50-85% of your 1 RM, 8-12 repetitions, resting 15-40 seconds between exercises.

Table 12.4 Weekly Preseason Schedule for Basketball Players

Day	Training programs	Guidelines
Daily	General warm-up Dynamic stretching Olympic form drills Static stretching	Slow jogging for 1/2 to 3/4 mile increasing the pace the final 100 yards of each 1/4 mile. Use dynamic stretching before completing the form drills. End each workout with a static stretching session.
Mon.	Sprint-assisted training	Follow the program in Chapter 10, table 10.1.
	Starting/Stopping drills	Follow the program in Chapter 11. Execute stops and starts from a defensive stance and offensive posture.
	Basketball speed endurance	Use repeated high-speed sprints following the program described in chapter 9. Use some backward high-speed sprints to develop the hamstring muscle group.
	Speed-strength training	Follow the program in Chapter 8.
Tue.	Aerobics	15-30 minutes of continuous work at your target heart rate.
	Basketball skill session	Integrate speed into your basketball drills. High-speed sprinting is the major objective; think speed and quickness as you work out. Include drills using the defensive stance.
	Basketball cutting and acceleration drills	Complete the drills in Chapter 11. Master the basic fakes and cuts with and without the ball and accelerate for 8-10 yards.
	Sprint-resisted training (Sport loading)	Follow the program in Chapter 8, tables 8.13 and 8.14. Use a weighted vest, harness, or parachute to execute power starts from a defensive stance and from an offensive posture with and without the ball.

Day	Training programs	Guidelines
	Plyometrics	Follow the program in Chapter 8, table 8.10.
	Short-all out sprints	4-10 repetitions of 10-20 yard sprints with a 30 second rest interval.
Wed.	Starting/Stopping drills	Follow the program in Chapter 11. Execute stops and starts from a defensive stance and offensive posture.
	Basketball speed-endurance	Use repeated high-speed sprints following the program described in Chapter 9. Use some backward high-speed sprints to develop the hamstring muscle group.
	Speed-strength training (Upper Body)	Follow the program in chapter 8.
Thur.	Aerobics	15-30 minutes of continuous work at your target heart rate
	Basketball skill session	Integrate speed into your basketball drills with high-speed sprinting as the major objective. Include drills using the defensive stance.
	Sprint-resisted training (Sport loading)	Follow the program in Chapter 8, tables 8.13 and 8.14, "Hill bursts" (2.5- to 7-degree stadium steps or hill) for 10 to 60 yards. Use a weighted vest, harness, or parachute to execute power starts from a defensive stance and from an offensive posture with and without the ball.
	Speed-strength training (Lower Body)	Follow the program in Chapter 8.
Fri.	Sprint-assisted training	Follow the program in Chapter 10, table 10.1. Use repeated sprints using the program in in chapter 9. Use backward sprints to develop the hamstring muscle group.

Day	Training programs	Guidelines
	Speed-strength training	Follow the program in chapter 8.
	Short-all out sprints	4-10 repetitions of 10-20 yard sprints with a 30 second rest interval.
Sat.	Aerobics	15-30 minutes of continuous work at your target heart rate.
	Starting/Stopping drills	Follow the program in Chapter 11. Execute stops and starts from BOTH a defensive stance and offensive posture.
	Basketball cutting and acceleration drills	Complete the drills in Chapter 11. Master the basic fakes and cuts with and without the ball and accelerate for 8-10 yards.
	Basketball skill session	Integrate speed into your basketball drills. High-speed sprinting is the major objective; think speed and quickness as you work out. Include drills using the defensive stance.
	Plyometrics	Follow the program in Chapter 8, table 8.10.
	Muscle endurance	Circuit weight training; complete three sets at 50-85% of your 1 RM, 8-12 repetitions, resting 15-40 seconds between exercises.

Table 12.5 Weekly Preseason Schedule for Soccer Players

Day	Training programs	Guidelines
Daily	General warm-up Dynamic stretching Olympic form drills Static stretching	Slow jogging 1/2 to 3/4 mile increasing the pace the final 100 yards of each 1/4 mile. Use dynamic stretching before completing the form drills. End each workout with a static stretching session.
Mon.	Sprint-assisted Training	Follow the program in Chapter 10, table 10.1.
	Starting/Stopping drills	Follow the program in Chapter 11. Use a standing and walking start.
	Soccer speed-endurance	Use repeated high-speed sprints following the program described in Chapter 9. Use some backward high-speed sprints on both a level surface and a slight incline to develop the hamstring muscle group.
	Speed-strength training	Follow the program in Chapter 8.
Tue.	Aerobics	15-30 minutes of continuous work at your target heart rate.
	Soccer skill session	Integrate speed into your soccer drills with sprinting as the major objective. Include drills that involve a walk and jog to a sprint for 10-30 yards emphasizing proper form and technique. Repeat with the ball.
	Soccer cutting and acceleration drills	Complete the drills in Chapter 11. Master the basic cuts and fakes used in soccer with and without the ball.
	Sprint-resisted training (Sport loading)	Follow the program in Chapter 8, tables 8.13 and 8.14. Use a weighted vest, harness, or parachute to execute power starts from a walking, jogging and 3/4 striding action.

Day	Training programs	Guidelines
	Plyometrics	Follow the program in Chapter 8, table 8.10.
	Short-all out sprints	4-10 repetitions of 10-20 yard sprints with a 30 second rest interval.
Wed.	Starting/Stopping drills	Follow the program in Chapter 11. Use a standing and walking start.
	Soccer speed-endurance	Use repeated high-speed sprints following the program described in Chapter 9. Use some backward high-speed sprints on both a level surface and a slight incline to develop the hamstring muscle group.
	Speed-strength (Upper Body)	Follow the program in Chapter 8.
Thur.	Aerobics	15-30 minutes of continuous work at your target heart rate
	Soccer skill session	Integrate speed into your soccer drills. High-speed sprinting is the major objective; think speed and quickness as you work out. Include drills using a walk and jog to a sprint for 10-30 yards emphasizing proper acceleration, form and technique. Repeat with the ball.
	Sprint-resisted training (Sport loading)	Follow the program in Chapter 8, tables 8.13 and 8.,14. Hill bursts" (2.5 to 7-degree stadium steps or hill) for 10 to 60 yards. Use weighted vests, harness, or parachutes to execute power starts from a walking, jogging and 3/4 striding action.
	Speed-strength (Lower Body)	Follow the program in Chapter 8.
Fri.	Sprint-assisted training	Follow the program in Chapter 10, table 10.1.

Day	Training programs	Guidelines
	Soccer speed endurance	Use repeated high-speed sprints following the program described in Chapter 9. Use some backward high-speed sprints on both a level surface and a slight incline to develop the hamstring muscle group.
	Speed-strength training	Follow the program in Chapter 8.
	Short-all out sprints	4-10 repetitions of 10-20 yard sprints with a 30 second rest interval.
Sat.	Aerobics	15-30 minutes of continuous work at your target heart rate.
	Starting/Stopping drills	Follow the program in Chapter 11. Use a standing and walking start.
	Soccer cutting and acceleration drills	Complete the drills in Chapter 11. Master the basic cuts and fakes used in soccer with and without the ball.
	Soccer skill session	Integrate speed into your soccer drills with sprinting is the major objective. Include drills that involve a walk and jog to a sprint for 10-30 yards emphasizing proper form and technique. Repeat with the ball.
	Plyometrics	Follow the program in Chapter 8.
	Muscle endurance	Circuit weight training; complete three sets at 50-85% of your 1 RM, 8-12 repetitions, resting 15-40 seconds between exercises.

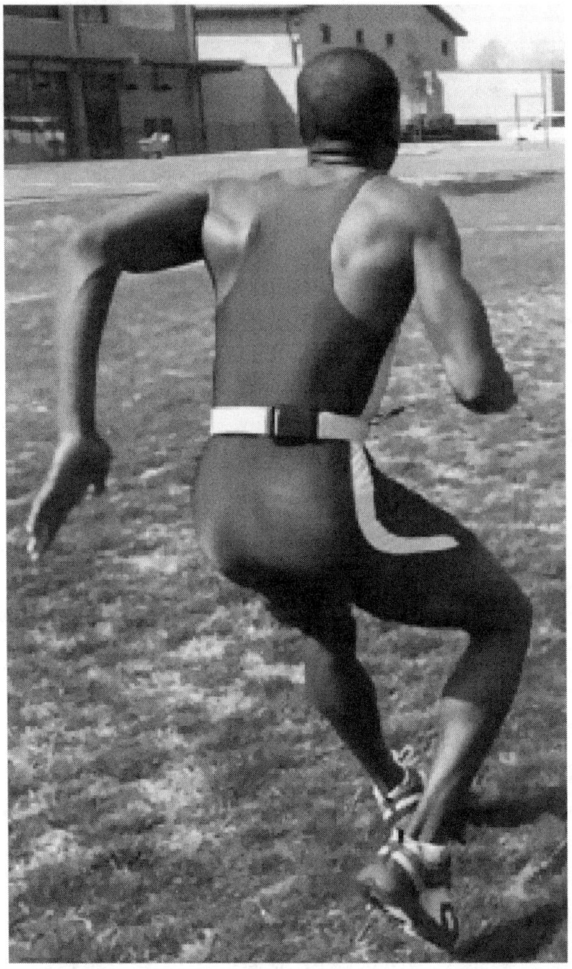

Figure 12.1 High-speed backward sprints

IN-SEASON MAINTENANCE PROGRAM

Although time becomes precious during the competitive season in most sports, it is not difficult to find the time to apply the correct maintenance loads to prevent loss of speed.

By the first day of the competitive season in team sports, athletes may be near their peak conditioning and speed performance levels. As the season progresses, limited practice time, skill and strategy sessions taking precedent, injuries, and little speed, power and strength training results in a "detraining" effect in every athlete. Detraining actually occurs faster than training gains and is noticeable in 1-2 weeks as sports skills requiring speed-strength are performed less efficiently. Research has revealed that speed-strength losses are a result of decreases in motor recruitment as the body is no longer capable of utilizing the same number of motor units. Losses in speed and quickness have also been documented. According to Tudor Bompa (1999), speed tends to be the first ability affected by detraining as the power capabilities of muscle contraction diminish.

The nervous system is also sensitive to detraining and the motor unit is one of the first to deteriorate. Soon, the amount of force generated declines since fewer motor units are recruited. Two weekly weight training sessions using exercises that involve the prime movers and core muscles (abs, lower back, hips), one weekly plyometric session and two 15-minute sprint-assisted sessions are recommended for team sport athletes to prevent loss of speed, power and strength.

Although the in-season maintenance program is secondary to the goals of the competitive season, it is a phase of training that requires attention to detail to design an effective program that can be completed without disrupting the practice session. *Coaches only need a slight adjustment and departure from the normal practice schedule to add a maintenance program.*

To make this adjustment, coaches should consider the following suggestions:

- Assign an assistant coach to the task of designing and incorporating a maintenance program.

- Commit a brief portion of each practice day to speed training.

- Eliminate traditional wind sprints from the practice schedule. Substitute interval sprint training, pickup sprints or hollow sprints that control the distance covered, number of repetitions, and the rest interval between sprints. By recording this information each workout, it is an easy task to make certain athletes are progressively doing more work each session and that speed endurance is being maintained or improved.

- Include testing at least twice per season in the major areas described in Chapter 2 to locate weaknesses that are restricting fast and quick movement and preventing athletes from reaching their genetic speed potential.

- Use two 15-minute sprint-assisted training sessions weekly to maintain stride rate and stride length.

- Use two strength-power training sessions weekly in the weight room.

- Use plyometric training no more than once weekly.
- Use the speed improvement maintenance programs in the proper order.

Table 12.6 below provides one example of how the in-season program would work in a scheduled practice session and places the maintenance training programs in a logical order. The extra time is well worth the effort and will prevent loss of conditioning and a decrease in individual and team performance as the season progresses.

Table 12.6 **Maintenance Loads During the Season**

Quality	In-season Maintenance Loads
Power Output (speed-strength)	One vigorous weight training workout weekly combined with plyometrics (in the weight room).
Speed	Two 15-minute sprint-assisted workouts weekly (5-8 towing pulls each session with full recovery between each repetition).
Speed-endurance	Two pickup sprint training workouts weekly to replace wind sprints. Careful record keeping on the distance covered, number of repetitions, and rest interval between repetitions and sets.
Flexibility	Daily sessions of dynamic stretching at the beginning of practice and static stretching following each speed-strength training workout and at the end of practice for 5-10 minutes.
Starting, Stopping, Cutting, Accelerating	Two 15-minute sessions using the drills specific to your sport.

PERIODIZATION

Coaches refer to a periodization program used by Michael Young. What type of periodization does he recommend for sprinters?

Michael Young (2001), former Assistant Track Coach at West Point, compares two common methods: the Eastern and Western Models of Periodization. A summary of the characteristics and effectiveness of both methods are listed in Table 12.7.

Table 12.7 Periodization: Eastern and Western Models

Characteristics	Eastern Model	Western Model
Begins with general low intensity exercise.	X	X
Planning occurs around the competitive schedule	X	X
Loads placed on the athlete are cycled throughout the week.	X	X
The primary objective is to reach peak sprinting condition for a major competitive event.	X	X
Each phase builds on the previous phase.	X	
Maximum intensity training, speed endurance training, and strength training are used year around, peaking during the competitive season.	X	
Speed endurance is developed year around by lengthening the distance over which maximum speed can be maintained.	X	
Athletes achieve maximum levels in one area of conditioning before moving to a different phase. *Example:* One month of general conditioning, followed by three months of speed-endurance training, three months of strength training, three months of power training, before concentrating on speed training as the competitive season approaches.		X
Maximum levels of each fitness component is first achieved before moving to another component.		X

The concept of periodization can be adapted to any sport or activity including sprinting. The same principles apply when a training program is being designed. Coaches should keep the terminology simple to avoid confusion. Terms such as macro cycle (1 phase or more training year), mesocycle (weeks of training), micro cycle (days of training), volume, intensity, training categories, peaking and active rest can be easily learned. Modern day athletes are surprisingly good at understanding and applying basic training principles in their workouts. The goal of a sprinter is SPEED. and the competition dates for near peak and peak performance are the important focus points. This information allows coaches and athletes to carefully design their training program.

Which of the two general models presented in Table 12-7 are most effective?

According to Young, who carefully analyzed each method, the Eastern Model is superior since it leads to better performance by permitting athletes to develop maximum levels of strength, speed endurance and speed at the same time. Since the Western Model involves peaking in some areas prior to the competitive event, it never results in peaking in all components at the right time.

TRACKING PROGRESS

To properly track progress, isolate the factors responsible for the improvement or lack of improvement, and identify the areas where you need to place more emphasis and work harder. Proper tracking involves careful record keeping in two areas: Test Score Results and the actual workout schedule completed.

Follow these simple steps in each of the two areas to make certain you are fully aware of exactly how you are training, what you are doing, how it is affecting speed test scores, and what needs to change to stay on course to improve speed for your sport.

Speed Profile Form

- Record initial test scores on the Speed Profile Form shown in Table 2.1. Make a copy of the form and place it on a clipboard.

- Retest in each area after completing the fourth workout week.

- Compare scores in each area for improvement. If no improvement has occurred, alter the workout by increasing the number of times a specific program is used and the intensity of that phase of the workout. If you now meet the standard where you were previously deficient and feel you no longer need as much effort, reduce the use and intensity and resort to the "maintenance load" specified in each training program to merely keep the gains that have occurred.

- At the close of the 8-week pre-season training period, retest once again in each area and make the comparisons and changes indicated above.

Workout Records

- Make two copies of the Workout Record Form in Table 12.8, place one on a clipboard and take it with you to each training session.

• Record the information requested in each speed improvement training program identified immediately after completing each separate training program in a workout. This information is now available for review and analysis to help understand why test score improvement in some areas may not have occurred or was less than anticipated. This record- keeping is also necessary to make certain you are applying the principle of progressive resistance exercise to each speed improvement training program and increasing the number of repetitions, distance covered, intensity, and altering the amount of rest interval between each repetition to complete more work (volume) and more work per unit of time (intensity) each session.

• Study Table 12.8 carefully until you understand how to record what you actually did each workout.

HOW THEY TRAINED

This Chapter closes with a tribute to the late Lloyd "Bud" Winter (1909-1985), former track coach at San Jose State College, President of the National Track Coaches of America, and Assistant Coach of the American track and field team at the 1960 Summer Olympics in Rome and one of the most successful coaches of all times. His San Jose State teams placed among the top ten on 14 occasions at the national collegiate championships. Coach Winter also wrote one of the first booklets ever on sprinting: *So You Want to Be a Sprinter*, by Lloyd C. "Bud" Winter; Fearon Publishers: Palo Alto, CA, ©1956. Now 50 years later, it is interesting to look at some of his coaching comments, verbal cues, and recommendations; many of which still apply today.

<u>On improving speed</u>

"Possibly your inherent quality may prevent you from becoming a great champion. But the truth is your speed can be improved,"

<u>On training to improve speed</u>

"A good sprinter will: 1) have high knee action, 2) have good foreleg reach, 3) run high on the toes (balls of feet), 4) have good arm action, 5) bound forward, not up, 6) maintain good forward lean, 7) run tall, with back straight, and 8) be relaxed (loose jaw--loose hands). These are not natural movements, so you must practice these exercises."

On Sprinting Form

"Keep the hips forward, back straight--the straight line from the back of the head to the heel."

"The secret of sprinting is to have a long stride that carries you low to the ground. Bound forward, not up; drive forward with the toes."

NOTE: The drive forward is with the balls of the feet. which is likely what was actually meant. Driving off the toes produces a slowing effect.

On Stride Rate

"There is not much we can do about leg speed except practice. Therefore, we must work on developing the most efficient stride--a long low one."

NOTE: The discovery that stride rate (steps per second) can be improved by training the neuromuscular system and increasing ground contact force has added another dimension to speed improvement in the past 35-40 years.

Table 12.8 **Workout Record form**

Name______________________ Age ____ Height ______ Weight ______

Sport ______________________ Position ____________

Starting date _______ second test date _______ third test date ________

Training area	Weeks 1 and 5	weeks 2 and 6	Weeks 3 and 7	Weeks 4 and 8	Total
Number of workouts	_______	_______	_______	_______	_______
	_______	_______	_______	_______	_______
Sprinting form Two-foot push-off and starting reps	_______	_______	_______	_______	_______
	_______	_______	_______	_______	_______
Completed	_______	_______	_______	_______	_______
	_______	_______	_______	_______	_______
	_______	_______	_______	_______	_______
Sprinting form drill sessions	_______	_______	_______	_______	_______
	_______	_______	_______	_______	_______
Completed	_______	_______	_______	_______	_______
	_______	_______	_______	_______	_______
	_______	_______	_______	_______	_______
Sprint-assisted training	_______	_______	_______	_______	_______
	_______	_______	_______	_______	_______
Completed	_______	_______	_______	_______	_______
	_______	_______	_______	_______	_______
	_______	_______	_______	_______	_______
Stop and start drills	_______	_______	_______	_______	_______
	_______	_______	_______	_______	_______
Completed	_______	_______	_______	_______	_______
	_______	_______	_______	_______	_______
	_______	_______	_______	_______	_______

Table 12.8 **(continued)**

Training area	Weeks 1 and 5	weeks 2 and 6	Weeks 3 and 7	Weeks 4 and 8	Total
Cutting and acceleration (reps)					
Distance, reps, rest					
Speed endurance training					
Completed					
Speed strength training					
Completed					
Sport loading					
Completed					
Plyometric training Completed					
Sprinting form training Completed					

CHAPTER 13

SPEED IMPROVEMENT FOR YOUNG ATHLETES

This chapter discusses the various sports speed training practices suitable for young boys and girls, identifies programs that are unsafe, and provides guidelines for coaches and parents involved in the training of preadolescent athletes.

GROWTH AND DEVELOPMENT

How is a young athlete's stage of development determined and used to provide a safe, effective speed training program?

The task is to make certain an athlete has reached a physiological age that permits safe involvement in either a modified speed improvement program for prepubescent and early adolescent athletes or the complete program for late adolescent and adult athletes presented in Chapters 1-12.

Preadolescent Athletes. Athletes who have not reached the age of puberty and show no signs of developmental changes can safely engage in some training programs such as flexibility training (stretching), form training, modified speed endurance training and limited speed-strength, sprint-resisted and sprint-assisted training. Programs such as plyometric training and heavy weight training are not recommended.

Early Adolescent Athletes. The beginning of adolescence involves the growth spurt and the onset of puberty. Rapid growth of the long bones (arms and legs) takes place and changes body proportions. In females, puberty begins with breast development, presence of pubic hair, followed by first menstruation; in males by the level of development of secondary sex traits such as facial hair, pubic and genital hair. There is also an increase in muscle mass in boys and body fat in girls. These changes usually take place between 10 1/2 - 12 years of age in females and 12 1/2 - 14 years of age in males, although some individuals will not reach this stage until 2-3 years later. Since boys and girls are more likely to be injured during this period, training programs must be carefully supervised.

Prior to the late adolescent period, young athletes should devote most of their time to skill development, learning proper starting and sprinting form, and practicing various forms of sprint-assisted training. A modified speed improvement program for early adolescent males and females prevents unnecessary injury, avoids interference with growth and development and lays the foundation for advanced training methods that will be used in the future.

Late Adolescent and Adult Athletes. The slowing or end of the growth spurt and the presence of secondary sex traits for several years suggests that the athlete is in the late adolescent or adult stage of growth and development and ready to respond to more vigorous training.

Age is a poor indicator of maturity at any stage of growth and development prior to the adult years and should only be used as a guide. Wrist X-ray and other tests may be done by a physician to more accurately determine the end of the growth spurt in both males and females. This normally occurs after age 13-14 in females and 15-16 in males although some individuals may not reach this stage for another 2-3 years.

At what age should a child begin to participate in sports?

Parents should allow the child to answer this question and avoid being too pushy or the child may reject a particular sport or activity. Family influences are important during the early years and a parent's interest and appreciation in sports is often transferred to the children. Chances of transfer are improved with the correct approach.

Whether a child pursues sports depends on ability and parental respect for individuality. The secret is to persuade and not command, lead and not pressure, nurture and not force. An interest in sports can be developed through a child's own curiosity, directed and encouraged through indirect family influences. Moments of interest, within a child's attention span, are used wisely by parents with no pressure to continue when the child chooses to do something else. A child who experiences early success is more likely to continue with that sport or activity. Pressure to continue when a child loses interest is counterproductive.

The Law of Readiness also prevents parents from starting a son or daughter too early in many sports. Until finer muscular movements are possible, some sports are virtually impossible.

How does "adolescent awkwardness" affect the performance of young athletes?

The concept of adolescent awkwardness refers to a period during the growth spurt called PHV (*peak height velocity*); the maximum rate of growth in height that is accompanied by a temporary disruption in motor performance. According to the Feis longitudinal study, PHV occurs in boys at a mean estimated age of 13.7 years and in girls at 11.8 years (Boche and Sun, 2003). Researchers have found a disruption in balancing abilities for up to 6 months and a decline on four of seven motor tasks in a significant number of boys during PHV. Although not everyone experiences a disruption, adolescent awkwardness does exist, but primarily among boys with 1.4 to 33.5 percent affected in some studies on items such as arm pull or static strength (1.4%), speed of limb movement (7.0 %), vertical jump (9.5%), sit and reach (18.7%), leg lift (26.1%), bent-arm hang (30.5%), and shuttle run (33.5%). Boys who showed performance declines were often the best performers at the beginning of peak height velocity.

Studies also indicate that these decreases in performance are only temporary, therefore, it is important to use caution in interpreting motor performance test scores during this critical growth period (Payne and Isaacs, 2007).

EARLY SPECIALIZATION

Isn't it important for young athletes to concentrate on one sport at as early an age as possible?

There are supporting arguments on both sides of the issue and the correct choice may depend more on the physiological and emotional development of the athlete than on chronological age.

Most experts feel that it is best to avoid specialization prior to age 15 or so, depending upon the stage of growth and development. Others argue for specialization as early as possible whenever the child is ready. Tudor Bompa, in his book *Total Training for Young Champions: Proven Conditioning Programs for Athletes Ages 6 to 18*, suggests a Multilateral Plan for various age groups that slowly prepares young athletes for specialization after building a basic skill and conditioning foundation. This foundation training is recommended until age 15. A summary of this approach is provided below.

Ages 6-10 (Initiation Period)---Children should be encouraged to participate in as many sports as possible using low intensity training programs with the emphasis on enjoyment. During this period, attention spans are short and the human body is rapidly changing and susceptible to soft tissue injuries that can seriously affect growth and development and health. Children are encouraged to try many different activities and develop the fundamental skills that are common to most sports such as throwing, kicking, catching, batting, jumping and running, and other basic traits such as coordination, flexibility, and balance. It is the formation of sound technique in these skills that prepare young athletes for later specialization in a sport of choice. These skills need much more attention than they currently receive in our nation's physical education programs. The trend to reduce and eliminate school P.E. programs must be reversed to improve the health of the nation and provide enough time for the formation of sound fundamental skills.

Ages 11-14 (Athletic Period)---The emphasis remains on fun competition and Foundation Training. Athletes are exposed to more complex drills and activities with the emphasis on "fun" rather than competition. Training intensity is increased slightly. Although still susceptible to injury, the body is somewhat more prepared for moderate foundation training in strength, muscular endurance (anaerobic training), and cardiovascular endurance. Core (hips, lower back, abdomen) and arm and shoulder development is initiated using body weight, light dumbbells and medicine balls. Heavy weights are avoided and workouts are supervised at all times.

Ages 15-18 (Specialization Period)---Emphasis shifts to specific exercises and drills aimed at high specialization performance development. As this stage progresses, emphasis moves move from a coaching to a training role. Careful supervision is needed to prevent "too much, too soon" and ensure proper conditioning progression. Athletes begin longer practice sessions as they work hard on perfecting the techniques of the sport. Mental training is also added.

Age 19 and above (High performance Period)---Exceptional performance results usually occur after athletes reach athletic maturation.

Studies show that the average age of Olympic athletes for most sports is 19-25: (Basketball - 24.7, Cycling - 23.4, Soccer - 24.1, Swimming - 21.6 for men and 18.9 for women, Volleyball - 25.2, Water Polo - 25.3, and Wrestling - 24.8).

Not all psychologists, physiologists, medical personnel and coaches are in agreement with this model. Evidence to the contrary does exist in some areas where it is extremely difficult to reach a high performance level when an athlete begins at a later stage of growth and development. Some experts argue for specialization to begin in the 11-14 age group. This is particularly true for gymnastics, golf, and tennis where early emphasis on proper technique and execution of the fundamental skills of the sport are critical. Moderate and heavy supplemental conditioning (other than aspects such as tennis stroking, drills, and play) are avoided until the next stage.

What is recommended as a general, realistic speed training program for preadolescent boys and girls?

This is the age to keep workouts fun, focusing on improving starting and sprinting form. Learning proper starting techniques (from a 4-point, 3-point, standing or moving start) and mastering form during acceleration and maximum speed carries over to every sport. Build a series of 5-6 form drills into each workout. These drills (butt kickers, wall slide, quick feet drills, cycling movement, down-and-offs, pull throughs, stationary high knee lifts, backward sprinting, bounding) are described in Part II: The 5-step Model, Chapter 11.

View early speed training as a long-term approach rather than focusing on short term speed improvement. Strive for a little improvement each week. Eventually this will lead to long lasting, big improvements. Regular testing also helps keep young athletes interested. There is no greater motivational device in sports than for a young athlete to improve their 20-yard or 40-yard dash test scores by a few tenths of a second after 3-6 months of training. Keep in mind also that conditioning programs to develop speed-strength and speed-endurance occur more slowly in prepubescent athletes and attempts to accelerate the process using heavy weights and lengthy workouts is dangerous and not recommended. Emphasis should be placed on slow skill development and slow improvement in conditioning and speed rather than who wins the game

INJURY PREVENTION AND THE YOUNG ATHLETE

What do the experts recommend to keep sports "fun" and our young athletes safe and injury free?

All parties agree that there is great need for change. According to sports medicine pediatricians, the number of injuries among the 45 million young athletes ages 6-18 who engage in competitive sports is steadily increasing. Each year, more and more children are participating in organized and recreational sports with many playing year around on more than one team simultaneously. This combination of early specialization and over training can lead to serious injury and burnout and actually affect a child's decision to participate in sports throughout life, sacrificing the health benefits, which is a key outcome of sports participation. To counter this trend, the *American Academy of Pediatrics Sports Medicine Council* has issued specific recommendations on intensive training and sports specialization. Recommendations are used in conjunction with the *American Academy of Pediatrics* policy statement on intensive training and sports specialization in young athletes. Since scientific evidence is not available in all areas, some findings are based on committee opinion.

Recommendations are designed to assist those who manage young athletes in identifying overtraining issues such as participation in endurance events, weekend tournaments, year-round training on multiple teams, and multipart involvement (Brenner, 2007).

The following training guidelines are recommended for young athletes:

- Use 1-2 days of rest each week. For adequate physical and psychological recovery, 1-2 days of inactivity are needed with no involvement in competition, sport-specific training, or competitive practice. This rest period ensures more complete recovery from vigorous training, improves the benefits of training, and reduces the chance of injury, illness and burnout.

- Restrict weekly training loads to an increase of no more than ten percent. "Too much, too soon" is a major cause of injury in sports. Slow, safe progression is needed for young athletes. This requires regular record keeping on the frequency (number of weekly training sessions), intensity (repetitions, sets, weight, speed) and duration (length of each workout session) to make sure progression is slow, safe and effective.

- Encourage athletes to take an annual break from the sport for 2-3 months. Getting away from year-around involvement in one sport greatly reduces the chances of overuse injuries. Age group athletes often participate for as long as 5-6 hours each day in weekend sports tournaments for soccer, basketball, baseball, softball, field hockey, rugby and tennis and are exposed to heat-related illness, nutritional deficiencies, overuse injuries, and burnout. A 2-3 month "break" each year provides both physical and psychological healing.

- Encourage preadolescent athletes to try a variety of sports and concentrate on skill acquisition, safety, sportsmanship and having fun. Less than one percent of age group athletes will ever compete at the professional level in any sport. Specializing too young can deprive an athlete of discovering which sport they are actually best suited for. In sprinting, the emphasis should be placed on mastering correct form and technique in the start, acceleration, the drive phase, and the stride cycle. Sound sprinting mechanics also aid performance in other sports making this aspect of training critical to every young athlete. Studies show that young athletes who participate in a variety of sports have fewer injuries and play sports longer than those who specialize before puberty.

- Allow participation on only one team during a season. Members of a traveling or select team should participate on that squad only and incorporate the guidelines in this section.

• Be alert to signs of burnout. Nonspecific muscle or joint problems, fatigue, poor academic performance, and decreases in motivation can be signals that the athlete needs help to counteract the problem.

Are female athletes more susceptible to injury?

Female athletes are 5-7 times more likely to sustain ACL (anterior cruciate ligament) and other knee injuries as males. Girls and women are also more susceptible to runner's knee, stress fractures, sprained ankles, arthritis in the knee, shoulder instability and frozen shoulder (adhesive capilitus). Dr. Laura Tosi, Director of the bone-health program of Children's National Medical Center in Washington, D.C. points out that women tend to have looser ligaments than men and are not able to pull in a straight line, which puts stress on the kneecap. Girls also do not bend their knees and hips as much as boys when they run, jump and turn. Girls tend not to "stay low to the ground" when sprinting as recommended for efficient and correct form. Although the anatomical structure of young girls and women is quite different and a part of the susceptibility issue, there is a lot that can be done to prevent these injuries and conditions.

Are there specific programs for girls and women that reduce the risk of injury in sports?

Although male and female athletes of all ages need to utilize an injury prevention program consisting of strength, flexibility, and sport-specific drills, this program is designed for female athletes. The PEP Program (Prevent injury, Enhance Performance), discussed in a *Parade* article uses what appears to be a very effective injury prevention program for female athletes. PEP was developed by the Santa Monica Orthopedic and Sports Medicine Group in conjunction with teams of physicians, physical therapists, athletic trainers and coaches and includes exercises that target areas identified as vulnerable by researchers. Each 20-minute session is designed to strengthen critical muscle groups and promote proper alignment during running, jumping, and turning. According to a recent study of 1435 female soccer players, PEP reduced non-contact ACL injuries by 70%.

This prevention program includes general warm-up, stretching, strengthening, plyometrics, and correct form and technique in executing sport specific movements that involve deficits in the strength and coordination of the stabilizing muscles around the knee joint. Correct posture, straight up and down jumps without excessive side-to-side movement, and soft landings are emphasized in three 20- minute sessions weekly. Specific features of the preventive program include:

• *Cross-training.* To avoid overuse injuries on repetitive movements such as running, jumping, and throwing.

• *Strengthening the hamstring muscles.* Hamstrings should be at least 75% as strong as the quadriceps since lower ratios leave athletes more susceptible to injury. Both male and female athletes tend to neglect the hamstrings since so many weight training exercises and actual movements in sports involve the quadriceps muscle group and so few focus on the hamstrings.

• *General Warm-up.* Walk and jog for 5-10 minutes.

• *Stretching.* PEP uses static stretching with a hold time of 30 seconds. The authors strongly recommend dynamic stretching at the beginning of all workouts and static stretching for improved range of motion (ROM) at the end of workouts. The PEP stretching program includes the calf stretch, quadriceps stretch, figure four hamstring stretch, inner thigh stretch, and hip flexor stretch (lunge forward with the right leg and drop the left knee to the ground, lean forward with the hips with hands on top of the right thigh, grasp the left ankle and pull the heel toward the buttocks).

• *Shuttle Run (side to side)*

• *Backward Running*

• *Strengthening (*Leg strength exercises). Walking Lunges--3 sets x 10 reps, Russian, Single Toe Raises - 30 reps x 2 reps, and Hamstring--3 sets x 10 reps Kneel on the ground with hands at your side as a partner holds your ankles. With a straight back, lean forward leading with your hips. The knee, hip and shoulder should be in a straight line as you lean toward the ground without bending at the waist.

• *Plyometrics.* Basic exercises only are performed on a soft surface (mats, field area) emphasizing a soft landing on the balls of the feet, rolling back to the heel with a bent knee and a straight hip (Lateral Hops over Cone-20 reps, Forward/Backward Hops--20 reps, Single Leg hops over cone - 20 reps, Vertical Jumps with headers--20 reps, Scissors Jump - 20 reps).

• *Agility.* Shuttle run with forward/backward running, diagonal runs (3 passes), and Bounding run (44 yards).

Hamstring injuries are common in sports requiring repeated sprints. How do athletes reduce their risk and recover from such an injury?

A stretch or tear of one of the three large muscles of the back of the thigh comprising the hamstring muscle group (biceps, semimembranosus, and semitendinosus) typically occurs when these muscles are contracting forcefully during the sprinting or jumping action. Some studies indicate the injury is also more likely to occur in sprinters and other athletes as they run the curves on a 400-meter track.

Athletes experience a burning or popping sensation followed by pain when walking, jogging, bending or strengthening the leg. Bruising may also be noticeable below the injured site in 2-3 days. Hamstring injuries generally occur at the proximal myotendinous junction. In the biceps femoris muscle, this junction extends over most of its entire length. Injury rarely occurs within the tendon itself.

- Grade 1 is a mild strain, with few muscle fibers being torn.
- Grade 2 is a moderate strain, with a definite loss in strength.
- Grade 3 is a complete tear of the hamstrings.

An *avulsion strain* is rare, but much more serious and occurs when the tendon tears and pulls a small part of the bone away with it. This is more common in younger athletes (14-18 year olds) who may have had a history of chronic hamstring tendinitis. If a young athlete complains of severe hamstring pain at the point of origin, avulsion strain should be suspected until it is ruled out by an X-ray or bone scan. Treatment of a severe case will require surgery.

In young athletes in the developmental stage, risk factors include inadequate warm-up, failure to use proper techniques of dynamic stretching immediately after the general warm-up period, muscle tightness, muscle imbalance (low hamstring to quadriceps ratio), incorrect muscle timing (muscle groups firing in the wrong order), muscle fatigue, and over training. Studies also show that the flexibility of the hamstrings and the eccentric and concentric muscle torque in the hamstrings and quadriceps muscles at different angular velocities are a factor. Sprinters who suffered a previous hamstring injury have significantly tighter hamstrings than uninjured sprinters. Uninjured sprinters had significantly higher eccentric hamstring torques at all angular velocities and higher concentric quadriceps and hamstring torques at 30 deg/sec but not at higher velocities. Sprinters with a history of hamstring injury have been found to be weaker in eccentric contractions and in concentric contractions at low velocities.

The exact cause of hamstring strains is still unknown and cannot be attributed to any single factor. One area of concern in team sports has been the belief that the common strength disparity between hip extensor and hip flexor muscles may play a role. Some coaches have even recommended a 1:1 ratio between the hamstrings and quadriceps although most have their athletes strive for hamstrings strength development to approximately 75-80 per cent of the quadriceps. Injuries are more likely a result of a multi factorial group of risk factors. Sprinting is a complicated, demanding skill that places supra-maximal loads on the hamstring muscle group. In fact studies show that the hamstrings may be the most active muscles during the sprinting gait cycle. During the forward leg swing phase, the hamstring activity increases. Once the terminal stage of the forward swing phase is complete, muscle activity continues to remain high as the hamstrings concentrically contract to extend the hip and flex the knee. Greater speeds of running have been found to be associated with longer periods of hamstring activity during the support phase. Researchers believe that this further validates the role of the hamstrings as hip extensors during the stance phase of running and sprinting.

Proper treatment calls for 2-3 days of ice packs for 20-30 minutes every 3-4 hours, elevating the leg with a pillow when resting, use of compression by wrapping the thigh with an elastic bandage, use of anti-inflammatory medication prescribed by a physician, and use of crutches until an athlete can walk pain free. A return to the sport and workouts occurs only after full range of motion and full strength returns without pain, linear jogging and sprinting occur without pain, 45 degree cuts can be completed without pain, and jumping on the injured leg can take place without pain. Rehabilitation exercises recommended by Pierre Rouzier (2004) for use both during the recovery and for prevention following recovery include the following:

Prone Leg Bends--Lie on the stomach with legs flat on the floor. Bend your knee and bring the heel toward your buttocks, then back down to the starting position. Complete 2-3 sets of 10 repetitions.

Standing Hamstring Stretch--From a standing position, place the heel of the injured leg on a chair approximately 15" high. Bend at the hips and lean forward to produce an easy stretch at the back of the thigh. Hold the stretch for 30-60 seconds, repeat 3 times.

Hamstring Stretch on the Wall--Lie on your back with the buttocks near a doorway and legs extended through the doorway. Raise the injured leg and rest the heel against the door frame. Hold the stretch you feel in the back of your thigh for 30-60 seconds, repeat 3 times.

Standing Calf Stretch--Place both hands on a wall at chest level. Place the injured leg 12-18" behind the front leg. Keep the injured leg straight and the heel flat on the floor as you lean into the wall. Bend the front knee until you feel a mild stretch in the back of the calf muscle of the injured leg. Hold for 30-60 seconds, repeat 3 sets.

Prevention involves use of a 15-25 minute general warm-up followed by dynamic stretching before each workout. Static stretching of the hamstring muscle group occurs at the close of each workout or practice session to increase range of motion.

Parents worry about heat-related illnesses during and after a workout in hot, humid weather. Once a workout is over, doesn't *body temperature drop immediately to ward off heat exhaustion or heat stroke?*

The post workout period is actually needed to assist the body in its cooling effort. As Gabe Mirkin, M.D. (http://www.DrMirkin.com) points out, you sweat more after exercise than while exercising. Body temperature also continues to rise, adding to the over heated condition. During exercise, about 70 percent of the energy that powers muscles is lost as heat, causing body temperature to rise. To prevent temperature from rising too high, the heart pumps the heat in the blood from muscles to the skin, increasing perspiration and the efficiency of the body's main cooling mechanism; evaporation of sweat. The amount of perspiration is controlled by the temperature of the blood flowing to the part of the brain called the hypothalamus. When body temperature rises, additional sweating occurs. During exercise, the heart beats rapidly to pump blood and bring oxygen to muscles and hot blood from the muscles to the skin where the heat can be dissipated. When exercise stops, the heart slows down, the amount of blood pumped to the skin decreases, the amount of sweat increases and temperature rises. At this point you can help by getting out of the sun, entering an air conditioned or cool area, drinking cold water and cold electrolyte drinks, and applying cool towels to the elbows, back of the knee, and neck areas.

Body temperatures commonly reach 101 F during workouts in a warm gym or weight room. At the extreme, marathon runners may finish the raise with temperatures considerably higher. One such runner supposedly developed a temperature of over 107 F. With a temperature of 102 F, muscle discomfort occurs that may produce a burning sensation, over 104 F results in shortness of breath, and temperatures over 105 F cause brain distress (headache, blurred vision, ringing in the ears, dizziness, nausea, and possibly unconsciousness).

The higher the temperature, the more difficult it becomes to dissipate heat and cool the body. The key to protecting yourself from heat stroke is to avoid acquiring unusually high core temperatures by drinking fluids and electrolyte solutions freely prior to exercise or competition (loading), drinking freely during the activity session, drinking before you are thirsty, wearing a visor type hat to allow the heat to dissipate through the head, changing wet clothing frequently, and using shade to protect yourself from the sun whenever possible.

PLAYING SPEED TEST BATTERY FOR YOUNG ATHLETES

The recommended testing program for preadolescent athletes is described below. Details of test administration and score analysis were presented in Chapter 2. Young athletes should ask a parent, friend or coach to help them complete these tests.

Test results will locate weakness areas that are preventing a young athletes from sprinting faster and help measure progress during the speed improvement training program.

What specific tests should young athletes use?

The tests listed below are recommended for preadolescent boys and girls.

- Stationary 120-yard dash with split times at the 20-, 40-, and 80-yard mark. This single test provides a stationary 40-yard dash time, flying 40-yard dash time, acceleration time, mph speed, speed endurance evaluation, and one-half of the data needed to determine how many steps are taken per second (stride rate). The standing start may be a better choice for young athletes since it is often faster than the 3-pt. or 4-pt. start because of the lack of strength development necessary to drive out of the crouch position.

- The First 3-Step Test. This is one of the most important tests for every athlete. Those who are capable of covering the most ground in the initial first 3 steps of a short sprint are more likely to be successful in their sport. Until age-group standards are available, it is important to acquire accurate baseline data.

- Stride Length. This test reveals the length of one stride and uncovers any muscle imbalances present between the right and left leg. It also provides the second part of the data needed to determine stride rate.

- Stride Rate (Steps taken per Second). Stride rate is determined from the flying 40-yard dash score and stride length score using the Matrix in Chapter 2, table 2.2.

- *Acceleration.* Acceleration time is determined by subtracting the flying 40-yard dash time from the stationary 40-yard dash. With a stationary 40 of 5.2 seconds and a flying 40 of 4.4, the acceleration time is 8/10 of a second. A difference of more than 7/10 of a second is POOR.

- Speed Endurance. Speed endurance is determined by subtracting the 80- 1 2 0 - yard time from the flying 40-yard time. This indicates the amount of slowing that occurred after a long sprint. Example: A flying 40-yard time of 4.4 and an 80-120-yard time of 4.9 seconds equals a 5/10 second slowing due to fatigue and earns a rating of POOR.

The NASE repeated 40-yard dash test measures "recovery time" and reveals the ability of athletes to make repetitive sprints throughout a game or match at the same high speed without slowing due to fatigue. For young athletes, five 20-yard dashes are completed at 10-30 second intervals (depending upon the average recovery time between sprints that actually occurs in a particular sport). There should be a difference of no more than 2/10 second among any of the five scores.

The following modified tests are suitable for early adolescents but are not recommended for prepubescent athletes

- Leg Strength/Body Weight Ratio. A modified 1RM test (maximum weight that can be lifted for only one repetition) is recommended. A safe approach is to find the amount of weight that allows an athlete to complete a maximum of 6 repetitions, then add 20 pounds to estimate the 1RM. Athletes should slowly progress until capable of leg pressing at least 2 X body weight. An athlete who weighs 150 pounds should strive to leg press 300 pounds.

- Single-Leg Kick Back. The single-leg kickback test measures the force exerted against an area similar to a starting block and the ground during the acceleration phase of sprinting. Find the 1RM safely as described for leg strength. At this age, the purpose of this test is to identify muscle imbalance between the right and left leg.

- Hamstring/Quadriceps Ratio. Find the 6RM safely for the double leg extension and double leg curl. Ideally, the double leg curl scores (Hamstrings) should be 70-75% of the leg extension (quadriceps) score.

- Standing Triple Jump. Scores should exceed 20 feet for middle school males and 15 feet for middle school females.

- Quick Feet Test. This test provides an indication of an athlete's potential to execute fast steps and quick movements. An acceptable score is 3.8 or less seconds (middle school males), and 4.2 for middle school females.

- Aerobic Fitness (1.0 mile walk/run).

Age	*Minimum standard for Boys*	*Minimum standard for Girls*
12	*10 minutes*	*12 minutes*
13	*9 minutes, 30 seconds*	*11 minutes, 30 seconds*
14-16	*8 minutes, 30 seconds*	*10 minutes, 30 seconds*
17-19	*8 minutes*	*9 minutes, 30 seconds*

- Body Composition. Skinfold measures, described in Chapter 2, will provide an estimate of each athlete's percent of body fat. Consult a physician for advice and avoid putting young athletes on a weight loss program.

What sport specific speed tests are recommended for young athletes in different team sports?

The tests listed below are valuable for the particular sport and provide baseline data for future comparison and improvement. The list does *not* include some key strength and power tests that are critical for older athletes and unsafe for young athletes.

Baseball, Softball	Crack of the bat to first base Crack of the bat to second Crack of the bat to third Base stealing: First to second base, Second to third base during a game
Basketball:	First 3-step test and a speed endurance test--5 repeated 20 yard dashes at 15 second intervals
Football,	First 3-step test, 10, 20, 40, 80, 120 yard dash (all in one sprint). Speed endurance (5 repeated 20-40 yard sprints at 25-30 second intervals)
Soccer, Lacrosse, Field Hockey Rugby	First 3-step test from a standing position and a jog, 10 and 20 yard sprint test, speed endurance (five 20-yard dashes at 15 second intervals), 1 1/2 mile run
Tennis	First 3-step test, speed endurance, five 10-yard sprints (each timed separately with no rest between any of the runs).

FOUNDATION TRAINING

Flexibility and Stretching

The stretching, flexibility, warm-up, cool-down, and core training, programs presented in Chapter 7 (Foundation Training) are safe and recommended for preadolescent athletes.

Conditioning Potential

How do coaches identify a young athlete's conditioning potential?

Conditioning potential refers to an athlete's ability to handle vigorous, intense training in their sport. Observation suggests that hereditary plays a role in this process. Some young athletes handle periods of rigorous training with ease while others cannot seem to tolerate repeated high intensity exercise. The good news is that coaches have learned how to bring even the least tolerable athlete to peak levels of conditioning with various motivational techniques, variation of drills and workout schemes, and mental-emotional stimulation.

Core strength and speed

What is core strength and how is it developed in young athletes?

Core training is designed to centralize the strength, flexibility, power and coordination of the body in the hips and torso. This is the body's center of mass and the point of stability for performance in sports. A strong, stable core (abdominals, hips and torso) provides the base for the body to drive in all directions. Flexible hips and a strong torso are essential to generate the power needed to perform in most sports.

For young athletes, this is the ideal time to work on all aspects of core training to further develop this foundation that contributes so much to strength, power, speed, agility, and the performance of athletic skills. Training focuses on movement patterns and stability (ability to control movement and force, not generate force). The Core Program Progression described by Cook (2003) is excellent and can easily be adapted to young athletes.

Core Board Squat Program. Toe touch squat, squat reach, deep squat and slide board

Core Board Hurdle Step. Double-leg stretch, slow motion mountain climber, dynamic lunge

Core Board Lunge Progression. Stride and twist, dynamic lunge

Core Board Straight Leg Raise Program. Single leg bridge, dip bridge, straight leg raise

Core training programs involving a wide variety of exercises and movements without the use of the core board are also effective.

Approximate Ambidexterity

The early years prior to adolescence are ideal for young athletes to develop near equal skill in their sport using both the dominant and recessive or non-dominant side. The program discussed in Chapter 7, Foundation Training, should be a regular part of youth training programs in all sports.

POWER OUTPUT TRAINING (SPEED STRENGTH)

Young Athletes and weight training

Are weight training workouts safe for young athletes?

Properly conducted strength training programs can be both safe and effective for young athletes. In fact, studies indicate that supervised programs result in a lower incidence of injury than other activities for young athletes. The additional strength acquired also provides protection from common musculoskeletal injuries that occur in power sports such as baseball, basketball, field hockey, football, gymnastics, soccer, and track and field.

Strength training programs for young athletes begin using only the body weight and slowly progress to conventional weight lifting that involves a variety of exercises, a high number of repetitions, and light to moderate weight. The main emphasis is placed on skill improvement, experiencing success, and enjoyment. The "no pain, no gain," high intensity approach has no place in this age group. Rather than focusing on the amount of weight a youngster can lift, emphasis is placed on mastering proper form and technique in each exercise. The purpose is to make certain each athlete experiences success, enjoys each workout, and develops enough interest in strength training to make it a lifetime activity.

Parents can help by providing a health history of preexisting injuries and ailments to the instructor and scheduling a meeting to discuss the basic approach to make certain that a safe, sound program philosophy is in place. Modern day strength coaches and physical educators are very well trained and will welcome your interest in their program.

Is weight training really necessary for young athletes?

Studies clearly show that elementary school-age children are extremely weak in the upper body and the abdominal area. A survey of 18,857 public school students at 187 schools revealed that 40 percent of boys, ages 6-12 and 70 percent of girls in that age group could not do more than one pull-up, and 45 percent of boys ages 6-14 and 55 percent of girls in that age group could not hold their chins over a raised bar for more than 10 seconds. These findings are "very poor" compared to children in other countries.

The *Power Lifting Federation* suggests young people begin weight training at around age 14 for males, slightly younger for females. Since every child is different, age is not a solid guide for determining physical and mental readiness. Parents should consult their physical education instructor, a professional trainer, or a physician for help in determining the physical maturity level and readiness for weight training. Preadolescent children who have not reached the age of puberty and show no signs of developmental changes will benefit less from weight training and could injure joints and soft tissue. A calisthenic program that uses one's own body weight will strengthen the upper body (shoulders, arms, and stomach) of these young athletes.

For early adolescents or those 14 years of age and older, *the American Society for Sports Medicine, the American Academy of Pediatrics, the Society of Pediatric Orthopedics, the National Athletic Trainer's Association, the U.S. Olympic Committee and the President's Council on Fitness and Sports* all support a safe, modified weight training program that is carefully supervised, involves 2-3 workouts weekly for no more than 30 minutes, uses a high number of repetitions (12-15), low to moderate weight, 8-10 exercises that are carried through the full range of motion, and slow progression by adding 1-2 pounds of weight to each exercise when 3 sets of 10-15 repetitions can be completed.

How much weight should a young athlete lift?

As soon as they enter the weight room, some young athletes have a keen interest in trying to lift as much weight as possible. Clearly, such attempts by prepubescent boys and girls can result in serious injury. Even with careful supervision, maximum effort lifting is strongly discouraged for this age group. There is no need to administer a 1RM test to begin an exercise program. For this age group, the task is to safely choose a starting weight that requires no more than 65 percent of their maximum for each exercise. In addition to the method described previously that used the 6RM to estimate the maximum weight one can lift in a leg strength test, coaches can also safely estimate the 1RM for any exercise by finding the number of repetitions it takes to reach muscle failure, then referring to table 13.1. If a program suggests 14-17 repetitions for a specific exercise, for example, this requires a starting weight that permits 14 repetitions before reaching muscle failure. Table 13.1 indicates that this is a the safe starting level requiring about 60% of the 1RM.

There is so much misinformation on weight training. What is myth and what is fact?

The NASE Weight Training Myth and Fact Sheet below dispels ten of the common myths about weight training.

Table 13.1 **Estimating the 1RM**

Repetitions	Approximate percent of 1RM (maximum weight that can be lifted one time)
1	100% of RM
2-3	95%
4-5	90%
6-7	85%
8-0	80%
10-13	70%
14-17	60%
18-21	50%

NASE MYTH AND FACT SHEET: WEIGHT TRAINING

Myth # 1 *Young children do not need strength training.*

Fact For over 50 years, test results of children in the U S have revealed poor upper body (arm and shoulder) and abdominal strength; considerably worse than European children. Strength in these areas is critical to adequate performance of daily chores, performance in a wide variety of physical education activities and sports, and in the prevention of soft tissue injuries. Widespread use of weight training and other strength training programs in physical education, recreation, and home fitness programs can easily eliminate the problem.

Myth # 2 *Strength training will stunt growth in children.*

Fact Properly supervised strength exercises do not place excessive pressure on the growth plates of children. In fact, such training favorably affects growth both during the preadolescent and the adolescent period.

Myth # 3 *Strength training is not safe for children.*

Fact Properly supervised programs provide an atmosphere every bit as safe as other activities engaged in by children.

Myth # 4 *Young children do not like strength training.*

Fact One of the problems with this type of training is that young children like it too much and, if left unsupervised, will engage in "horse play" and attempts to lift as much weight as possible. With sound leadership, this motivation can be channeled into very positive results.

Myth # 5 *Strength cannot be increased in young athletes.*

Fact Strength gains do occur in young male and female athletes who engage in weight training.

Myth #6 *Strength training is suitable for young athletes and not other children.*

Fact Strength training is suitable for everyone and all young boys and girls can receive the benefits discussed in this section.

Myth #7 *Strength training will make you inflexible.*

Fact Strength training actually improves flexibility providing athletes go through the full range of motion on each exercise and stretch before and after each workout.

Myth #8 *Strength training will convert fat to muscle.*

Fact Fat and muscle are separate tissue types. One cannot be converted to the other. When more calories are expended that consumed, fat cells shrink. Strength training does burn calories and contribute to this process.

Myth # 9 *Strength training has few health benefits.*

Fact Strength training adds muscle mass, increases resting metabolism, and is a key factor in maintaining muscle mass and controlling body weight. The *American Heart Association* indicates that it improves heart and liver function, reduces coronary disease risk factors and enhances glucose metabolism. Studies also show that strength training improves bone mineral density and decreases the risk of osteoporosis. All this in addition to increased strength and endurance, less lower back pain, improved appearance, body image and self concept.

Myth #10 *Older men and women should not use weight training.*

Fact Older coaches and parents of coaches, ages 50-90, need weight training to prevent loss of muscle mass, prevent the slowing of metabolism, to increase strength and endurance, to maintain independence, to complete daily chores, and to enjoy life.
Although the skeletal muscles of the elderly respond more slowly to strength training, muscle mass can be maintained and even increased

at any age. Without a strength training program, muscle atrophy occurs along with loss of strength and endurance and gains in body fat and weight.

PLYOMETRIC TRAINING

Should preadolescent athletes engage in plyometric training?

The plyometric exercise program described in Part III, Chapter 8 is NOT recommended for preadolescent athletes although some age group coaches have successfully used a well controlled, modified program. If a modified program is used, the following restrictions must be applied:

- The total number of jumps, hops and bounds must be limited to no more than 50 each workout with the emphasis on quality, not quantity.
- No more than two 15-minute sessions should be used weekly.
- At the first sign of shin pain, ankle, knee, or low back pain, the program should be discontinued.
- Proper footwear with good ankle and arch support and a non-slip sole (basketball or aerobic shoe) should be enforced.
- The workout must take place on soft, grass areas, padded artificial turf, or wrestling mats; never on asphalt or gymnasium floors.
- A general warm-up and stretching program is required before each plyometric workout.
- All depth jumping from boxes or benches should be avoided.
- Only low intensity and medium intensity jumps (beginning program) should be used.

Low Intensity Jumps

Squat Jump--From an upright position, hands behind the neck, drop downward to a one-half squat position before exploding upward as high as possible. Land and immediately explode upward again.

Split Squat Jump--Same as above except landing occurs with one leg extended forward and the other behind the center of the body (lunge position).

Double-leg Ankle Bounce--With arms extended to the sides, jump upward and forward using the ankles. Execute the next jump upon landing.

Lateral Cone or Bench Jump--Stand to one side of a cone or bench, jump laterally to the other side, jumping back to the starting position immediately upon landing.

Medium Intensity Jumps

Pike Jump--Begin in an upright position with both arms to the side, feet shoulder-width apart. Complete a vertical jump and bring both fully extended legs in front of the body and reach out with both hands to touch the toes (pike position). Go into the next jump immediately upon landing.

Double-Leg Tuck Jump--From the starting position described above, complete a vertical jump and grasp the knees while in the air, releasing the grasp before landing and immediately going into the next jump.

Standing Jumps: Standing Triple Jump--From the standing broad jump position, use a two-foot takeoff to jump forward as far as possible, landing on the right foot; then immediately jump forward and land on the left foot. Finish with one last jump off the left foot landing on both feet. This is identical to the triple jump in track except for the use of a two-foot takeoff.

Standing Jumps: Standing Long Jump--Use the initial jump described above with maximum arm swing, exploding into the next repetition upon landing.

Standing Jumps: Single-Leg Hop--From a standing broad jump position with one leg slightly forward, rock to the front foot and jump as far and high as possible driving the lead knee up and out. Land in the starting position on the same foot and continue jumping for the number of repetitions specified.

Double-leg Bound--From the standing broad jump position, thrust both arms forward as the knees and body straighten and the arms reach for the sky.

Double-and-Single-leg Zigzag Hop--Place ten cones 20 inches apart in a zigzag pattern. Jump with the legs together in a forward diagonal direction over the first cone keeping the shoulders facing straight ahead. Immediately upon landing, change direction to move diagonally over the second cone, continuing over 10 cones. Repeat using one leg at a time.

Alternate Leg Bound--Stand upright with one foot slightly ahead of the other. Push-off with the back leg as you drive the lead knee up to the chest and try to attain as much height and distance as possible. Continue immediately by repeating this action with the other leg.

Running Bound--Run forward and jump as high as possible on each step, emphasizing height and high knee lift.

SUSTAINED POWER OUTPUT (Speed Endurance Training)

Should preadolescent athletes in team sports engage in speed endurance training?

To compete in any sport, preadolescent athletes must be capable of making repeated sprints in their sport with little slowing due to fatigue. At times, an athlete may also need to sprint 60 - 80 yards with minimum slowing the final 20 yards or so. This requires an adequate level of speed endurance (anaerobic fitness). The speed endurance training programs presented in Chapter 9 can be adapted and safely used for young athletes.

The object is not to push young athletes to complete exhaustion, but to progressively increase the number of short sprints they can complete each workout over a period of 6-8 weeks.

NEUROMUSCULAR TRAINING

Should preadolescent athletes use neuromuscular training?

Training the nervous system is critical for athletes of all ages. These exercises expose both the nervous and muscular systems to higher muscle contraction rates.

With proper supervision, young athletes can safely choose from four basic methods discussed in Chapter 10. The recommended choices for this age group include carefully supervised towing with surgical tubing, towing with the Ultra Speed Pacer, downhill sprinting and high speed stationary cycling. Two short 15-20 minute workouts weekly are recommended with strict supervision

SPRINTING FORM AND TECHNIQUE

The proper techniques of starting, accelerating and sprinting presented in Chapters 3 and 4 apply to athletes of all ages. Young athletes should also follow the form and technique training program described in Chapter 11.

What is the best time for athletes to master proper starting and sprinting form for their sport?

The preschool and early elementary school years are the most favorable for learning correct sprinting form. After age 7 or 8 children have lost a unique opportunity to learn to sprint correctly. Although you can "teach an old dog new tricks," it is much more difficult to eliminate faulty form after bad habits have been used for so many years. The preadolescent and early adolescent period is an ideal time to develop proper form and correct form errors that will hinder speed in the future.

BIBLIOGRAPHY

Suggested Reading and Viewing

Allerheligen, W.B. 1994. Speed development and plyometric training. In T.R. Baechle (Ed). *Essentials of Strength Training and Conditioning* (314-344). Champaign, IL: Human Kinetics.

Alter, Michael J. 1998. *Sport Stretch.* Champaign, IL.: Human Kinetics.

Baechle, T., Ed. 1994. *Essentials of Strength Training and Conditioning.* Champaign, IL.: Human Kinetics.

Baker, D. 1995. Selecting the appropriate exercises and loads for speed-strength development. *Strength and Conditioning Coach* 3 (2: 8-16).

Bell, Sam. 2000. Drills which lead to better sprint performance. In *Sprint and Relays: Contemporary Theory, Technique and Training.* 5th Ed., Mt. View, CA: Tafnews Press, p-91.

Benardot, Dan. 2006, *Advanced Sports Nutrition.* Champaign, IL: Human Kinetics.

Berkun, Scott. 2005. *The Art of Project Management.* Sebastopol, CA: O'Reilly Media, Inc.

Bivens, S., & Leonard II, W. M. 1994. Race, centrality, and educational attainment: An NFL perspective. *Journal of Sport Behavior 17,* 1-8.

Bompa, Tudor O. 1999. *Periodization Training for Sports.* Champaign, IL: Human Kinetics

Bompa, Tudor, and Cornacchia, Lorenzo. 1999. *Serious Strength Training: Periodization for Building Muscle Power and Mass* . Champaign, IL.: Human Kinetics.

Bondarchuk, Anatoliy. 2007. Transfer of Training Michigan, USA. *Ultimate Athlete Concepts.*

Bosco, C., H. Rosko, and J. Hirvonem. 1986. The effects of extra-load conditioning on muscle performance in athletes. *Medicine and Science in Sport and Exercis*e 18(4):415-419.

Bosch, Frans., and Klomp, Ronald. 2005. *Running: Biomechanics and Exercise Physiology in Practice.* London: Elsevier Churchill Livingstone.

Bosco, Carmelo. 1999. *Strength Assessment with Bosco's Test.* Italian Society of Sport Science, Rome.

Bosen, K.O. 1979. Spring. Experimental speed training. *Track Technique*, 2382-2383.

Brenner, Joel S. 2007. Council on Sports Medicine and Fitness. Overuse injuries, over training, and burnout in child and adolescent athletes. *Pediatrics 2007;119; 1242-1.*

Brown, Lee E., and Ferrigno, Vance A., Editors, 2005. *Training for Speed, Agility and Quickness: 195 Drills* Champaign, IL: Human Kinetics.

Brown, Lee E., 2007. *Strength Training.* Champaign, IL: Human Kinetics.

Bruggemann, G.P. Koszewski, D. & Muller, H. 1999. *Biomechanical Research Project Athens 1997: Final Report,* International Athletics Foundation. Meyer & Meyer Sport, Oxford, UK

Calais-Germain, Blanche. 1993. *Anatomy of Movement (Revised Edition)* Seattle, Washington: Eastland Press.

Chu, Donald A. 1998. *Jumping Into Plyometrics.* Champaign, IL: Human Kinetics.

Chu, Donald A., 1999. *Explosive Power and Strength.* Champaign, Ill.: Human Kinetics

Chumanov, E.S, BC Heiderscheit, & D.G. Thelen (2007). The effect of speed and influence of individual muscles on hamstring mechanisms during the swing phase of sprinting. *Journal of Biomechanic*s 40 3555-3562.

Coh, M. and K Tomazin (2005). Biomechanical characteristics of female sprinters during the acceleration phase and manual speed phase. *Modern Athlete and Coach.* 43(4), 3-9.

Coleman, Gene, et. al. 2004. Changes in running speed in game situations during a season of major league baseball. An International Electronic Journal, Volume 7 Number 3 June, *Sports Physiology.*

Colvin, Geoff. 2009. *Talent Is Overrated: What Really Separates World-Class Performers from Everybody Else* New York. New York. Bantam Publishing.

Cook, Gary. 2003. *Athletic Body in Balance*. Champaign, IL: Human Kinetics.

Cometti, Gilles. 1988. ***La Pliometrie***. Universite De Bourgogne.

Costill, D. L., J. Daniels, W. Evans, and W. Fink, G. Krahenbuhl, and B. Salin (1976) Skeletal muscle enzymes and fiber comparisons in male and female track athletes. *Journal of Applied Physiology*. 40, 149-154.

Counsilman, J.H. and B.E. Counsilman. 1994. *The New Science of Swimming*. 2nd ed. Englewood Cliffs, NJ: Prentice-Hall.

Coyle, Daniel. 2009. *The Talent Code: Greatness Isn't Born. It's Grown. Here's How.* New York. New York: Penguin Group.

Cunningham, M. Pure speed training. *Coaches review.* 72(2), 26-28.

Curwin, Sandra. & Stanish, William D. M.D. and Mandel, Scott. 2000. *Tendinitis: Etiology and Treatment,* New New York, New York: Oxford University Press.

Davids, Keith, Button, Chris, Bennett, Simon. 2008. *Dynamics of Skill Acquisition: A Constraints-Led Approach.* Champaign, Illinois: Human Kinetics.

Delecluse, C., 1997. Influence of strength training on sprint running performance: Current findings and implications for training. *Sports Medicine* 24(3): 147-156.

Delecluse, C., Van Coppenolle H., Goris M., Diels, R. 1990. Analysis of the front and rear foot action in the sprint start. In Bruggemann, G.P., and Ruhl, J.K. (Eds) *Techniques in Athletics Conference Proceedings* Volume 2, pp. 402-406.

Dintiman, George B. 1964. The effects of various training programs on running speed. *Research Quarterly* 35: 456-63.

______. 1966. The relationship between the leg strength/body weight ratio and running speed. The *Bulletin of the Connecticut Association for Health, Physical Education, and Recreation* 11:5.

______. 1970. *Sprinting Speed: Its Improvement for Major Sports Competition.* Springfield, Illinois: Charles C. Thomas, Publishers.

______. 1974. *What Research Tells the Coach about Sprinting.* AAHPERD.

______. 1976. *How to Run Faster.* Richmond, VA: Champion Athlete Publishing Co.

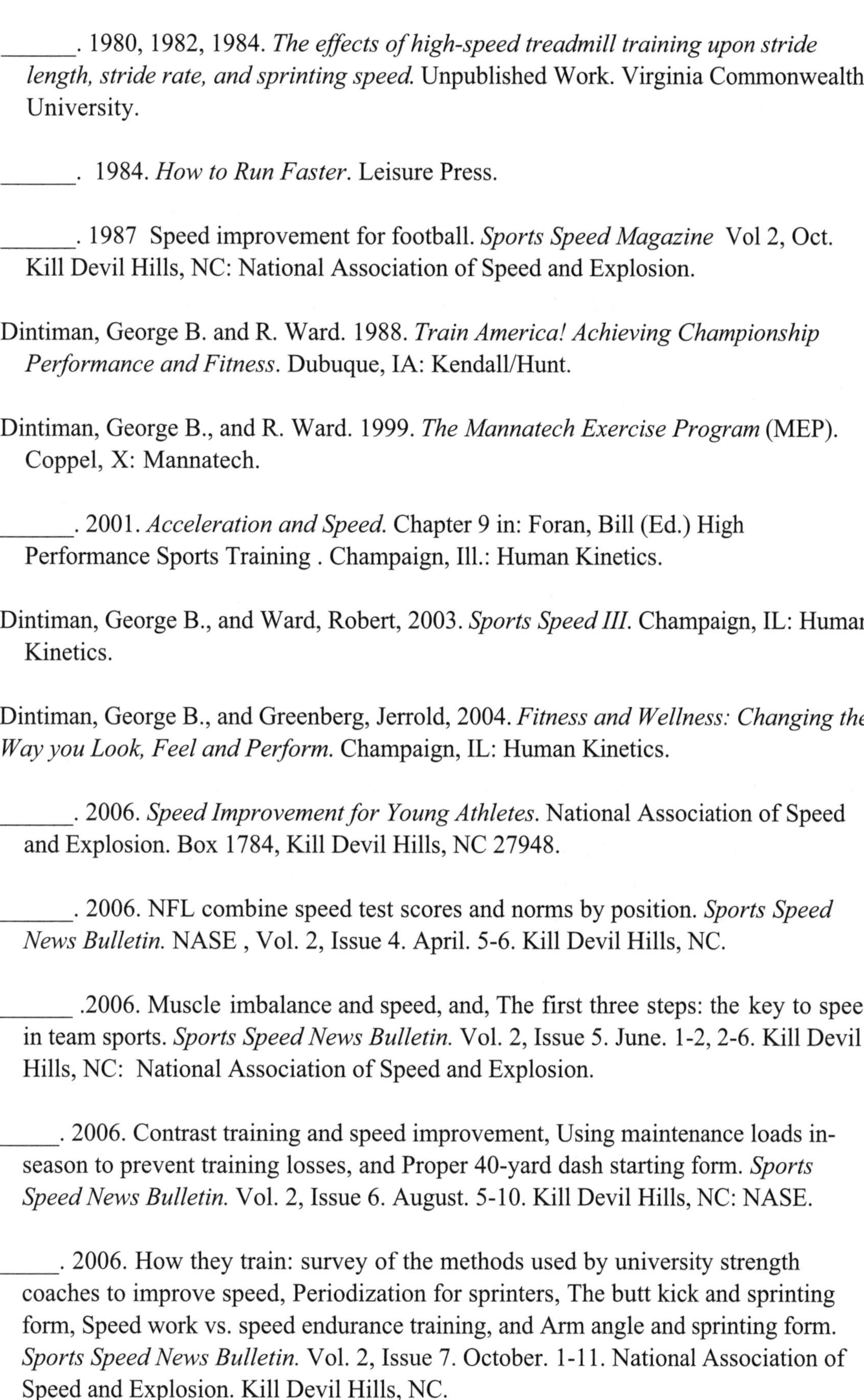

______. 1980, 1982, 1984. *The effects of high-speed treadmill training upon stride length, stride rate, and sprinting speed.* Unpublished Work. Virginia Commonwealth University.

______. 1984. *How to Run Faster*. Leisure Press.

______. 1987 Speed improvement for football. *Sports Speed Magazine* Vol 2, Oct. Kill Devil Hills, NC: National Association of Speed and Explosion.

Dintiman, George B. and R. Ward. 1988. *Train America! Achieving Championship Performance and Fitness*. Dubuque, IA: Kendall/Hunt.

Dintiman, George B., and R. Ward. 1999. *The Mannatech Exercise Program* (MEP). Coppel, X: Mannatech.

______. 2001. *Acceleration and Speed.* Chapter 9 in: Foran, Bill (Ed.) High Performance Sports Training . Champaign, Ill.: Human Kinetics.

Dintiman, George B., and Ward, Robert, 2003. *Sports Speed III.* Champaign, IL: Human Kinetics.

Dintiman, George B., and Greenberg, Jerrold, 2004. *Fitness and Wellness: Changing the Way you Look, Feel and Perform.* Champaign, IL: Human Kinetics.

______. 2006. *Speed Improvement for Young Athletes.* National Association of Speed and Explosion. Box 1784, Kill Devil Hills, NC 27948.

______. 2006. NFL combine speed test scores and norms by position. *Sports Speed News Bulletin.* NASE , Vol. 2, Issue 4. April. 5-6. Kill Devil Hills, NC.

______ .2006. Muscle imbalance and speed, and, The first three steps: the key to speed in team sports. *Sports Speed News Bulletin.* Vol. 2, Issue 5. June. 1-2, 2-6. Kill Devil Hills, NC: National Association of Speed and Explosion.

_____. 2006. Contrast training and speed improvement, Using maintenance loads in-season to prevent training losses, and Proper 40-yard dash starting form. *Sports Speed News Bulletin.* Vol. 2, Issue 6. August. 5-10. Kill Devil Hills, NC: NASE.

_____. 2006. How they train: survey of the methods used by university strength coaches to improve speed, Periodization for sprinters, The butt kick and sprinting form, Speed work vs. speed endurance training, and Arm angle and sprinting form. *Sports Speed News Bulletin.* Vol. 2, Issue 7. October. 1-11. National Association of Speed and Explosion. Kill Devil Hills, NC.

_____. 2007. When to start your child in sports, The effectiveness of drills as a speed improvement technique. *Sports Speed News Bulletin.* Vol. 3, Issue 8. January. 3, 8-9. National Association of Speed and Explosion. Kill Devil Hills, NC.

_____. 2007. Comparative speed of humans and animals, How they train - Bill Bates in 1986. *Sports Speed News Bulletin.* Vol. 3, Issue 9. March. 3, 9. National Association of Speed and Explosion. Kill Devil Hills, NC.

_____. 2007. Understanding fast and slow twitch fiber, Developing faking and cutting skills in running backs, How they train: Speed training concepts at the University of Massachusetts. *Sports Speed News Bulletin.* Vol. 3, Issue 10. May. 1-4, 7-9. National Association of Speed and Explosion. Kill Devil Hills, NC.

_____. 2007. Off-season speed improvement for football, basketball, baseball and soccer. *Sports Speed News Bulletin.* Vol. 3, Issue 11. July. 9-11. National Association of Speed and Explosion. Kill Devil Hills, NC.

_____. 2007. Realistic speed training for young athletes. *Sports Speed News Bulletin.* Vol. 3, Issue 13. November. 11. National Association of Speed and Explosion. Kill Devil Hills, NC.

_____. 2008. Baseball and speed, Ground contact forces and speed, Core strength and speed, Verbal cues and speed. *Sports Speed News Bulletin.* Vol. 4, Issue 14. January. 1-8. National Association of Speed and Explosion. Kill Devil Hills, NC.

_____. 2008. Sprint-strength training, Form and technique: foot placement. *Sports Speed News Bulletin.* Vol. 4, Issue 15. March. 4-6. National Association of Speed and Explosion. Kill Devil Hills, NC.

_____. 2008. All the right moves: agility training and speed, Stride rate and stride length. *Sports Speed News Bulletin.* Vol. 4, Issue, 16. May. 1-6. National Association of Speed and Explosion. Kill Devil Hills, NC.

_____. 2008. Improving playing speed: What we know and don't know, Crack of the bat to first, Warm-up to speed up. *Sports Speed News Bulletin.* Vol. 4, Issue 17. July 1-11. National Association of Speed and Explosion. Kill Devil Hills, NC.

_____. 2008. Sprint supremacy and the USA, Lactic acid and sprinting in team sports, Verbal cues and sprinting form, and Metabolic syndrome and retired NFL linemen. *Sports Speed News Bulletin.* Vol. 4, Issue 18. September. 1-11. National Association of Speed and Explosion. Kill Devil Hills, NC.

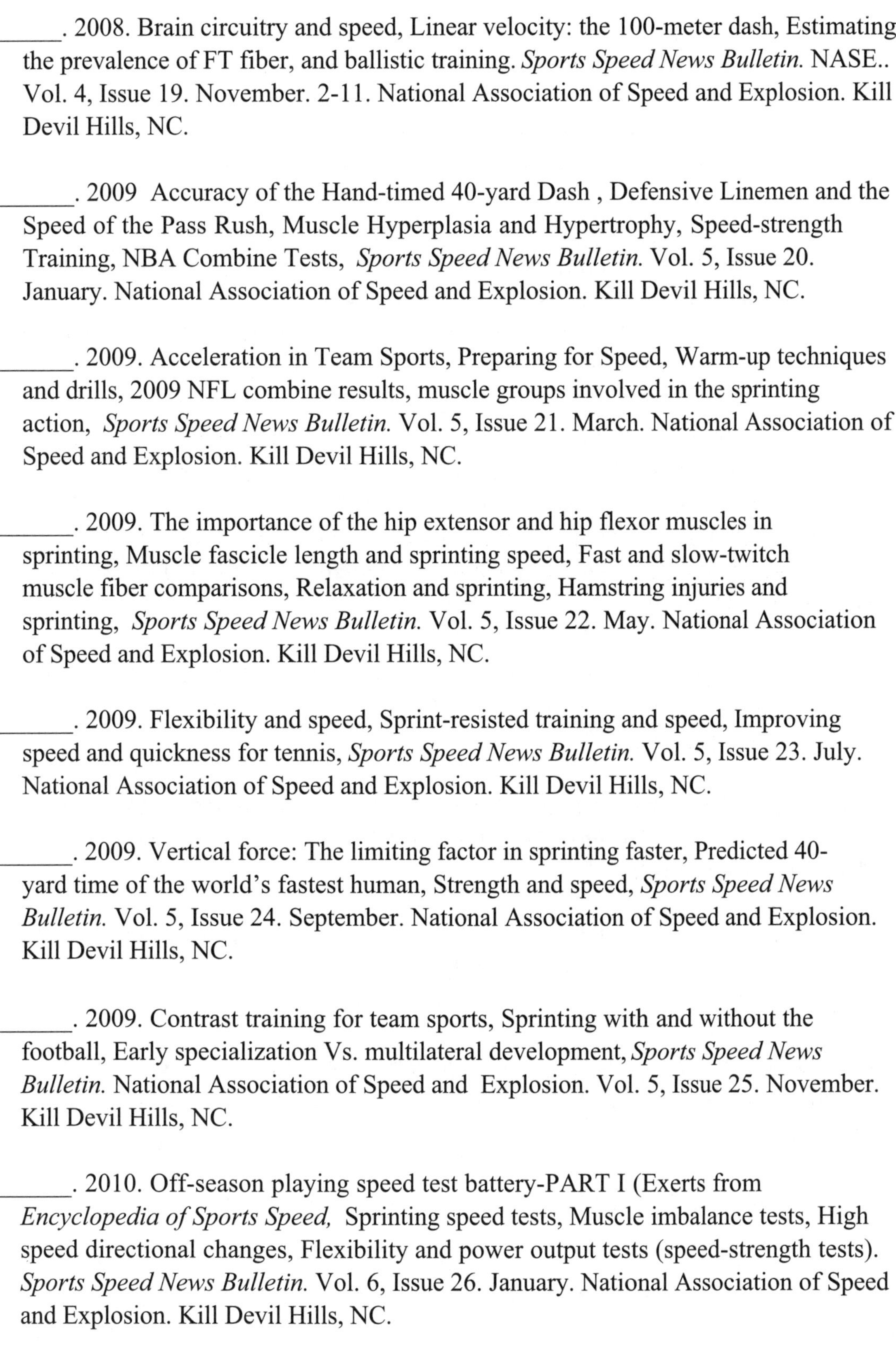

_____. 2008. Brain circuitry and speed, Linear velocity: the 100-meter dash, Estimating the prevalence of FT fiber, and ballistic training. *Sports Speed News Bulletin.* NASE.. Vol. 4, Issue 19. November. 2-11. National Association of Speed and Explosion. Kill Devil Hills, NC.

______. 2009 Accuracy of the Hand-timed 40-yard Dash , Defensive Linemen and the Speed of the Pass Rush, Muscle Hyperplasia and Hypertrophy, Speed-strength Training, NBA Combine Tests, *Sports Speed News Bulletin.* Vol. 5, Issue 20. January. National Association of Speed and Explosion. Kill Devil Hills, NC.

______. 2009. Acceleration in Team Sports, Preparing for Speed, Warm-up techniques and drills, 2009 NFL combine results, muscle groups involved in the sprinting action, *Sports Speed News Bulletin.* Vol. 5, Issue 21. March. National Association of Speed and Explosion. Kill Devil Hills, NC.

______. 2009. The importance of the hip extensor and hip flexor muscles in sprinting, Muscle fascicle length and sprinting speed, Fast and slow-twitch muscle fiber comparisons, Relaxation and sprinting, Hamstring injuries and sprinting, *Sports Speed News Bulletin.* Vol. 5, Issue 22. May. National Association of Speed and Explosion. Kill Devil Hills, NC.

______. 2009. Flexibility and speed, Sprint-resisted training and speed, Improving speed and quickness for tennis, *Sports Speed News Bulletin.* Vol. 5, Issue 23. July. National Association of Speed and Explosion. Kill Devil Hills, NC.

______. 2009. Vertical force: The limiting factor in sprinting faster, Predicted 40-yard time of the world's fastest human, Strength and speed, *Sports Speed News Bulletin.* Vol. 5, Issue 24. September. National Association of Speed and Explosion. Kill Devil Hills, NC.

______. 2009. Contrast training for team sports, Sprinting with and without the football, Early specialization Vs. multilateral development, *Sports Speed News Bulletin.* National Association of Speed and Explosion. Vol. 5, Issue 25. November. Kill Devil Hills, NC.

______. 2010. Off-season playing speed test battery-PART I (Exerts from *Encyclopedia of Sports Speed,* Sprinting speed tests, Muscle imbalance tests, High speed directional changes, Flexibility and power output tests (speed-strength tests). *Sports Speed News Bulletin.* Vol. 6, Issue 26. January. National Association of Speed and Explosion. Kill Devil Hills, NC.

______. 2010. Off-season playing speed test battery-PART II: (Exerts from *Encyclopedia of Sports Speed*, Sustained power output test (speed endurance), aerobic fitness, quickness tests, muscle imbalance tests, flexibility tests, body composition, strength curve testing, On-field analysis. *Sports Speed News Bulletin.* National Association of Speed and Explosion. Vol. 6, Issue 27. March. Kill Devil Hills, NC.

______. 2010. The 100-meter dash: summary training recommendations from start ` to finish, Horizontal speed at touchdown during the sprinting action, Eye focus and performance, What Research Tells the Coach About Sprinting: Biological limits to running speed, *Sports Speed News Bulletin.* NASE.. Vol. 6, Issue 28. May.

______. 2010. The NFL combine: do test results predict success in the NFL, Foot spacing for the 40-yard dash, Body temperature during and after exercise in hot weather, What research tells the coach about sprinting,: Effects of resisted training, Does stretching improve sprinting speed? *Sports Speed News Bulletin.* NASE.. Vol. 6, Issue 29. July. National Association of Speed and Explosion. Kill Devil Hills, NC.

Dowson M. N., Nevill M. E., Lakomy H. K., Nevill A. M. and Hazeldine R. J. 1998. Modeling the relationship between isokinetic muscle strength and sprint running performance. *J Sports Sci* 16: 257-265.

Drabik, Jo'zef. 1996. *Children and Sports Training: How your Future Champions Should Exercise to Be Healthy, Fit and Happy*, Island Pond, Vermont: Stadion Publishing Company, Inc.

Ebbehow, N.E., F.R. Hansen, M.S. Harreby, and C.F. Lassen. 2002. Low back pain in children and adolescents: prevalence, risk factors and prevention. Ugeskr *Lfaeger* 164(6): 755-758.

Ebben. W.P., J.A. Davis, and R.W. Clewien. 2008. Effect of the degree of hill slope on acute downhill running velocity and acceleration. *Journal of Strength and Conditioning.* 22(3), 898-902.

Emmna, Thomas, 2007. *Peak Conditioning for Young Athletes* Monterey, CA: Coaches Choice Publishers.

Enoka, Roger M. 2008. *Neuromechanics of Human Movement.* 4th Edition Champaign, Illinois: Human Kinetics.

Faigenbaum, Avery and Westcott, Wayne. 2000. *Strength and Power for Young Athletes.* Champaign, IL: Human Kinetics

Farrey, Tom. 2008. *Game On: The All-American Race to Make Champions of Our Children* New York: ESPN Books.

Figoni, S., C.B. Christ, and B.H. Mossey. 1988. Effects of speed, hip, knee angle, and gravity on hamstring to quadriceps torque ratios. *Journal of Orthopedics Sports and Physical Therapy* 9(8):287-291.

Foran, Bill (Ed.). 2001. *High Performance Sports Training* . Champaign, Ill.: HKP.

Frederick, E.C., Hagy, J.L. 1986. Factors affecting peak vertical ground reaction forces in running. *International Journal of Sport Biomechanics*, **2**, 41-49.

Gabbard, Carl. Leblanc, Elizabeth., and Lowy, Susan. 1987. *Physical Education for Children: Building the Foundation.* Englewood Cliffs, New Jersey: Prentice-Hall.

Gambetta, Vernon A. 2007. *Athletic Development.* Champaign, IL: Human Kinetics.

Gambetta, Vernon A. 2002. *The Gambetta Method (2nd edition): Common Sense Training for Athletic Performance.* Sarasota, FL: Gambetta Sports Training.

Garhammer, J. 1991. A comparison of maximal power output between elite male and female weight lifters in competition. *Interntl Journal of Sports Biomechanics* 7:3-11.

Gottschall, Jinger S., and Bradley M. Palmer. 2002. The acute effects of prior cycling cadence on running performance and kinematics. *The Locomotion Laboratory.* University of Colorado, Boulder, CO, USA.

Grace, T., E.R. Sweetser, M.A. Nelson, L.R. Ydens, and B.J. Skipper. 1984. Isokinetic muscle imbalance and knee joint injuries. *Journal of Bone and Joint Surgery* 66A:734.

Greenberg, Jerrold and Dintiman, George B.. 2009. *Managing Athletic Performance Stress: Getting the Mind Out of the Way.* Kill Devil Hills, NC: NASE.

Grimshaw, P.A., R. Tong, and K. Grimmer. 2002. Lower back and elbow injuries in Golf. *Sports Medicine.* 32(10):655-666.

Guskiewicz, K., Lephart, S., Burkholder, R. 1993). The relationship between sprint speed and hip flexion/extension strength in collegiate athletes. *Isokentics and Exercise Science* Vol. 4, No. 21993.

Gustavsen R, Streeck R: 1993. *Training Therapy: Prophylaxis and Rehabilitation (How It Works (Ziff-Davis/Que).* New York: Thieme Medical Publishers.

Guthrie, Mark, 2008, *Coaching Track and Field Successfully,* Champaign, IL: HKP.

Hannaford, Carla. 1995. *Smart Moves: Why Learning Is Not All in Your Head.* Great Ocean Publishers: Arlington, Virginia.

Hanson, Derek M., 2009. Where you look can affect how you look: running mechanics and gaze control. *Ausuts.*

Harre, Dietrich. 1992. *Principles of Sports Training: Introduction to the Theory and Methods of Training.* Berlin, GDR: Sportverlag.

Headly, D., 2000. Radar technology as a tool for the sprint coach. *Track Coach* Vol. 165, p.5257.

Herman, D. 1976. The effects of depth jumping on vertical jumping and sprinting speed. *Unpublished master's thesis.* Ithaca, NY: Ithaca College.

Hudson, A.J. 1968. The acute effects of prior cycling cadence on running performance. *Brain.* 91, 571-582.

Huxley, H.E. 2004. Fifty years of muscle and the sliding filament hypothesis. *European Journal of Biochemistry* 27(8):1403-1415.

Inglis, Robert, 2000. Training for acceleration in the 100m sprint. *Sprint and Relays: Contemporary Theory, Technique and Training.* 5th Ed., Mountain View, CA: Tafnews Press, pgs. 35-39.

Issurin, Vladimir. 2008. *Advanced Athletic Training.* Michigan, USA. Ultimate Athlete Concepts.

Issurin, Vladimir. 2008. *Block Periodization* Michigan, USA. Ultimate Athlete Concepts.

Jackson, K.M. 1979. Fitting of mathematical functions to biomechanical data. *Journal of Biomechanical Engineering,* 26, 122-124.

Jakalski, Ken, 2000. Parachutes, Tubing and Towing. *Sprint and Relays: Contemporary Theory, Technique and Training.* 5th Ed., Mountain View, CA: Tafnews Press, pgs. 95-100.

Kellman, Michael, Editor. 2002. *Enhancing Recovery: Preventing Under Performance in Athletes*. Champaign, Illinois: Human Kinetics.

Klinzing, J. 1984. Improving sprint speed for all athletes. *NSCA Journal* 6(4):32-33:

Komi, P. V. Editor (Second Edition). 2003. Strength and Power in Sport: Olympic Encyclopedia of Sports Medicine. *The Encyclopedia of Sports Medicine.* London: Blackwell Scientific Publications.

Korchemny, R. 1985. Evaluation of sprinters. *NSCA Journal* 7(4):38-42.

Kozlov, V. Muravyev, 1992. Muscles and the Sprint. *Fitness and Sports review International* (Vol. 27, #8, 192-195.

Kraemer, W.J., N.A. Ratamess. 2005. Hormonal responses and adaptations to resistance exercise and training. *Sports Medicine* 35:336-361.

Kraemer, William, and Fleck, Steven, 1993. *Strength Training for Young Athletes* Champaign, Ill.: Human Kinetics.

Kraemer, William J. and Hakkinen, Keijo. Editors. 2002. *Strength Training for Sport.* London, England: Blackwell Science, Ltd.

Kreighbaum, Ellen and Barthels, Katharine M. 1996. *Biomechanics: A Qualitative Approach for Studying Human Movement.* Fourth edition. Boston, Allyn and Bacon.

Kumagai, Kenya, Abe Takashi, William F. Brechue, Tomoo Ryushi, Susumu Takano, and Masuhiko Mizuno. 2000. Sprint performance is related to muscle fascicle length in male 100-m sprinters. *Appl Physiol* 88, 811-816.

Kurz, Thomas., 2001. *Science of Sports Training: How to Plan and Control Training for Peak Performance.* Island Pont, Vt: Stadion Publishing Company.

Laird, D.E. 1981. Comparison of quadriceps to hamstring strength ratios of an intercollegiate soccer team. *Athletic Training* 16:666-667: 1981.

Leierer, S. 1979. A guide for sprint training. *Athletic Journal* June, 105-106.

Lopez, Victor, 2000. An approach to strength training for sprinters. *Sprint and Relays: Contemporary Theory, Technique and Training.* 5th Ed., Mountain View, CA: Tafnews Press, pgs. 58-63.

Luhtanen, P., and P.V. Komi. Mechanical factors influencing running speed. In *Biomechanics* VI-B, 23-29: 1978, edited by E. Asmussen and E. Jorgensen. Baltimore: University Park Press.

Mach, Gerard. 1980. *Sprints & Hurdles.* Canadian Track & Field Association, Ontario.

Majdell, R., & Alexander, M.J.L. 1991. The effect of overspeed training on kinematic variables in sprinting. *Journal of Human Movement Studies* **21**, 19-39.

Mann, Ralph, 2007. *The Mechanics of Sprinting and Hurdling.* Dr. Ralph Mann 3622 Famiglia Drive, Las vegas, NV 89141.

Mann, R. Speed development. 1984. *NSCA Journal* 5(6):12-20, 72-73:

Markovic, G., Jukic,I., Milanovic, D. and Metikos, D. 2007. Effects of sprint and plyometric training on muscle function and athletic performance. *Journal of Strength and Conditioning Research* 21, 543 – 549.

Marlow, Bill. 1966. *Sprinting and relay racing.* British Amateur Athletic Board. 70 Brompton Road, London, SW3 1EE).

McFarlane, B. 1985. Developing maximal running speed. *Track and Field Quarterly Review* 83(2), 4-9.

McKensie, Robin, 2006. *Treat Your Lower Back.* Lower Hutt, New Zealand: Spinal Publications Ltd.

Mero, A., & Komi, P.V. 1985. Effects of supra maximal velocity on biomechanics variables in sprinting. *International Journal of Sport Biomechanics,* **1**, 240-252.

Mero, A., Komi, P.V, Rusko, H., & Hirvonen, J. 1987. Neuromuscular and anaerobic performance of sprinters at maximal and supra maximal speed. *International Journal of Sport Biomechanics* 8, 55-60.

Mero, A., Komi, P.V., & Gregor, R.J. 1992. Biomechanics of sprint running: a review. *Sports Medicine.* 13, 376-392.

Mero, A. 1988. Acceleration in the sprint start. *Track Technique* No 105, pg. 3359-3360.

Moore, J., and G. Wade. 1989. Prevention of anterior cruciate ligament injuries. *NSCA Journal* 11(3):35-40.

Moyer-Mileur, LJ, 2003. *Human Growth Assessment and Interpretation*, edited by Roche, Alex F. Roche and and Shumel Sun, Cambridge University Press.

Mujika, Inigo. 2009. *Tapering and Peaking for Optimal Performance* Champaign, Illinois: Human Kinetics.

National Association of Speed and Explosion, 2008. NASE *National Conference on Improving Playing Speed for Sports Competition.* 4 DVDs. NASE, Box 1784, Kill Devil Hills, NC 27948.

Newton, Robert U. 1997. *Expression and Development of Maximal Muscle Power.* Doctoral Dissertation, Southern Cross University.

Noakes, Tim, MD. 2003. *Lore of Running.* Fourth Edition. Champaign, Illinois: Human Kinetics.

Novacheck TF. 1998. The biomechanics of running. *Gait Posture* 7: 77-95.

Olbrecht, Jan. 2000. *The Science of Winning: Planning, Periodizing and Optimizing Swim Training.* Swim Shop, Luton, England.

Parker, M.G., D. Holt, E. Bauman, M. Drayna, and R.O. Ruhling. 1982. Descriptive analysis of bilateral quadriceps and hamstring muscle torque in high school football players. *Medicine and Science in Sports and Exercise* 14:152.

Pauletto, B. Let's talk training: periodization-peaking. *NSCA Journal* 8(4):30-31: 1986.

Payne, Gregory V., and Larry Isaacs, (2007) *Human Motor Development: A Lifespan Approach.* 7th edition. McGraw-Hill Publishing Co.

Peterson, M.D., M.R. Rhea, and B.A. Alvar. 2004. Maximizing strength development in athletes: a meta-analysis to determine the dose-response relationship. *Journal of Strength and Conditioning Research* 18(2):377-382.

Plagenhoef, S., Evans, F.G., & Abdelnour, T. 1983. Anatomical data for analyzing human motion. *Research Quarterly for Exercise and Sport* 54, 169-178.

Plagenhoef, S. and L. McBryde. 1994. Application of anatomical strength curves to function and rehabilitation. *Southwest Ergonomic Systems.*

Platonov, Vladimir N. and Bulatova, Marina M. *Preparacion Fisica (Coleccion: DePorte y Entrenamiento) (Spanish Edition)* 2006. Fourth Edition. Barcelona, Spain. Editorial Paidotribo.

Prampero, S. Fusi, L. Sepulcri, J. B. Morin, A. Belli, and G. Antonutto. 2005. Sprint running: a new energetic approach *J. Exp. Biol* July 15: 208(14): 2809 - 2816.

Radcliffe, James. *High Powered Plyomerics.* 1999. Champaign, ILL: HKP.

Rapaso, Vasconcelos A. 2000. *Planificacion y Organizacion del Entrenamiento Deportivo (Spanish Edition).* Barcelona, Spain. Editorial Paidotribo.

Rogers, J. 1967. A study to determine the effect of the weight of football uniforms on speed and agility. *Master's Thesis.* Springfield, IL: Springfield College.

Ross, Ross. 2005. *Underground Secrets to Faster Running.* Bear Powered Publishers.

Rouzier, Pierre MD 2004. *The Sports Medicine Patient Advisor.* SportsMedPress.

Sandwick, C.M. 1967. Pacing machine. *Athletic Journal* Jan. 36-38.

Sayers, A.L., et. al. (2008). The effect of static stretching on phases of sprint performance in elite soccer players. *Journal of Strength and Conditioning Research.* 22(5), 1416-1421.

Schlinkman, B. 1984. Norms for high school football players derived from Cybex data reduction computer. *Journal of Orthopedics Sports and Physical Therapy* 5:410-412.

Schmolinsky, G. (Editor). 1993. Track and Field: *The East German Textbook of Athletics.* Toronto: Sport Books Publishing.

Shrier, I. & Gossal (2000). Myths and truths of stretching. *The Physician and Sportsmedicine.* 28(8), 57-63.

Silvers and Mandelbaum. 2007. ACL Injury in the Female Athlete. *Br J Sports Med* 0: bjsm.2007.037200v1 .

Singh, M., Irwin, D., & Gutoski, F.P. 1976. *Effect of high speed treadmill and sprint training on stride length and stride rate.* Paper presented at the International Congress on Physical Activity Sciences. Quebec City.

Smith, Mike 2005, *High Performance Sprinting.* Ramsbury, Marlborough, Wiltshire SN8 2HR: The Crowwood Press LTD.

Spassov, A. 1989. Bulgarian training methods. Paper presented at the symposium of the *National Strength and Conditioning Association.* Denver, CO.

Starkes, Janet L. and Ericsson, K. Anders. Editors. 2003. *Expert Performance in Sports: Advances in Research on Sport Expertise.* Champaign, Illinois: Human Kinetics.

Starzynski, Tadeusz. And Sozanski, Henryk. 1999. *Explosive Power and Jumping Ability for All Sports.* Island Pond, VT: Stadion Publishing Company.

Tansley, J. 1980. Tow training. *Track and Field Quarterly Review* 80(2), 45-46.

Tellez, Tom. 2011 Mechanics of Sprinting. *Notes*:

Thomas, L. 1984. Isokinetic torque levels for adult females: effects of age and body size. *Journal of Orthopedics Sports and Physical Therapy* 6:21-24.

Tinning, R., & Davis, K. 1978.. The effectiveness of towing in improving sprinting speed. *Australian Journal for Health, Physical Education and Recreation* March, 19-21.

Unitas, John and Dintiman, G. B. 1982. *The Athlete's Handbook: How to become a champion in any sport.* Englewood Cliffs, NJ: Prentice-Hall.

USA Track and Field, 2000. *USA Track and field Coaching Manual*, Champaign, IL: Human Kinetics.

Verkhoshansky, Y. V. 1996. Quickness and velocity in sports movements. New Studies in Athletics 11(2-3): 29-37.

Verhoshansky, Yuri, 2000. Recommended methods of speed development for elite athletes. *Sprint and Relays: Contemporary Theory, Technique and Training.* 5th Ed., Mountain View, CA: Tafnews Press, pgs. 79-82.

Vickers, J. N. 2007. *Perception, cognition and decision training: The quiet eye in action.* Champaign, IL., Human Kinetics.

Vittori, Carlo in collaboration with Plinio Castrucci, Ida Nicolini, Ennio Preatoni. Corse Di Velocita. 1983. *Atleticastudi. Fidal – Centr Studi & Ricerche*, Anno XIV, May/June.

Vizard, Frank (Editor) Popular Mechanics, *2008. Why a Curve ball Curves: The incredible science of sports.* New York: Hearsts Books.

Volek, J.S. 2004. Influence of nutrition on responses to resistance training. *Medicine and Science in Sports and Exercise* 53436(4):689-696.

Ward, P.E., and R.D. Ward. 1991. *Encyclopedia of Weight Training.* Laguna Hills, CA: QPT.

Ward-Smith AJ. 2001. Energy conversion strategies during 100 m sprinting. *J Sports Sci* 19: 701-710.

Weyand P.G., D.B. 1991-1999. Sternlight, M.J. Bellizzi MJ and S. Wright. 2000. Faster top running speeds are achieved with greater ground forces not more rapid leg movements. *J Appl Physiol 89(5)*

Wiedmann, Klaus and Gunter Tidlow, 1995. Relative activity of hip and knee extensors in sprinting: implications for training. *New Studies in Athletics.*

Wilt, Fred. Editor. Second Edition. 1973. *How They Train Volume III: Sprinting And Hurdling*. Tafnews Press. Los Altos, California.

Winter, Lloyd C., 1956. *So You Want to Be a Sprinter.* Fearon Publishers: Palo Alto, CA.

Yessis, Michael. and F. Hatfield. 1986. *Plyometric Training: Achieving Explosive Power in Sports*. Fitness Systems.

Young, M. (2001). *Review of Training Theories on Periodization for Sprinters.* Retrieved from ELITETRACK Web Site: elitetrack.com/articles/sprint theories.

Young W, McLean B and Ardagna J. 1995. Relationship between strength qualities and sprinting performance. *J Sports Med Phys Fitness* 35: 13-19.

Young WB, McDowell MH and Scarlett B.J. 2001. Specificity of sprint and agility training methods. *J Strength Cond Res* 15: 315-319.

VIDEOS

Coaching Speed. 1998. Champaign, IL.: Human Kinetics Publishers.

Speed Improvement for Soccer by Dr. George B. Dintiman and Dr. Larry Isaacs, 1995. *National Association of Speed and Explosion*, Box 1784, Kill Devil Hills, NC 27948; Web site: naseinc.com

Speed and Explosion: by Bob Ward and George Dintiman, 1987 and 1995. With Tom Landry, Bob Hayes, Tony Dorsett, Randy White, Doug Donley, Bill Bates and Brian Baldinger. *NASE,* Box 1784, Kill Devil Hills, NC 27948.

GLOSSARY

adenosine triphosphate (ATP) A high energy compound for cells; with limited storage available, it must be generated quickly during high intensity anaerobic exercise.

adipose tissue Fatty tissue.

aerobic Aerobic means "with oxygen' and describes exercise that develops the cardiovascular-respiratory system and is performed in the presence of oxygen using fat as the major source of fuel.

Afterburn The extra calories burned for 30 minutes to several hours after an exercise workout is completed as resting metabolism remains elevated above baseline.

agonist muscles A muscle or muscle group in a state of contraction with reference to its opposing muscle (antagonist).

amenorrhea Absence of at least three consecutive menstrual cycles when they are expected to occur.

amino acids The basic component of most proteins.

anaerobic High intensity activity, such as sprinting, performed in the absence of oxygen, using glucose as the major source of fuel.

anaerobic threshold The point at which blood lactate accumulation (OBLA) begins during anaerobic exercise.

anorexia nervosa An eating disorder found most often in women that involves lack of appetite and motivation to eat to the point of self-starvation and dangerous weight loss.

antagonistic muscles A muscle or muscle group in a state of relaxation with reference to its opposing contracting muscle (agonist).

back side mechanics The phase of sprinting that dominates during the start and acceleration with powerful thrusts pushing against the ground; with the upper leg vertical, back side mechanics are in play if the foot is recovered behind the butt.

ballistic stretching Flexibility exercises that employ bouncing and jerking movements at the extreme range of motion.

ballistics A training technique designed to improve the ability of delivering, resisting, redirecting and yielding force.

basal metabolism The number of calories burned while the body is at rest but not sleeping

blood glucose The form of sugar in which carbohydrate is carried in the blood.

BP Blood pressure

body composition The relative amounts of fat and lean tissue.

BMI Body mass index

bulimia An eating disorder, found more often in women, including athletes, that involves eating binges followed by self-induced vomiting or the use of laxatives to expel the unwanted food.

caloric balance When caloric intake equals caloric expenditure at which point no weight loss or weight gain occurs.

calories A large calorie is equal to 1,000 small calories; 1 calorie is the amount of heat required to raise the temperature of 1 kilogram (about 1 quart) of water 1 degree Celsius.

carbohydrate loading (super compensation) A 5-7 day nutritional procedure designed to increase carbohydrate stores in preparation for an event lasting 1-3 hours. Carbohydrate intake is reduced to near zero for 2-3 days and exercise intensity and volume is increased (depletion stage) before reducing exercise efforts and beginning a high high carbohydrate diet for 3-4 days (loading phase) to raise glycogen stores in skeletal muscles and the liver.

cardiac output The volume of blood pumped by the heart per minute (stroke volume or amount of blood ejected per beat X heart rate).

cartilage A fibrous connective tissue between the surfaces of movable and immovable joints.

cellulite The name commonly given to fat that accumulates on the legs and buttocks of over fat individuals; from a medical point of view, no different than fat in other parts of the body other than the dimply appearance it presents.

CHO Carbohydrate

citric acid energy cycle The aerobic energy pathway fueled primarily by fat, small quantities of glucose fragments, and certain amino acids.

combat breathing The proper mechanics of breathing using the mouth and nose through the diaphragm during vigorous activity.

cool-down The 5-10 minute period immediately following a long aerobic exercise session or heavy anaerobic workout; involves activity that allows the body to return slowly to normal resting metabolism such as slow walking, jogging, or slow movement in the workout activity.

complete protein A food source, such as meat, milk, and eggs, that contains all amino acids in the correct proportion.

complex carbohydrates (polysaccharides) Starch and fiber; chains of sugar molecules (three or more) found in fruits, vegetables, and grains.

contralateral muscle imbalance Speed-strength and power differences in the same muscle groups on the right and left side of the body.

contrast training Alternative use of sprint-assisted training and sprint-resisted training in the same workout session.

CP Creatine phosphate; a substrate present in muscle tissue that is broken down into its component parts (creatine and phosphate) to provide phosphates for the production of ATP.

dietary fiber The undigested portion of complex carbohydrates (fruits, vegetables and grains).

dietary reference intakes (DRIs) Generic term that refers to three reference values: adequate intake for a nutrient (AI), the tolerable upper intake level (UL) representing the highest intake level without toxicity, and the estimated average requirement (EAR) of half of all healthy people in a population.

dynamic stretching Use of specific movements of an activity or sport such as jogging in place, throwing motions, butt kickers, and other activities that move joints through the full range of motion; used as a stretching session immediately following the general warm-up period.

ergogenic aids Substances (pharmacological, nutritional, physiological, mechanical, or psychological) that can increase physical performance, commonly by eliminating fatigue substances.

essential fat The amount of fat required for normal physiological functioning of the body.

fast-twitch, glycolytic muscle fiber (Type 11b) White muscle fiber used in anaerobic activity that contracts rapidly and explosively but fatigues quickly due to poor blood supply.

fast-twitch oxidative oxidative muscle fiber (Type 11a) An intermediate fast twitch fiber similar to Type 11b that does not fatigue as quickly, has a higher capillary density, and more aerobic and less anaerobic capacity.

FIT Frequency, intensity, time

flexibility The range of motion around a joint.

flight distance Distance the center of gravity (COG) travels in the non-support phase of a single stride. Determined by angle of impulse, velocity at take-off, relative height of COG at take-off, air resistance, and acceleration due to gravity,

flying 40-yard dash A test that determines maximum (mph) speed by timing a 40-yard segment after a runner has reached full speed.

front side mechanics Shifting ground contact efforts to the front of the body at the end of the acceleration phase of sprinting by making certain the foot lands under the center of gravity.

glucagon A natural hormone secreted by the pancreas when blood glucose levels are low causing a release of stored liver glycogen into the blood stream.

gluconeogenesis The process of making glucose from non carbohydrate substances.

glycemic index An index rating the effects of various foods on the rate and amount of increase in blood glucose levels.

glycolysis energy cycle The anaerobic pathway fueled primarily by glucose

HR Heart rate

Insoluble fiber The indigestible portion of food after it has been exposed to the body's enzymes.

health-related fitness An adequate or above average level of achievement on exercise field test scores in components such as cardiorespiratory endurance, muscular strength and endurance, flexibility, and body composition that has been tied to the prevention of certain diseases and disorders, high energy, and a high level of wellness.

heme and non-heme iron Heme iron is derived from red meats and other foods of animal original and is easily absorbed; non-heme iron is found in fruits, vegetables and grains and is not easily absorbed although absorption is enhanced by eating foods high in vitamin C.

hollow sprints A speed endurance training program using two sprints interrupted by a hollow period of recovery that includes walking or jogging; a 40-yard jog, 50-yard sprint, and 40-yard walk for recovery.

hyperplasia New cell formation such as the adding new fat cells.

hypertrophy An increase in the size of existing cells such as muscle fibers.

hypervitaminosas The toxic side effects that result from the consumption of excess vitamins.

hyponatremia Abnormally low concentrations of sodium ions in the circulating blood; resulting from excessive perspiration, too little sodium intake and high water intake in hot, humid weather that alters the water-sodium ratio.

insulin A hormone secreted by the pancreas when blood glucose levels are high to help lower and regulate blood sugar levels.

interval sprint training An anaerobic training routine that manipulates four elements: the intensity of exercise, the duration or length of each workout, the number of repetitions completed per workout, and the rest interval between each repetition.

isometric Increased tension on a muscle at a constant overall length without muscle shortening such as when attempting to move an immovable object.

isotonic The shortening of a connecting muscle against a constant load; such as lifting weights.

kcal Kilocalories

kinetic energy Energy use during motion and exercise movement.

lactic acid A normal intermediate in the oxidation and metabolism of sugar; build-up during anaerobic activity leads to muscle fatigue.

landing distance Distance COG is away from the landing foot.

lean body mass The non fatty component of the body.

ligament Fibrous bands that hold bones together.

maximum effort training A series of all-out, anaerobic high speed exercises, such as sprinting in place, until the athlete is no longer able to continue.

maximum oxygen consumption (VO2 max) The optimal capacity of the heart to pump blood, of the lungs to fill with larger volumes of air, and of the muscle cells to use oxygen and remove waste products produced during aerobic metabolism.

megavitamin intake Consuming 10 to 100 times the DRI for a particular vitamin; imposes a danger of serious toxicity problems.

MET Multiples of basal metabolic rate, one MET equals the energy needs for resting metabolism.

metabolic specificity Training a specific energy system (citric acid cycle or glycolysis cycle).

muscle fibers Bundles of tissue composed of cells.

myofibrils Thin protein filaments that interact and slide by one another during a muscle contraction.

muscular endurance The muscle's ability to continue sub maximal contractions against resistance.

muscle imbalance Unequal strength and power in opposing muscle groups (agonist and antagonist) or when comparing muscle groups on the right side of the body to the left side.

muscular strength The amount of force a muscle can exert for one repetition (the 1RM-repetitions maximum)

NASE First three-step test Measures the total distance covered in three steps (to the nearest inch) and the time to cover the distance (to the nearest 1/100 of a second) from a standing, moving, three-point or four-point starting position.

NASE repeated sprint test A series of 6-10 consecutive 40-yard dashes completed at 30-second intervals.

neuromuscular specificity Training a specific muscle group.

olympic lifts Clean, jerk, and snatch.

overspeed training See sprint-assisted training.

oxygen debt The difference between the actual amount of oxygen needed for an exercise task and the amount taken in.

periodization The structuring of training into phases according to competition schedules with each phase striving for a specific goal to achieve peak performance for key games and events.

PC Phosphocreatine

pick-up sprints A speed endurance training program involving a gradual increase from a jog to a striding pace, to a maximum effort sprint, to a recovery activity; a 25-yard jog, stride for 25 yards, a 25-yard sprint, finishing with a 25-yard walk.

playing speed The actual speed needed and utilized to perform various tasks in a sport during competition.

plyometrics A series of hopping, jumping, and bounding movements for the lower body and swinging, push-offs, catching, throwing, and arm swings for the upper body to increase muscle strength and power (speed-strength).

power output The maximum amount of force an athlete can generate over a short period of time; such as the force that can be applied against the ground during the pushing action of each step in sprinting.

preconditioning period A period of several weeks used to prepare the body gradually for more vigorous workouts or testing.

PNF Proprioceptive neuromuscular facilitation; a two-person stretching technique used at the end of a workout that involves the use of steady pressure by a partner at the extreme range of motion in each exercise followed by steady resistance to the pressure.

power Force X velocity

protein sparing Consuming sufficient amounts of dietary carbohydrates and fat each day to prevent the conversion of dietary and lean muscle protein to glucose.

prime muscle movers Four muscle groups associated with fast sprinting: quadriceps, plantar-flexors, hamstrings, and dorsi-flexors

progressive resistance exercise (PRE) The theory of gradually increasing the amount of resistance to be overcome, the number of repetitions and sets in each exercise, and the amount of total exercise intensity and volume each workout.

resisted training Refers to sprint-resisted methods of sport loading such as use of weighted vests, sleds, and band resistance.

ROM Range of motion

RM (Repetition maximum); maximum amount of weight that can be lifted for just one repetition using a particular muscle group.

set point A theory indicating that each individual has an ideal weight (the set point) that the body will attempt to maintain and defend against pressure to change.

simple carbohydrates (monosaccharides and disaccharides) Sugars; chains of sugar molecules (one or two) found in concentrated sugar and the sugar that occurs naturally in food.

slow twitch oxidative muscle fiber (ST) Red muscle fiber used in endurance sports and aerobic activity that contracts and fires slowly and is equipped metabolically for long duration without fatigue.

soft tissue Tissue other than bone.

specificity of training Use of various exercises that closely mimic the actual movements and muscle involvement of the sport for which an athlete is training.

speed endurance The ability to complete repeated short sprints in a sport as well as a long sprint of 100 yards or more with minimal or no slowing due to fatigue.

sport loading Training that involves adding resistance to the body while running and sprinting in the form of weighted vests, a sled, a slight incline, or stadium stairs.

sprint-assisted training A training program, such as towing, downhill sprinting, and high-speed stationary cycling, that forces an athlete to sprint faster by taking longer and faster steps than they can take without assistance.

sprinting velocity Stride length X stride frequency.

sprint-resisted training Also called sport loading; the method adds weight or resistance to athletes during high speed sprinting drills.

sport loading Refers to the use of resistance during the start, acceleration and sprinting action such as uphill sprinting, stair case sprinting, weighted vests, and sleds.

standing triple jump A test similar to the triple jump in track and field, except that the athlete uses a two foot take-off from a stationary position to begin the jump.

static stretching Flexibility exercises used at the end of a workout to increase range of motion in various joints by holding a position of maximum stretch for 30 seconds in each exercise.

stretch reflex. When a muscle spindle is stimulated by a rapid stretching movement, a sensory neuron from the spindle innervates a motor neuron in the spinal column. This motor neuron causes a contraction of the muscle that was stretched.

steroids Synthetic versions of the male hormone testosterone.

stride length Distance traveled by the center of gravity between each foot contact. in sprinting.

stride rate The number of steps taken per second.
]
stride time The time to complete one stride (time of support and non-support).

stroke volume The amount of blood ejected per heart beat.

subcutaneous tissue The layer of adipose (fat) tissue directly beneath the skin.

sustained power output The ability to apply force over an extended period of time such as a 60-220 yard sprint.

take-off distance Distance the COG travels between the landing point and point where ground contact is broken.

target heart rate The minimum rate to which the heart must be elevated and sustained at that level for 30 minutes or more during continuous aerobic activity to improve the cardiovascular and respiratory system and receive health-related benefits.

tendon Fibrous band that attaches some muscles to bones to permit movement when the muscles contract.

triple extension Exercises affecting the joints and muscles of the hip, knee, and ankle that are involved in the force of the pushing action away from the ground during the start, acceleration, and maximum speed phases of sprinting.

triglycerides Most lipids (fats), which contain three fatty acids and a glycerol molecule; stored as adipose tissue (groups of fat cells).

USDA United States Department of Agriculture

warm-up The preparation of the body for vigorous activity through large muscle group movement such as fast walking, jogging, or calisthenics until core temperature rises 1-2 degrees and perspiration is evident.

yielding phase The rapid loading of muscles in a plyometric exercise or movement such as cocking the wrist just before the contraction phase of throwing a ball.

INDEX

Note: The first number in each listing indicates the chapter. The second and third numbers represent the chapter page. For example: 2.5 refers to Chapter 2, page 5; 8.19-24 refers to Chapter 8 pages 19-24.

C

D

E

F

ABOUT THE AUTHORS

George Blough Dintiman received his B.S. from Lock Haven University, M.S. from New York University and Doctorate from Columbia University. He is an internationally recognized authority on speed improvement for team sports, author of 51 books, four videos, and over 175 articles on speed, conditioning, fitness, nutrition, weight control, and health. He is cofounder and President of the National Association of Speed and Explosion (naseinc.com), a major certification body in speed and explosion for team sport coaches, strength and conditioning coaches, athletic trainers, personal trainers, and undergraduate and graduate students preparing in the fields of physical education, coaching, personal training, health, AT, and PT. The NASE, located in Kill Devil Hills, NC is dedicated to one objective: improving speed in short sprints for sports competition. Dr. Dintiman has trained athletes of all ages and consulted in the NFL, NBA, MLB, and MLS. He remains active in the research and training of athletes for the improvement of speed in short sprints for team sport competition.

Dr. Dintiman set numerous rushing and scoring records at Lock Haven University, breaking practically every record in existence by the end of his career in 1957, several still remain in 2011. He was a draft choice of the Baltimore Colts (NFL) and selection of the Montreal Alouettes (CFL), a star for the University basketball team scoring 42 points in a college and 56 in a high school game, and captained the Track Team competing in the 100-meter dash, high and low hurdles, and high jump. He was also an outside center on the Richmond Rugby Club for 9 years in the 70s.

Dr. Dintiman served as head basketball coach at Inter American University of Puerto Rico from 1959-1965 (two undefeated teams, five league championships). While in Puerto Rico, he also coached their professional team, the Athleticos de San German; and formed and coached the First Intercollegiate Football Team in the history of Puerto Rico in 1964. Football continues to flourish in 2011. He then moved on to coach at Southern Connecticut State University (1965-68).

Dr. Dintiman has received numerous honors and awards and was recently inducted into the Inaugural Class of the Lock Haven University Football Hall of Fame in 2010, and the Pennsylvania Sports Hall of Fame, Capital Area Chapter, in 1993. Dr. Dintiman has two daughters, one son, and three grandchildren and resides on the Outer Banks of North Carolina where both he and his wife, Carol Ann, are avid fitness participants in tennis, cycling, kayaking and weight training.

Bob Ward received his BA from Whitworth University, MS from University of Washington and a PED from Indiana University. During his collegiate days he was an NAIA All-American in Football and a competitor for his college track team in the NAIA National Track and Field Meet in the Shot and Discus. Dr. Ward established himself as a successful coach on the High school and collegiate levels. As the Head Track Coach at Fullerton Community College, his team won the California State Championships in 1974. During this time, he worked with the Elite Throwers USOC Program.

Coach Ward is best remembered for his position as Head Strength and Conditioning Coach and Sports Scientist for "America's Team" – the Dallas Cowboys--a position he held for 14 years (1976-1989). Ward's impressive coaching career with the Cowboys included 10 Winning Seasons, 2 Super Bowls, Championship in 1977-78, Super Bowl win in 1977, and a Pro Bowl Win in 1983. During his 14 years with the Cowboys, Ward completed extensive research with his athletes on predicting success in the NFL. He designed the ProTrain Computer Program, as well as invaluable equipment for training athletes. He codeveloped, with Dr Ralph Mann, an On-Field Analysis (OFAS), computer graphic game analysis system for football (NFL, All Star Games). Bob also brought his Martial Arts Training to the NFL in the form of a Sports Martial Arts System for training all position in football. Randy White, All Pro Defensive Tackle and Bob produced the video, *Creating Big Plays*.

Since leaving the Dallas Cowboys in 1989, Ward has been an active member of the Strength and Conditioning Community. He has consulted with NFL teams using the Computer Graphic Player Analysis Football (On-Field Analysis), served as the Director of Sports Science and Nutrition for Mannatech International (1994-2001), and Director of Sports Sciences for AdvoCare, also serving on their Sports Council (2001-2009). Ward currently works with the SPORTS SCIENCE NETWORK (www.sportsscience.com), and BLAZINGTHUNDER SPORTS (Robotic Machines-Assessment and Training in Sport and Health).

Dr. Ward reentered Masters Track & Field competition in 1998, and has amassed additional honors that include World & USA Champion in the Throws Pentathlon (World Records 70-74 – 75-79), (75-79), Hammer Throw, Curl Squat, "Outstanding Single Performance" in 2003 -USATF Masters. In addition, he has received the following awards for his performance: Whitworth University Heritage Hall of Fame, USA Strength and Conditioning Coaches Hall of Fame in 2003, CSCCa LEGEND AWARD 2008, and in 2009 was inducted into USATF Masters Hall of Fame.

QUICK ORDER FORM

(Make a copy and mail, e-mail or fax OR telephone your order to 252.441.1185)

Encyclopedia of Sports Speed: Improving Playing Speed for Sports Competition ©2011, 400 pgs. $39.95

The most comprehensive book ever written on all aspects of speed improvement for sports competition by Dr. George B. Dintiman, international authority on speed improvement and Bob ward, former Dallas Cowboy Conditioning Coach. Information based on hundreds of scientific studies is provided in a practical manner that coaches and players can apply to their sport. Includes training techniques and programs to improve speed in short sprints for football, baseball, basketball, field hockey, lacrosse, rugby, soccer, softball, tennis, and other sports. Over 400 pages, 75 photos and illustrations.

Encyclopedia of Sports Speed: e-Book $19.95

Purchase online at naseinc.com

- -

Name ____

Address ____

City ________________________ State _____ Zip Code ____________

Telephone __________ E-mail address __________________________

Method of Payment:

___ Check or money order enclosed
___ Visa ___ Master Card

OR purchase online at our secure web site at naseinc.com

Acct. # ________________________ Expiration Date ______________
3-digit Number on back of card ______________________________
(Name and address above must apply to your credit card)

PLEASE SEND __ COPIES OF *Encyclopedia of Sports Speed* at $39.95 + $4.00 for shipping

QUICK ORDER FORM

(Make a copy and mail, e-mail or fax OR telephone your order to 252.441.1185)

Encyclopedia of Sports Speed: Improving Playing Speed for Sports Competition ©2011, 400 pgs. $39.95

The most comprehensive book ever written on all aspects of speed improvement for sports competition by Dr. George B. Dintiman, international authority on speed improvement and Bob ward, former Dallas Cowboy Conditioning Coach. Information based on hundreds of scientific studies is provided in a practical manner that coaches and players can apply to their sport. Includes training techniques and programs to improve speed in short sprints for football, baseball, basketball, field hockey, lacrosse, rugby, soccer, softball, tennis, and other sports. Over 400 pages, 75 photos and illustrations.

Encyclopedia of Sports Speed: e-Book $19.95

Purchase online at naseinc.com

- -

Name ______________________________

Address ______________________________

City ____________________ State _____ Zip Code ____________

Telephone __________ E-mail address ____________________

Method of Payment:

___ Check or money order enclosed
___ Visa ___ Master Card

OR purchase online at our secure web site at naseinc.com

Acct. # ____________________ Expiration Date ______________
3-digit Number on back of card ______________________________
(Name and address above must apply to your credit card)

PLEASE SEND __ COPIES OF *Encyclopedia of Sports Speed* at $39.95 + $4.00 for shipping.

NOTES

NOTES

NOTES

NOTES

NOTES

NOTES

NOTES